Concise Paediatrics

Second Edition

Concise Paediatrics

Second Edition

Edited by

Rachel U Sidwell MBChB DA MFRCP MRCPCH
Dermatology Registrar
Chelsea and Westminster Hospital
London, UK

Mike A Thomson MBChB DCH FRCP FRCPCH
Consultant Paediatric Gastroenterologist
Sheffield Children's Hospital Foundation NHS Trust
Sheffield, UK

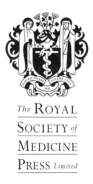

The ROYAL
SOCIETY *of*
MEDICINE
PRESS *Limited*

Published by the Royal Society of Medicine Press Ltd
1 Wimpole Street, London W1G 0AE, UK
Tel: +44 (0)20 7290 2921
Fax: +44 (0)20 7290 2929
E-mail: publishing@rsm.ac.uk
Website: www.rsmpress.co.uk

British Library Cataloguing in Publication Data
A catalogue record for this book is available from the British Library

ISBN 978-1-85315-836-0

Distribution in Europe and Rest of World:

Marston Book Services Ltd
PO Box 269, Abingdon
Oxon OX14 4YN, UK
Tel:+44 (0)1235 465 500
Fax: +44 (0)1235 465 555
Email: direct.order@marston.com

Distribution in the USA and Canada:

Royal Society of Medicine Press Ltd
c/o BookMasters, Inc
30 Amberwood Parkway
Ashland, Ohio 44805, USA
Tel: +1 800 247 6553 / +1 800 266 5564
Fax: +1 419 281 6883
Email: order@bookmasters.com

Distribution in Australia and New Zealand:

Elsevier Australia
30–52 Smidmore Street
Marrickville NSW 2204, Australia
Tel: +61 2 9517 8999
Fax: +61 2 9517 2249
Email: service@elsevier.com.au

Typeset by Phoenix Photosetting, Chatham, Kent
Printed and bound in Great Britain by Bell & Bain Ltd, Glasgow

Contents

Contributors

Chapters are shown in italics

Siobhán Carr MRCP MSc FRCPCH
Consultant Respiratory Paediatrician, St Bartholomew's and The Royal London Hospitals, London, UK
Respiratory disorders

Robert C Coombes BSc FRCPCH
Consultant Neonatal Paediatrician, Sheffield Children's Hospital NHS Trust, Sheffield, UK
Neonatology

Peter Cuckow FRCS (Paed)
Consultant Paediatric Urological Surgeon, Great Ormond Street Hospital for Children NHS Trust and University College Hospital, London, UK
Surgical conditions

Claire Daniel BSc FRCOphth
Consultant Ophthalmologist, Moorfields Eye Hospital NHS Foundation Trust, London, UK
Ophthalmology

James SA Green LLM FRCS (Urol)
Consultant Urological Surgeon, Whipps Cross University Hospital, London, UK
Surgical conditions; Emergencies, accidents, non-accidental injury and the law

Ian M Hann MD FRCP FRCPCH FRCPath
Professor of Paediatric Haematology and Oncology, Great Ormond Street Hospital for Children NHS Trust and UCL Institute of Child Health, London, UK
Oncology

John I Harper MD FRCP FRCPCH
Professor of Paediatric Dermatology, Great Ormond Street Hospital for Children NHS Trust, London, UK
Dermatology

Paul T Heath FRACP FRCPCH
Consultant in Paediatric Infectious Diseases, St George's Healthcare NHS Trust, London, UK
Infectious diseases

Nigel Klein BSc MRCP PhD
Professor of Immunology and Infectious Diseases, Great Ormond Street Hospital for Children NHS Trust and UCL Institute of Child Health, London, UK
Immunology

Melissa M Lees MRCP DCH MSc MD FRACP
Consultant in Clinical Genetics and Honorary Senior Lecturer, Great Ormond Street Hospital for Children NHS Trust and UCL Institute of Child Health, London, UK
Genetics

Ahmed F Massoud MRCP MRCPCH MD
Consultant Paediatrician and Endocrinologist, Northwick Park Hospital, London, UK
Endocrinology, growth and puberty

Anthony J Mikalski FRCPCH PhD
Consultant Paediatric Oncologist, Great Ormond Street Hospital for Children NHS Trust, London, UK
Oncology

Mike Potter MA PhD FRCP FRCPath
Consultant Paediatric Haematologist, The Royal Marsden NHS Foundation Trust, London, UK
Haematology

Robert J Sawdy BSc MRCOG PhD
Consultant Obstetrician and Specialist in Maternal and Fetal Medicine, Poole Hospital NHS Foundation Trust, Poole, UK
Neonatology

Rod C Scott ChB PhD MRCP MRCPCH
Senior Lecturer in Paediatric Neurology, Great Ormond Street Hospital for Children NHS Trust, London, UK
Neurological and neuromuscular disorders

Rachel U Sidwell MBChB DA MFRCP MRCPCH
Dermatology Registrar, Chelsea and Westminster Hospital, London, UK
All chapters

Mike A Thomson MBChB DCH FRCP FRCPCH
Consultant Paediatric Gastroenterologist, Sheffield Children's Hospital Foundation NHS Trust, Sheffield, UK
Gastrointestinal disorders; *Liver disorders*; *Emergencies, accidents, non-accidental injury and the law*

Michael Waring BSc FRCS (ORL-HNS)
Consultant Otolaryngologist, St Bartholomew's and The Royal London Hospitals, London, UK
Ear, nose and throat disorders

Nick Wilkinson MBChB MRCP MRCPCH DM
Consultant Paediatric Rheumatologist, Nuffield Orthopaedic Centre NHS Trust, Oxford, UK
Rheumatic and musculoskeletal disorders

Callum J Wilson DCH Dip O&G FRACP
Metabolic Consultant, Starship Children's Health, Aukland, New Zealand
Metabolic disorders

Paul JD Winyard MA MRCP MRCPCH PhD
Senior Lecturer in Paediatric Clinical Science, Great Ormond Street Hospital for Children NHS Trust and UCL Insitute of Child Health, London, UK
Renal disorders

Robert WM Yates BSc FRCP
Consultant Paediatric Cardiologist, Great Ormond Street Hospital for Children NHS Trust, London, UK
Cardiology

Preface

Following feedback, this fully revised, second edition of Concise Paediatrics retains the ethos of the popular and successful first edition: to provide a succinct, easy-to-access reference work, filling the gap between larger paediatric reference works and undergraduate books, the latter of which often do not contain enough detail. Each chapter has been extensively updated and there are new chapters on ENT and ophthalmology. The editors have tried to retain a pithy and user-friendly style, using many lists, boxes and annotated diagrams for ease of learning. Concise Paediatrics, Second Edition is particularly focused on those contemplating MRCPCH and DCH higher examinations, but, as well as being useful for medical students, it is also a useful quick reference for practitioners and for those more advanced in their training. This book aims to provide thorough background knowledge of the subject and will help to give inspiration for further exploration in the field of paediatrics.

We would like to thank all those who helped with this book. In particular we are indebted to the contributing authors and specialists for providing valuable, up-to-date knowledge and experience, which add to the quality of the book. A big thank you also to Rachel's husband, James Green, and to her father, Duncan Sidwell for their support. Finally, we would like to thank Peter Richardson, Sarah Ogden, Mark Sanderson and the team at the Royal Society of Medicine Press for all their help.

Best of luck!

Rachel and Mike

1
Genetics

- *Clinical application of genetics*
- *Basic cell genetics*
- *Mutations*
- *Techniques for DNA analysis and mutation detection*
- *Chromosomal disorders*

- *Single gene defects (Mendelian inheritance)*
- *Factors affecting inheritance patterns*
- *Multifactorial inheritance*
- *Dysmorphology*

CLINICAL APPLICATION OF GENETICS

Genetics is a rapidly advancing and fascinating field of medicine, which has particular relevance in paediatrics. Increasingly, medical genetics is becoming central to our understanding of many diseases, and not just rare disorders. A large proportion of paediatric admissions are due to genetic diseases, as are a large proportion (50%) of paediatric deaths.

GENETIC COUNSELLING

This involves:

- Making or confirming a diagnosis
- Discussing the natural history of the disorder and relevant management
- Discussing risks to other family members of developing or passing on the disorder
- Options for screening and prenatal diagnosis

GENETIC SCREENING

Genetic screening is the search in a population for individuals possessing certain genotypes (variations of a specific gene) that:

- Are known to be associated with disease or predisposition to disease, or
- May lead to disease in their offspring

Disorders such as thalassaemia are amenable to population screening as the test can be performed by a buccal smear or blood test; the carrier frequency is common in specific populations; gene carriers themselves are not at increased risk of disease; and a specific prenatal test can be offered to couples identified to be at risk.

Genetic carrier testing is the search in at-risk individuals for a specific genotype known to be associated with disease in that family.

PRENATAL DIAGNOSIS

This involves both **screening tests** that give a probability of disease and **diagnostic tests** that give a definite diagnosis.

- **Screening tests** include the antenatal nuchal ultrasound scan (USS), which identifies a pregnancy at increased risk of Down syndrome, and then definitive testing via a chorionic villus biopsy (CVS) or amniocentesis may be offered.
- **Diagnostic tests** include DNA analysis of a fetal sample for DNA changes known to be associated with disease in that family, e.g. analysis of the cystic fibrosis gene in a CVS sample, where both parents are known to be carriers of the disorder.

Reasons for antenatal testing

1. To reassure parents in a normal pregnancy
2. To identify an affected fetus in a high-risk family
3. To allow parents to make an informed decision about continuation of the pregnancy where an anomaly is identified
4. To enable optimal medical management (in utero and after birth), e.g. to arrange for the baby with a congenital cardiac anomaly to be born in a hospital where the cardiologist is aware and able to manage the problem

Prenatal screening and diagnostic tests

Prenatal screening tests	
• Nuchal ultrasound scan (USS)	(11–14 weeks)
• Fetal anomaly USS	(20–24 weeks)
• Maternal blood sampling for α-FP, β-hCG	(14–15 weeks)
Prenatal diagnostic tests	
• Chorionic villus sampling (CVS)	(11–14 weeks)
• Amniocentesis	(> 16 weeks)
• Percutaneous umbilical blood sampling	(> 20 weeks)
Testing of genetic disorders in at-risk families	
• Heterozygote screening in at-risk families, e.g. cystic fibrosis gene analysis	
• Pre-symptomatic testing in adult-onset disorders, e.g. Huntington disease, breast cancer	
• Carrier testing for at-risk relatives in X-linked disorders, e.g. Duchenne muscular dystrophy	
• Family history of chromosomal disorder, e.g. translocation	

GENE THERAPY

This is the treatment of genetic disease via **genetic alteration** of the genome of cells of individuals with a genetic disease. Although this is an exciting area which may in the future provide treatment for genetic disorders, success to date has been limited. Many clinical trials are in progress. Most techniques involve inserting a functioning normal gene into somatic cells to programme the cell to produce the normal gene product.

Currently gene therapy is being used in somatic cells and *not* in germline cells (which could result in the future generation being affected).

Diseases in which gene therapy is being investigated

Disease	Gene inserted	Somatic cells into which gene inserted
Cystic fibrosis	CFTR	Airway epithelial cells
Duchenne muscular dystrophy	Dystrophin	Muscle
Haemophilia B	Factor IX	Hepatocytes and skin fibroblasts
Severe combined immunodeficiency	ADA	T cells

BASIC CELL GENETICS

The gene is the basic unit of inheritance. Humans are estimated to have around 30 000 structural genes, i.e. that code for proteins. Genes are made of deoxyribonucleic acid (DNA) and are organized within chromosomes in the cell.

Somatic cells	Contain 22 pairs of **autosomes**	**46** chromosomes altogether
(*Diploid*)	(One pair of **sex chromosomes**)	
Gametes	Contain 22 **autosomes**	**23** chromosomes altogether
(*Haploid*)	(One **sex chromosome**)	

DNA COMPOSITION

DNA is a double helix composed of:

1. Sugar–phosphate backbone (the pentose sugar *deoxyribose* and a phosphate group)
2. Nitrogenous base
   Pyrimidines: Cytosine (C) and thymidine (T)
   Purines: Adenine (A) and guanine (G)

   A always pairs with T
   C always pairs with G } **Complementary** base pairing

- The sugar–phosphate backbone has a 5′ and a 3′ end
- A **nucleotide** = a unit of one base, one deoxyribose and one phosphate group
- The DNA is coiled tightly to make up **chromosomes**
- The gene sequence is made of **exons** (code for proteins) interspaced with **introns**
- Three bases make up a **codon**, which codes for one amino acid (via the **genetic code**)
- The sequence of amino acids determines the protein product

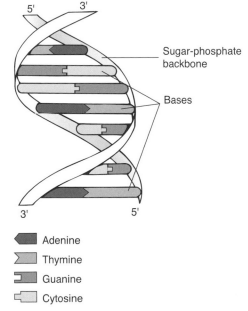

Figure legend:
- Adenine
- Thymine
- Guanine
- Cytosine

Figure 1.1 Structure of DNA

DNA REPLICATION

This occurs in a sequence:

1. DNA helix splits to form two single strands
2. New complementary base pairs, i.e. C with G, and T with A, are added to the single strands at the 3′ end (so the new DNA replication grows from 5′ to 3′). **DNA polymerase** enzyme adds the new nucleotides.

NB: Along a gene, the 5′ direction is 'upstream' and the 3′ direction is 'downstream'.

Forming proteins from DNA

1. **Transcription**. The DNA sequence is transcribed into **messenger RNA** (mRNA). (mRNA is a single strand like DNA but with a uracil (U) base replacing all the T bases, and a ribose sugar instead of a deoxyribose sugar.) **RNA polymerase** initiates this process. All the introns are removed, so the mRNA is made only of exons. The mRNA then moves from the nucleus to the cytoplasm.

2. **Translation.** The mRNA is translated into a protein in the ribosomes (organelles in the cytoplasm). **Transfer RNA** (tRNA) attaches to the mRNA. Each tRNA is a clover shape with a three base pair (anticodon) at one end, which attaches to the mRNA, and a three base pair at the other which codes for one amino acid (via the genetic code). Thus a sequence of amino acids is formed which will form a protein.

THE CELL CYCLE

New cells are constantly created. The cell cycle is a continuum of the cell's life, made up of:

1. Interphase. Most of the cell's life, **replication of DNA** and cell contents occur here
2. Division. The cell divides into two:

   Diploid cell creation: **Mitosis** (nuclear division)
   Cytokinesis (cytoplasmic division)

   Haploid cell creation: **Meiosis**

NB: After the S phase of the cell cycle, the DNA has already replicated, so the cell contains two identical copies of each of the 46 chromosomes. The identical copies are joined together at a centromere and are called **sister chromatids**, making up one chromosome. Because the chromosomes are studied in metaphase of mitosis when they are most condensed, we actually always look at DNA that has replicated, the sister chromatids joined together and appearing as 46 separate chromosome bodies.

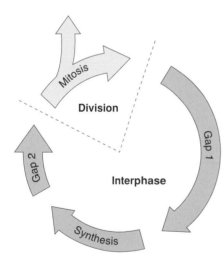

Figure 1.2 The cell cycle

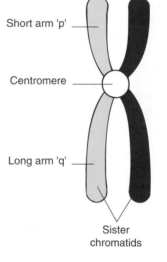

Figure 1.3 Chromosome (composed of two identical chromatids). There are two copies of this chromosome in each cell (one from the mother and one from the father).

MUTATIONS

A mutation is a change in the DNA sequence within a specific gene which leads to an alteration of gene function.

- Mutations in germline cells (cells that produce gametes) generally result in genetic diseases

- Mutations in somatic cells (normal body cells) may result in cancer (if they occur early on in the developing zygote, they may result in mosaics)

Genes differ among individuals due to polymorphisms, and differing sequences for the same gene are called **alleles**. If someone has the same allele on both members of a chromosome pair, they are **homozygous**. If the alleles have different gene sequences, the person is **heterozygous**.

A **locus** is the position of a gene on a chromosome.

The **genotype** is the alleles present at a given locus.

A **polymorphism** is a variation in DNA sequence found with a frequency of at least 1% in the normal population.

TYPES OF SINGLE GENE MUTATION

These are not visible under the microscope and are studied by **molecular genetic** techniques. Examples of single gene mutations:

- **Point mutation.** One base pair is substituted by another. They may cause one amino acid to change to another (**missense mutation**) which may alter the structure of the protein product, or produce a stop codon (**nonsense mutation**) where no protein product may be produced
- **Insertions** or **deletions** of one or more base pairs. The most common cystic fibrosis mutation, D508, is a 3 base-pair deletion at position 508 of the CFTR gene. Since codons are made of 3 base pairs, alterations in base pairs not in a multiple of three can exert their effect by altering all the downstream codons, and therefore the amino acid sequence (**frameshift mutation**)
- **Whole gene duplications**, e.g. Charcot–Marie–Tooth disease (three copies of PMP22 encoding myelin)
- **Splice site mutations**. These result in abnormal splicing of introns and exons thus altering the mRNA
- **Expanded repeats**. Some genes are coded by triplet repeats, where the gene sequence is made up by a repetitive pattern of the same 3 base-pairs. An increase in the normal tandem repeat can lead to an alteration in the gene product, e.g. Fragile X syndrome

CAUSES OF MUTATIONS

- Spontaneous mutations (occur naturally during DNA replication)
- Induced mutations (by mutagens):   Ionizing radiation, e.g. X-rays
      Non-ionizing radiation, e.g. UV light
      Chemicals, e.g. nitrogen mustard, aflatoxin B1
- Defective DNA repair is seen in certain diseases, which consequently have a high rate of tumour formation, e.g. xeroderma pigmentosa, Fanconi anaemia, ataxia telangiectasia, Bloom syndrome.

Bloom syndrome

Autosomal recessive, chromosome 15q defect. A syndrome involving increased number of chromosomal breaks, with a sensitivity to UV radiation and increased risk of malignancy.

Features include:

Skin	Butterfly distribution facial rash of telangiectasia and erythema with sun exposure
	Bullae on lips, hands and forearms
Dysmorphism	Malar hypoplasia
	Short stature
	Syndactyly, polydactyly, short lower limbs
Immunity	Low antibody levels (IgG, IgM and IgA), recurrent infections

TECHNIQUES FOR DNA ANALYSIS AND MUTATION DETECTION

CYTOGENETIC TECHNIQUES

Karyotype and chromosome banding

A karyotype is an ordered display of the chromosomes, which are studied during the metaphase part of mitosis. Staining techniques bring out the **chromosome bands** that may be viewed under the light microscope. Structural chromosome rearrangements may be identified.

Normal karyotypes: 46, XX (female)
                         46, XY (male)

Fluorescent *in situ* hybridization (FISH)

This is a technique using fluorescently-labelled DNA probes that are hybridized with a specific DNA sequence within the chromosome region being studied. They are then viewed under a fluorescence microscope to detect submicroscopic deletions, e.g. in Williams syndrome, and duplications, e.g. in Pelizaeus Merzbacher disease, and to define chromosome rearrangements, e.g. translocations.

MOLECULAR GENETIC TECHNIQUES

Polymerase chain reaction (PCR)

This is a technique to replicate a short specific DNA sequence, making millions of copies, suitable for analysis.

1. Double-stranded DNA is denatured to single strands by heating
2. Primers are added and the DNA cooled to enable the primers to anneal to the single DNA strands. (The primers are selected because they will attach next to the region of interest on the DNA)
3. DNA polymerase is added so the primers are extended along the target DNA, and thus two extra copies are made

The cycle is repeated, with doubling of the DNA occurring at each repeat cycle.

Restriction fragment length polymorphisms (RFLPs)

These are varying length fragments of DNA that are used to detect DNA polymorphisms in individuals. Bacterial enzymes known as restriction enzymes, e.g. EcoR1, cut the DNA at recognized sequences known as restriction sites. If a polymorphism or mutation exists within the DNA sequence cut by the restriction enzyme, the DNA will not be cut at this point and the DNA length will vary from the expected length and may be detected by gel electrophoresis. Once a variation is detected, DNA sequencing of the DNA region will determine the precise gene change.

Southern blotting

A technique to detect relatively large mutations (insertions, deletions and rearrangements) by separating and ordering fragments of DNA. Test DNA is digested by restriction enzymes, e.g. EcoR1, into RFLPs, these fragments are separated by *size* with gel electrophoresis. The DNA is transferred to a nylon membrane and a labelled probe is hybridized to the DNA fragments which show up as dark bands.

DNA sequencing

This is determination of the actual order of nucleotides of a strand of DNA. PCR is first used to amplify the region of test DNA, which is then sequenced using automated methods with fluorescent labels and laser detection. Mutations are detected by comparing this sequence to the DNA sequence of an unaffected individual.

DNA chips

This is a quick, accurate computer-based method to detect mutations. DNA chips are computer chips that contain arrays of different oligonucleotides. The oligonucleotides consist of both normal DNA sequences and those that contain known genetic mutations. Fluorescently-labelled test DNA is hybridized to the DNA chips, and it is observed whether it hybridizes to normal or to mutated oligonucleotides.

GENE MAPPING TECHNIQUES

Linkage analysis

This is the use of DNA markers to track a gene through a family and to help map a gene. Using linkage analysis, a specific chromosomal region is identified in which the gene is located (the region may contain several million DNA base pairs).

Closely located pieces of DNA (linked DNA) are less likely to be separated by the crossing over process in meiosis and thus are more likely to be inherited together. Linkage analysis is a complex process based on probabilities. The principle is that the chromosomes of a family with an inherited disease are marked with many DNA markers. A DNA marker that is near the disease allele will generally be inherited with the disease allele, the linkage is detected and thus the region containing the gene is identified.

Candidate genes

Once a chromosome region has been identified by linkage analysis, the genes in this area are determined (either by sequencing or using databases) and **candidate genes** are analysed to see if they are the gene responsible for the disorder in question. A gene may be a candidate for a disease either because of its position on the chromosome or because it is known to act in a way that could cause the condition. Identified candidate genes are then sequenced to see if a mutation in them gives rise to the disease.

CHROMOSOMAL DISORDERS

Chromosomal disorders are abnormalities in the:

- **Number**, e.g. trisomy or
- **Structure** (chromosome rearrangements)

of chromosomes which are large enough to be viewed under the light microscope. The phenotype results from an excess or deficiency of genes rather than from a mutation in a specific gene.

ABNORMALITIES OF CHROMOSOME NUMBER

Polyploidy is extra whole sets of chromosomes:
Triploidy (69,XXX)
Tetraploidy (92,XXXX) } Both lethal in humans

Aneuploidy is missing or extra individual chromosomes:
Monosomy (only one copy of a particular chromosome)
Trisomy (three copies of a particular chromosome)

Non-disjunction is the commonest cause of aneuploidy and is the failure of chromosomes to separate (dis-join) normally during meiosis.

Down syndrome (trisomy 21)

This is the most common autosomal trisomy.

Maternal age	Approximate risk of Down syndrome
All ages	1:650
30	1:1000
35	1:365
40	1:100
45	1:50

Clinical features

General	**Hypotonia** (floppy baby), relatively small stature, hyperflexible joints
CNS	Developmental delay, Alzheimer (later)
Craniofacial	Brachycephaly, mild microcephaly
	Upslanting palpebral fissures (Mongolian slant to eyes), **epicanthic folds**, myopia, acquired cataracts
	Brushfield spots (speckled irises)
	Small ears, mixed hearing loss, glue ear, small nose
	Protruding tongue, dental hypoplasia
	Short neck, (risk of atlantoaxial subluxation with anaesthetics)
Hands and feet	Short fingers, 5th finger clinodactyly, **single palmar crease** (NB: present in 1% of normal population), wide gap between 1st and 2nd toes (sandal gap)
Cardiac	Congenital heart disease (40%): AVSD, VSD, PDA, ASD. Valve prolapse > 20 years
Respiratory	Increased chest infections
Blood	Increased incidence of leukaemia
Endocrine	Increased incidence of hypothyroidism
Skin	Loose neck folds (infant), dry skin, folliculitis in adolescents
Hair	Soft, fine. Straight pubic hair
Genitalia	Small penis and testicular volume. Infertility common

Mechanisms of trisomy 21

1. Non-disjunction (95%)

Karyotype: 47,XY+21

This occurs where two chromosome 21s do not separate at meiosis. The extra chromosome is maternal in 90% of cases and the incidence increases with maternal age.

After having a child with Down syndrome the risk of recurrence is 1:200 under 35 years and twice the age-specific rate if over 35 years.

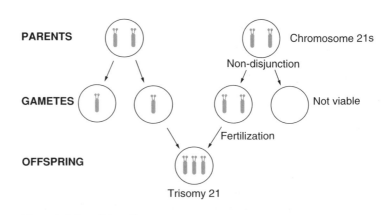

Figure 1.4 Non-disjunction

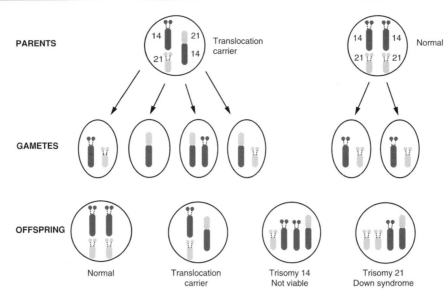

Figure 1.5 Robertsonian translocation

2. **Robertsonian translocation** (4%)

Common karyotype: 45,XY,14,21, +t (14q21q)

Here a chromosome 21 is translocated onto another chromosome (14, 15, 21 or 22). This may arise as a new mutation, but in a quarter of these cases one of the parents will have a balanced translocation (see p. 11)

The risk of recurrence is:

- 10–15% if the mother is a translocation carrier
- 2.5% if the father is a translocation carrier
- 100% if a parent has the translocation 21:21
- < 1% if neither parent has a translocation

3. **Mosaicism** (1%)

These children have some normal cells and some trisomy 21 cells.

Karyotype: 47,XY+21/46,XY, i.e. 47,XY+21/46,XY

This results from non-disjunction occurring during mitosis *after* fertilization.

Edwards syndrome (trisomy 18)

Karyotype: 47,XY,+18

Clinical features

General	Low birthweight, fetal inactivity, single umbilical artery, skeletal muscle and adipose hypoplasia, mental deficiency
Craniofacial	Narrow bifrontal diameter, short palpebral fissures, low-set abnormal ears, small mouth, micrognathia, epicanthic folds, cleft lip and/or palate

Hands and feet	**Overlapping** of index finger over 3rd and 5th finger over 4th
	Clenched hand, small nails, **rocker-bottom feet**
Trunk and pelvis	Short sternum, small nipples, inguinal or umbilical hernia, small pelvis
Genitalia	Cryptorchidism (male)
Cardiac	VSD, ASD, PDA, bicuspid aortic and/or pulmonary valves
Other organs	Right lung malsegmentation or absence, renal and gastrointestinal abnormalities

50% die within the first week, and only 5–10% survive the first year. Recurrence risk is low unless parental translocation is present.

Patau syndrome (trisomy 13)

Karyotype: 47,XY,+13

Clinical features

General	Low birth weight, single umbilical artery
CNS	**Holoprosencephaly** with varying degrees of incomplete forebrain development
	Seizures, severe mental retardation
Craniofacial	Wide fontanelles, microphthalmia, colobomas, retinal dysplasia
	Cleft lip and/or **cleft palate**
	Abnormal low-set ears
Skin	Parieto-occipital **scalp defects**
Hands and feet	Single palmar crease, polydactyly
Cardiac	(80%) VSD, PDA, ASD
Genitalia	Cryptorchidism (male), bicornuate uterus (female)

Most of these children die within the first month (around 80%). Recurrence risk is small unless one of the parents has a balanced translocation.

Turner syndrome (monosomy of the X chromosome)

Karyotype: 45,X0

Clinical features

General	**Short stature**, loose neck folds in infants
CNS	Mild developmental delay, hearing impairment
Gonads	**Ovarian dysgenesis** with hypoplasia or absence of germinal elements (90%)
Lymph vessels	**Congenital lymphoedema** (puffy fingers and toes)
Craniofacial	Abnormal ears (often prominent), narrow maxilla, small mandible
	Short webbed neck, low posterior hairline
Skeletal	**Broad chest** with **widely spaced nipples**
	Cubitus valgus
Nails	**Narrow hyperconvex** nails
Skin	Multiple pigmented naevi
Renal	Horseshoe kidney, double renal pelvis
Cardiac	Bicuspid aortic valve (30%), coarctation of the aorta (10%), aortic stenosis, mitral valve prolapse

These children may be given growth hormone, and oestrogen replacement (if necessary) at adolescence.

This is generally a sporadic event and the paternal sex chromosome is the most likely one to be missing. NB: Mosaicism is not uncommon and results in milder manifestations.

Klinefelter syndrome

Karyotype: 47,XXY

Estimated to affect 1:500 males.

Clinical features

Features are very variable. This syndrome may be identified as an incidental finding, or may present with behavioural difficulties or as infertility in an adult.

Skeletal	Tall and slim, long limbs, low upper:lower segment ratio
Genitalia	Relatively small penis and testes in childhood, most enter puberty normally
	Primary infertility secondary to azoospermia, reduced secondary sexual characteristics, gynaeco-mastia (33%)
CNS	Mild learning problems

Testosterone therapy may be given if deficient.

47,XYY syndrome

Incidence 1:840 males, though seldom detected as most are phenotypically normal.

Clinical features

CNS	Learning difficulties, poor fine motor coordination, speech delay common
	Behavioural problems (hyperactivity, temper tantrums)
Growth	Accelerated growth in mid-childhood
Craniofacial	Prominent glabella, large ears
Skin	Nodulocystic teenage acne
Skeletal	Long fingers and toes, mild pectus excavatum

CHROMOSOME REARRANGEMENTS

These are partial chromosome abnormalities, and may result from a number of causes.

Translocations

This is the interchange of genetic material between non-homologous chromosomes. There are two types:

- **Reciprocal translocations**. Two breaks on different chromosomes occur and so genetic material is exchanged between the two chromosomes. A carrier of a **balanced translocation** is usually of normal phenotype because they have the normal chromosome complement. However, their offspring may have an **unbalanced translocation**, resulting in a partial trisomy or monosomy, e.g. 6p trisomy, 4p monosomy
- **Robertsonian translocation** (results in altered chromosome numbers – see Down syndrome). The long arms of two acrocentric chromosomes fuse together to make one long chromosome, and their short arms are lost. This only occurs between chromosomes 13, 14, 15, 21 and 22 because these are acrocentric (have very small short arms that contain no essential genetic material.) It can result in Down syndrome for the offspring of a carrier of the Robertsonian translocation

Deletions

Deletion of a portion of the chromosome occurs, e.g. cri du chat syndrome (46,XY, del[5p]). Microdeletions (smaller deletions now visible microscopically using new techniques such as high-resolution banding and FISH, or by molecular techniques) include Williams syndrome (chromosome 7) and DiGeorge syndrome (chromosome 22, see p. 30).

Cri du chat syndrome (deletion 5p syndrome)

This is caused by a partial deletion of the short arm of chromosome 5.

Clinical features

General	Low birth weight, slow growth, **cat-like cry**
CNS	Hypotonia, mental retardation
Craniofacial	Microcephaly, hypertelorism, epicanthic folds, down-slanting palebral fissures, abnormal low-set ears
Hands	Single palmar crease (81%)
Cardiac	Variable congenital heart disease (30%)

Williams syndrome

This is due to a microdeletion of the chromosomal region 7q11.23 including the elastin gene.

Clinical features

Craniofacial	Medial eyebrow flare, depressed nasal bridge, epicanthic folds
	Blue eyes, **stellate pattern iris,** periorbital fullness
	Prominent lips (fish-shaped)
CNS	Mental retardation, friendly manner, **'cocktail party' speech**
	Hypersensitivity to sound
Skeletal	Short stature, hypoplastic nails, scoliosis, kyphosis, joint limitations
Cardiac	Supravalvular aortic stenosis, peripheral pulmonary artery stenosis, VSD, ASD, renal artery stenosis
Renal	Nephrocalcinosis, pelvic kidney, urethral stenosis

Duplications

Three copies of a portion of the chromosome are present, e.g. Charcot—Marie—Tooth disease.

SINGLE GENE DEFECTS (MENDELIAN INHERITANCE)

Single gene traits are also called Mendelian traits, after Gregor Mendel the 19th century Austrian monk who formed some basic genetic principles from experiments with peas. The inheritance of single gene disorders is based on the principles that genes occur in pairs (alleles), only one allele from each parent is passed onto the offspring, and an allele may act **dominantly** or in a **recessive** manner. There are many factors and exceptions that complicate this pattern.

A **pedigree** of family members is constructed to understand the inheritance of a particular condition.

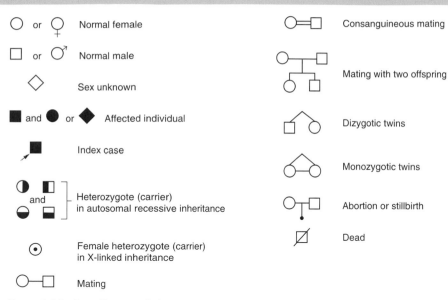

Figure 1.6 Basic pedigree symbols

AUTOSOMAL DOMINANT AND AUTOSOMAL RECESSIVE INHERITANCE

Autosomal dominant inheritance (AD)	Autosomal recessive inheritance (AR)
Often structural defects Single allele exerts an effect (thus heterozygotes and homozygotes manifest the disease) Transmission pattern is vertical (disease seen in successive generations) Offspring of an affected parent have a 50% chance of inheriting the disease (see Fig. 1.7)	Often metabolic conditions Phenotype only manifests if both alleles are abnormal Transmission pattern is horizontal (seen in multiple siblings but not parents) Offspring of two carriers have a 25% chance of inheriting the disease and a 50% chance of being an asymptomatic carrier (see Fig. 1.8) Consanguinity increases the chances of a child with a recessive disorder
Examples Marfan syndrome Achondroplasia Polyposis coli Noonan syndrome Familial hypercholesterolaemia Otosclerosis	*Examples* Cystic fibrosis Galactosaemia Homocystinuria Phenylketonuria Congenital adrenal hyperplasia Friedreich ataxia

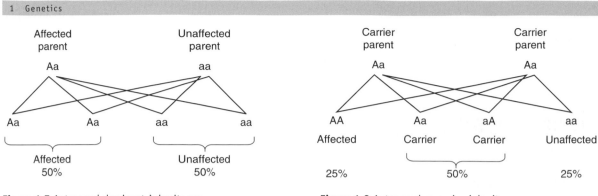

Figure 1.7 Autosomal dominant inheritance

Figure 1.8 Autosomal recessive inheritance

Marfan syndrome

Autosomal dominant, mutations in fibrillin (*FBN1*) gene on chromosome 15q21.1. There is a very wide variability of expression, and multiple mutations exist so screening cannot be performed. Linkage analysis can be used in families with multiple members affected to identify probable carriers.

Clinical features

Skeletal	Tall, thin habitus, muscle hypotonia and joint laxity
	Decreased upper:lower segment ratio
	Arachnodactyly, pes planus, pectus excavatum, **scoliosis**, kyphosis
	High arched palate
Eyes	Upward lens subluxation, myopia, retinal detachment
Cardiovascular	Dilatation of ascending aorta, dissecting aortic aneurysm, mitral valve prolapse

The cardiac complications are the commonest cause of death.

Noonan syndrome

Autosomal dominant condition, often sporadic.

Clinical features

CNS	Mild mental retardation (25%)
Craniofacial	**Ptosis, epicanthic folds**, hypertelorism, downslanting palpebral fissures, strabismus, nystagmus, low nasal bridge, low set abnormal ears, prominent upper lip
	Low posterior hairline, **short webbed neck**
Skeletal	Short stature, **shield chest**, pectus excavatum, pectus carinatum, **cubitus valgus**
Cardiac	**Pulmonary valve stenosis**, cardiomyopathy, PDA, VSD, ASD,
	Branch stenosis of pulmonary arteries
Genitalia	Small penis, cryptorchidism
Other	Bleeding diathesis due to a variety of defects

X-LINKED RECESSIVE INHERITANCE

Diseases caused by genes on the X chromosome are X linked, and are usually recessive. The Y chromosome is very small and contains few known genes.

X inactivation

This is a random inactivation in females of one of the X chromosomes in each cell. The inactivated chromosome is a dense chromatin mass called a **Barr body**. The theory of X inactivation is the **Lyon hypothesis**.

This explains why X-linked disorders are variably expressed in the female (because females have X-mosaicism).

X-linked recessive disorders
Affect males Carrier females *may* be affected (due to Lyonization) Sons of female carriers have a 50% chance of being phenotypically affected Daughters of female carriers have a 50% chance of being a carrier There is no father–son transmission Daughters of affected males have a 100% chance of being carriers

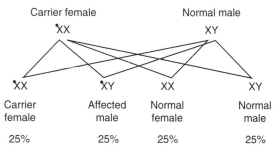

Figure 1.9 X-linked recessive inheritance

X-LINKED DOMINANT DISORDERS

These are uncommon. The disorder may be lethal in males and seen only in females (who have one normal X chromosome which modifies expression of disease), e.g. incontinentia pigmentii.

Examples of X-linked disorders	
X-linked recessive	**X-linked dominant**
Haemophilia A Colour blindness Duchenne muscular dystrophy G6PD deficiency	Familial hypophosphataemic rickets Incontinentia pigmentii

MITOCHONDRIAL DISORDERS

Mitochondria contain their own chromosomes which are *maternally derived*. A few diseases are the result of mitochondrial mutations. These have (not strictly Mendelian) inheritance through the maternal line. Examples are the mitochondrial myopathies, e.g. MELAS and MERRF (see p. 285 metabolic chapter).

FACTORS AFFECTING INHERITANCE PATTERNS

- **New mutation.** This is frequent in some conditions, e.g. achondroplasia. No previous family history of disease is seen (especially significant in autosomal dominant disorders)
- **Germline mosaicism.** A mutation that affects all or some of the germ cells of one parent. Thus a condition that may appear as a one-off mutation recurs in subsequent siblings
- **Imprinting and uniparental disomy**
- **Premutation**
- **Reduced penetrance.** Some individuals who have inherited the disease do not manifest it phenotypically, e.g. retinoblastoma. They can transmit the gene to the next generation
- **Variable expression.** Some individuals manifest the gene mildly and some severely, e.g. tuberose sclerosis
- **Non-paternity.** The genetic picture is confused because the apparent father is not the biological father (relatively common)

- **Anticipation**. This is the development of more severe expression of disease through successive generations. It is seen in diseases caused by genes with trinucleotide repeats. The number of repeats increases through generations and correlates with severity of disease

Examples of diseases associated with trinucleotide repeat expansions		
Disease	**Repeat sequence**	**Parent in which expansion occurs**
Myotonic dystrophy	CTG	Either parent Congenital form via mother
Fragile X syndrome	CGG	Mother
Huntington disease	CAG	Father > mother

PREMUTATION

Some diseases are caused by an expansion in the number of triplet repeats seen within the gene. Triplet repeats are found at many places across the genome and the normal number of repeats may vary between individuals. However, a repeat number above a certain size may make the gene unstable (**premutation**) and more likely to expand further, to a size that interferes with the function of the gene (**full mutation**). An example of premutation is fragile X syndrome.

Fragile X syndrome (FRAXA)

Clinical features

Learning difficulties	(Milder in females)
Dysmorphic facies	Large ears, long face
Other	Macro-orchidism (large testicular volume), hypermobile joints

Genetics

- An X-linked dominant condition with premutation and expansion occurring via the mother
- Seen in approximately 1:1250 males and 1:2500 females
- The term fragile X comes from the fact that the X chromosomes have a fragile site and may develop breaks when cultured in a medium deficient in folic acid
- The gene for fragile X syndrome (*FMR1*) contains a CGG repeat at one end
- Normal individuals have 5–50 copies of this repeat, those with fragile-X syndrome have >200–1000 repeats (a **full mutation**)
- People with an intermediate number of repeats (50–200) carry a **premutation** and are seen in **normal transmitting males** and their **female offspring**
- An expansion in the number of repeats occurs when a premutation is passed through the female line, resulting in a larger premutation or in the **full mutation** size
- Expansions from the premutation to the full mutation do not occur in male transmission. This explains why premutation carrier males do not give the disease to their daughters but the daughters' children may be affected and this becomes *more* likely through successive generations
- Most males with a full mutation will have the clinical signs of the condition. About one-third of females with a full mutation will be clinically affected. (The lower penetrance in females is thought to be due to X inactivation in females)

IMPRINTING AND UNIPARENTAL DISOMY

Genomic imprinting is the differential activation of genes depending on which parent they were inherited from. Examples are Prader–Willi, Angelman syndrome and Beckwith–Wiedemann syndromes.

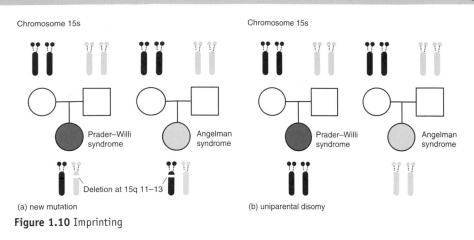

Figure 1.10 Imprinting

Prader–Willi and Angelman syndromes

Prader–Willi syndrome	Angelman syndrome (happy-puppet syndrome)
Neonatal hyopotonia	Ataxia
Learning difficulties	Microcephaly
Obsession with food	Severe learning difficulties
Obesity	Happy personality
Micropenis	Epilepsy
	Characteristic facies (broad smile)

Genetics

- Both disorders result from loss of a gene at chromosome 15q11–13.
- **Failure to inherit** the active gene causes the syndrome.
- Failure to inherit the paternal copy → Prader–Willi (paternal deletion or maternal UPD)
- Failure to inherit the maternal copy → Angelman syndrome (maternal deletion or paternal UPD)

The absence of the active gene may result from:

1. **New mutation.** Normal parental chromosomes. Gene deletion from one parent
2. **Uniparental disomy.** Normal parental chromosomes. The child inherits both copies from one parent. Thus the normal number of copies is present but there is an **effective deletion** of the copy from one of the parents. The resulting syndrome depends on which copy is missing

Beckwith–Wiedemann syndrome

Autosomal dominant, variable expression and incomplete penetrance. A minority are caused by paternal uniparental disomy (two copies inherited from the father), with Beckwith–Wiedermann syndrome resulting from **over-expression** of the gene product.

Gene located at 11p15.5, with the maternal copy normally inactivated (imprinted). Imprinting occurs in the insulin-like growth factor 2 (IGF_2) gene on chromosome 11. IGF_2 is active only in the paternal copy, i.e. imprinted in the maternal copy. Therefore a double dose of IGF_2 will occur with inheritance of both paternal copies, or loss of maternal imprint (so the maternal gene is activated). The high levels of IGF_2 are thought to result in the clinical features.

Clinical features

Pregnancy	Polyhydramnions, large for gestational age
Growth	**Macrosomia**, thick subcutaneous tissue, large muscle mass
	Advanced bone age when infantile
Craniofacial	**Macroglossia**, prominent eyes, port wine stain central forehead and upper eyelids
	Ear creases on ear lobule
Organ	Large kidneys, fetal adrenocortical enlargement, pancreatic hyperplasia, hepatosplenomegaly, large ovaries, cliteromegaly, cardiomegaly
Other	**Infantile hypoglycaemia**, neonatal polycythaemia, **Wilms tumour**, **hepatoblastoma** (5–10% risk), **hemihypertophy**, umbilical hernia, **omphalocoele**

MULTIFACTORIAL INHERITANCE

Characteristics affected by both genetic and environmental factors are **multifactorial**. Many quantitative traits are multifactorial, e.g. blood pressure, height, and are distributed in a symmetrical (Gaussian) fashion.

Many diseases are inherited in a multifactorial fashion and are present only if a liability threshold is reached, e.g. pyloric stenosis, cleft lip and palate, neural tube defects.

Recurrence risks for these diseases are based on empiric data, e.g.:

Risk of cleft lip $\pm$ cleft palate is 1:700 live births

Recurrence risk after one affected child is 3–4%

Recurrence risk after two affected children is around 10%

Congenital defects incidence
Major (2–3% newborns) — of functional or cosmetic importance
Minor (5–7% newborns) — *not* of functional or cosmetic importance
The aetiology of congenital defects is usually unknown or multifactorial. There is an identified genetic component in 30%, and environmental causes are infrequent.

DYSMORPHOLOGY

This is the study of abnormal physical development (**morphogenesis**) occurring during embryogenesis, resulting in congenital defects. There are four pathogenic processes.

1. Malformation

A primary defect resulting from intrinsic abnormal development during embryogenesis, e.g. polydactyly, cleft lip. Causes include:

- Chromosomal abnormalities
- Single gene defects
- Multifactorial

2. Dysplasia

A primary defect involving abnormal organization of cells into tissues, e.g. haemangioma.

3. Deformation

A secondary alteration of a previously normally formed body part by mechanical forces. These can be extrinsic or intrinsic. Causes include:

Extrinsic:	Oligohydramnios
	Abnormal presentation, e.g. congenital dislocation of the hip
	Multiple pregnancy
	Uterine abnormalities
Intrinsic	Congenital muscular dystrophy
	Congenital skeletal defects

Arthrogryphosis is a picture of prenatal joint contractures resulting from a variety of causes including fetal crowding (oligohydramnios, twins), external constraints (uterine abnormalities) and intrinsic neuromuscular, skeletal or connective tissue defects.

4. Disruption

A secondary defect resulting from extrinsic breakdown of an originally normal developmental process. Causes include:

- Teratogens
- Intrauterine infection
- Maternal disease
- Limb defect resulting from a vascular event

> **Syndrome** is a pattern of multiple primary malformations due to a single aetiology, e.g. trisomy 18
> **Sequence** is a primary defect with secondary structural changes, e.g. Potter phenotype, Pierre–Robin sequence

TERATOGENS

Teratogens are agents external to the fetus that induce structural malformations, growth deficiency and/or functional alterations during prenatal development.

Human teratogens

Drug	Potential effect	Critical period
Warfarin	Nasal hypoplasia	6–9 weeks
	Bone defects (chondrodysplasia punctata)	
	Intracerebral and other fetal haemorrhage	> 12 weeks
Phenytoin	Craniofacial dysmorphism, hypoplastic nails and fingers	< 12 weeks
Sodium valproate	Neural tube defects	< 30 days
Carbamazepine	Neural tube defects	< 30 days
Isotretinoin	Spontaneous abortion, hydrocephalus, other CNS defects, conotruncal heart defects, small or missing thymus, micrognathia	All pregnancy
Cocaine	Placental abruption, Intracranial haemorrhage Premature delivery Omphalocoele	> 12 weeks

continued

19

Drug	Potential effect	Critical period
Lithium	Polyhydramnios, pulmonary hypertension, Ebstein anomaly and other cardiac defects	< 8 weeks
Thalidomide	Limb hypoplasia, ear abnormalities	5–9 weeks
Diethylstilboestrol	Uterine abnormalities, vaginal adenocarcinoma, male infertility	< 12 weeks
Alcohol	**Fetal alcohol syndrome:** (Rare in the UK)	< 12 weeks
	Craniofacial: Long philtrum, flat nasal bridge Midfacial hypoplasia, micrognathia Upturned nose, ear deformities Eye malformations, cleft lip and palate	
	CNS: Microcephaly and developmental delay Growth retardation	
	Other: Cardiac, renal and limb abnormalities	

MATERNAL ILLNESS AND ASSOCIATED IMPACT ON THE INFANT

Maternal illness	Malformation/disorder
Diabetes mellitus	Organomegaly, transient neonatal hypoglycaemia, see p. 257 Caudal regression syndrome (sacral agenesis) Doubled risk of any congenital anomaly Hypoplastic left colon, renal vein thrombosis CHD, hypertrophic subaortic stenosis
Phenylketonuria	CHD, microcephaly, mental retardation (only if high maternal phenylalanine levels during pregnancy), see p. 277
Placental antibody transfer	
Rhesus disease	Fetal anaemia
Lupus erythematosis	Neonatal lupus, congenital heart block
Hyperthyroidism	Transient neonatal thyrotoxicosis
Autoimmune thrombocytopenia	Transient neonatal thrombocytopenia
Myasthenia gravis	Transient neonatal disease and arthrogryphosis

FURTHER READING

Connor M, Ferguson-Smith M *Essential Medical Genetics*, 5th edn. Oxford: Blackwell Science, 1997

Jones KL *Smith's Recognizable Patterns of Human Malformations*, 6th edn. Philadelphia: WB Saunders, 2005

Larson WJ *Essentials of Human Embryology*, Churchill Livingstone, New York, 1998

Sadler TW *Langman's Medical Embryology*, 10th edn. New York: Lippincott, Williams & Wilkins, 2006

2

Immunology

- Components of the immune system
- Clinical features in immunodeficiency
- Inherited immunodeficiencies
- Acquired immunodeficiency

COMPONENTS OF THE IMMUNE SYSTEM

The immune system is subdivided into **innate** and **specific** responses, though there is much interaction between the two.

INNATE IMMUNITY

This involves the elements of the immune system that produce an immediate, non-specific response. The main components involved are:

Phagocytes

Mononuclear phagocytes	**Monocytes** (blood), **macrophages** (tissues), **Kupfer cells** (liver)
Polymorphonuclear granulocytes	**Neutrophils** (granulocytes) (95%)
(PMNs)	**Eosinophils** (2–5%)

- These cells employ phagocytosis (cellular ingestion) of foreign material
- Opsonization (coating the antigen with antibody and complement) helps ingestion and killing
- Neutrophils live 2–3 days only. They have granules containing antibiotic proteins, enzymes, e.g. lysozyme, and lactoferrin
- Particularly active against bacteria and fungi
- Eosinophils produce cytotoxic granules, which are released onto the surface of large organisms (they can employ phagocytosis). Active against large parasitic infections

Other cells

Basophils and mast cells	Involved in inflammation, parasite immunity and immediate hypersensitivity
	Stimulated by antigens (with IgE) to *degranulate* and release vasoactive substances including histamine
	Basophils are in the circulation and mast cells in the tissues
Antigen presenting cells (APCs)	Present antigens to B and T cells
Platelets	Involved in inflammation and blood clotting
Endothelial cells	Involved in the distribution of leucocytes

Complement

The complement system involves > 20 glycoproteins which are activated in a cascade.

There are three pathways of activation:

1 and 2. **Classical (and lectin) pathway.** Activation via C1q + immune complex (**specific immunity**). (Lectin is antibody independent)

3. **Alternative pathway.** Activation via microorganism surface and factors B, D and then properdin (**innate immunity**)

All three result in activation of C3 (to C3a and C3b), and then the final common pathway C5 to C9. Involved in eradication of organisms (via opsonization, activation of leucocytes and target cell lysis), inflammation and immunoregulation (self from non-self).

Soluble mediators

These soluble messengers mediate inflammation and promote uptake by phagocytosis (opsonization). They signal their target cells to divide, activate or focus on an area of the body.

Cytokines (those produced by lymphocytes are **lymphokines**):

Interferons (IFNs)	Viral infections. INF-α, INF-β, INF-γ
Interleukins (ILs)	IL-1 to IL-17. Many functions, direct cells to differentiate and divide
Colony stimulating factors (CSFs)	E.g. G-CSF (granulocyte-colony stimulating factor)
	GM-CSF – differentiation and division of stem cells
Others	E.g. Tumour necrosis factors (TNF-α, TNF-β), transforming growth factor-β (TGF-β),

Antibodies – see below.

Acute phase proteins, e.g.
C-reactive protein (CRP)

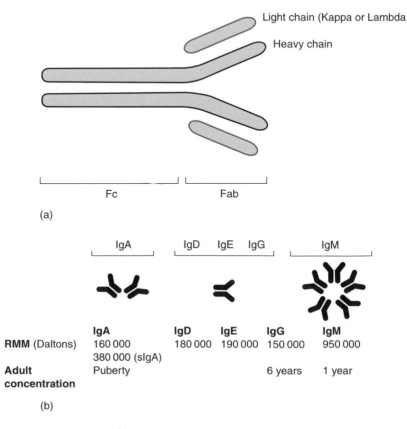

Figure 2.1 (a) Antibody composition. (b) Immunoglobulin structure

SPECIFIC IMMUNITY

This system involves lymphoid tissue and circulating leucocytes that mount a specific response to an antigen. The main lymphoid organs are:

Primary lymphoid tissue – bone marrow and fetal liver (make B cells), thymus (make T cells)._

Secondary lymphoid tissue – lymph nodes, spleen and mucosal-associated lymphoid tissue MALT, e.g. tonsils, Peyer's patches.

Leucocytes have molecules on their surface known as **clusters of differentiation (CD)**, identified using monoclonal antibodies, which are used for identifying subpopulations.

T Lymphocytes

T-Helper cells (TH)	CD4 on their surface. See antigens with MHC class II molecules
Th1 subset:	Secrete IL-2 and IFN-γ
	Cytotoxicity and inflammation (protect against intracellular organisms, e.g. viruses, bacteria, parasites)
Th2 subset:	Secrete IL-4, IL-5, IL-6, IL-10
	Stimulate B cells (protect against free-living organisms, i.e. humoral immunity)
T-Cytotoxic cells (TC)	CD8 on their surface. See antigens with MHC class I molecules
	Kill other cells
	Down-regulate immune responses.

B Lymphocytes (5–15%)

These produce immunoglobulins (antibodies) and have these on their surface. When activated they become **plasma cells** which make antibody. Carry markers CD19, CD20, CD22 and CD72–78. Carry MHC Class II antigens for interactions with T cells.

Antibodies

These are serum glycoproteins that are specific to particular antigens. The type of heavy chain determines the class.

IgG	Crosses the placenta (adult levels at birth, transient fall at 3–6 months, adult levels by 6 years)
	Antibody of secondary response
	There are four subclasses:
	IgG1, IgG3 – produced in response to many viruses and tetanus toxin
	Complement activation
	IgG2, IgG4 – produced in response to polysaccharide antigen, e.g. pneumococcus
IgM	Major antibody of primary response (elevated in acute infection). Complement activation
	Seen in the fetus only in intrauterine infection (does not cross the placenta)
IgA	Secretory (sIgA) important in protection of mucosal surfaces, e.g. respiratory tract, gut
IgE	Involved in type 1 hypersensitivity and against helminthic parasites
IgD	Present on B cell membranes, precise function unknown

Natural killer (NK) cells (15%)

CD56 and CD16 surface markings.

Eliminate tumour and virus-infected cells using cytotoxic means.

Lymphokine-activated killer (LAK) cells are cells (NK and certain T cells) that have been activated by IL-2 and particularly target tumour cells.

IMMUNE ACTIVATION AND INTERACTION

The mechanisms of activation and interaction are integral to the immune system and involve:

Antigen presenting cells

- Langerhans' cells (skin), interdigitating cells (IDCs; lymph node) and germinal centre dendritic cells (GCDC; lymph nodes) – present to **Th cells**. (These have class II MHCs)
- Follicular dendritic cells (FDCs) (lymph nodes, spleen, MALT) – present to **B cells**
- Macrophages
- B cells – present to **T cells**

Activation of T and B cells

T and B cells are activated by binding to their specific antigens.

B cells – Bind to native antigens but many need T cells to become activated (many activated B cells then become plasma cells).

T cells – Recognize antigen in association with MHC molecules on antigen-presenting cells.

HUMAN LEUCOCYTE ANTIGENS (HLA)

The HLA molecules are encoded for by a set of genes known as the **major histocompatibility complex (MHC)** on the short arm of chromosome 6.

The MHC genes code for HLA antigens (cell surface glycoproteins) which are present on all tissues and help to identify self from non-self. There are two classes of molecules:

1. **Class I** HLA-A, B, and C – on all cells except erythrocytes and trophoblast cells

2. **Class II** HLA-DP, DQ and DR – on T and B cells, monocytes and dendritic cells; inducible on endothelial and epithelial cells

HLA antigens are important in organ transplantation, where they need to be matched.

Several diseases are associated with specific HLA types (which are being subclassified):

A3	Haemochromatosis		B18	Hodgkin disease
B5	Behçet syndrome		B27	Ankylosing spondylitis
B8	Tuberculoid leprosy			Juvenile rheumatoid arthritis
				Psoriatic arthritis
B8, DR3	Myaesthenia gravis			Reiter syndrome
	Addison disease			Reactive arthritis
	Graves disease			Acute anterior uveitis
	SLE			
	Sjögren syndrome		Bw47	Congenital adrenal hyperplasia
	Membranous GN		DR7, DR2	Goodpasture syndrome
	Chronic active hepatitis			Multiple sclerosis
	Dermatitis herpetiformis			Narcolepsy
B8, DQ8	IDDM		DR7	Minimal change GN
DR4	Rheumatoid arthritis			
B8, DR3, DR7, DQw2	Coeliac disease			

HYPERSENSITIVITY REACTIONS

Reaction	Mediators	Histology	Test	Disease/condition
Type I Immediate	Free Ag + IgE, mast cells	Vasodilatation Oedema	Skin prick RAST	Anaphylactic shock Atopic diseases
Type II Antibody-dependent cytotoxic	Cell surface Ag + IgG, ± complement ± K cells	Target cell damage	Coombs' test Indirect immuno-fluorescence Precipitating Abs Red cell Agglutination	Transfusion reactions Autoimmune haemolytic anaemia Haemolytic disease of the newborn ITP
Type III immune complex	Immune complex deposition IgG, IgM, IgA, complement polymorphs	Acute inflammation Vasculitis	Skin test (Arthus reaction) Immune complexes detection (IMF, RIA)	Autoimmune, e.g. SLE, nephritis Low-grade persistent infections, e.g. viral hepatitis Environmental antigens, e.g. farmer's lung
Type IV delayed	Cell bound Ag + T cells, lymphokines, macrophages	Perivascular inflammation Caseation and necrosis (TB)	Skin test, e.g. tuberculin test – induration and erythema Patch test	Pulmonary TB Contact dermatitis GvHD Insect bites

Skin tests

Type I (prick test) A wheal and flare develop within 20 min and resolve in 2 h

Type III (intradermal or SC injection) A wheal develops over hours (maximal at 5–7 h) and resolves over 24 h (Arthus reaction)

Type IV (intradermal or patch test) An indurated area develops within 2–4 days and resolves over several days

Urticaria and angio-oedema

This is swelling of the skin and mucosa due to capillary leakage. Mechanism may be immunologically- (IgE or complement) or non-immunologically mediated (direct mast cell release, prostaglandin inhibitors). There is release of histamine ± bradykinin causing vasodilatation.

Clinical features

Urticaria Intermittent skin wheals, may itch, last 12–14 h (dermal swelling from leaking capillaries), recurrent crops may occur. **Chronic urticaria** if lasts > 6 weeks

Angio-oedema Swelling mouth, eyes, genitalia, GIT, upper respiratory tract (submucosal and subcutaneous involvement)

Causes

Cause is not often found.

Ingestion Foods, e.g. cow's milk, drugs

Contact Insects, plants

Infections	Viral, bacterial, parasitic
Physical	Cold, sun, heat, mechanical force
Cholinergic urticaria	Sweating (exercise, hot water, anxiety)
Systemic disease	Leukaemia, collagen-vascular disease
Genetic	Hereditary angio-oedema (see p. 25), urticaria pigmentosa

Management

- Self-limiting disease, usually resolves over weeks or months
- Avoid known triggers
- Antihistamines (H1 $\pm$ H2-receptor blockers)
- Adrenaline (severe reaction, anaphylaxis)

Atopy

Atopic individuals have the following:

- A predisposition to form IgE-mediated (type 1) reactions to common environmental allergens
- Susceptibility to asthma, hay fever (allergic conjunctivitis + rhinitis) and atopic eczema
- A family history of atopy

See p. 131 (asthma) and p. 291 (atopic dermatitis).

INFECTIONS ASSOCIATED WITH SPECIFIC IMMUNODEFICIENCIES

Deficiency	Organisms	
Humoral (antibody)	Bacteria	Staphylococci, streptococci, haemophilus, *M. catarrhalis*, mycoplasma, campylobacter
	Viruses	Enteroviruses
	Protozoa	*Giardia lamblia*
Cellular (T cell)	Bacteria (intracellular)	Myobacteria, listeria, legionella
	Viruses	CMV, HSV, RSV, measles, EBV, VZV
	Fungi	Candida, aspergillus
	Protozoa	*Pneumocystis jejuni* (formerly *carinii*), toxoplasmosis
Combined (cellular and humoral)	Bacteria	Intracellular and extracellular
	Viruses	CMV, HSV, measles
	Fungi	Candida
	Parasites	Cryptococcus, cryptosporidium
	Protozoa	*Pneumocystis jejuni* (formerly *carinii*), toxoplasmosis, giardia
Neutrophils	Bacteria	Staphylococcus, Gram-negative bacteria
	Fungi	Candida, aspergillus
Complement	Bacteria	Neisseria

CLINICAL FEATURES IN IMMUNODEFICIENCY

HISTORY

| Infections | Frequent, unusual severity, opportunistic, involving multiple sites, poor response to therapy, atypical symptoms and signs |

	Unusual organisms
	Recurrent skin infections, abscesses, sinopulmonary infections, periodontitis, chronic candidiasis
Autoimmune features	Arthropathy, rash
Family history	Neonatal deaths (particularly male)
	Immunodeficiency, parental tonsillectomy
	Consanguinuity
Other	Adverse reaction to vaccines, rashes
	Persistent diarrhoea, prolonged wound healing

EXAMINATION

Faltering growth	
Dysmorphism	
Lymphoid tissue	May be absent or enlarged, e.g. lymph nodes, tonsils, thymus
Skin	Eczema, petechiae, infections, granulomas, telangiectasia
Hepatosplenomegaly	
Eyes	Retinal abnormalities, conjunctival telangiectasiae
CNS	Ataxia

INVESTIGATIONS

Initial

FBC and film	Neutrophils, lymphocytes, monocytes, eosinophils, basophils, platelets (count and appearance)
Immunoglobulins	IgG, IgM, IgA, IgD, IgE
	IgG subclasses
Antibody response to vaccines	E.g. diphtheria, tetanus, Hib, polio
Isohaemagglutinins	(IgM to red cell antigen)
Complement	C3, C4, CH100, THC (total haemolytic complement)
Neutrophil function tests	Nitroblue tetrazolium dye reduction (NBT test)
Lymphocyte subsets	
HIV testing	
Ultrasound scan	Thymus, liver, spleen

Specific

Cell mediated

Quantitative	T cell subsets (CD3, CD4, CD8, CD4:CD8 ratio, etc.)
	NK cells (CD16 and CD56)
	Monocytes (CD14)
Functional	
General	Mitogen, e.g. phytohaemagglutinin stimulation (PHA) anti-CD3
Specific	Antigen specific assays
	E.g. Candida, PPD stimulation
	Mixed lymphocyte reaction
	Response to IL-2 stimulation
	Class II expression (DR expression)
	Activation status (CD25, IL-2 receptor)
	Adenosine deaminase (ADA) purine nucleotide phosphorylase (PNP) enzyme activity
	Surface expression of CD40 ligand and CD3 intensity

Humoral

Quantitative	B cell markers (CD19, CD20)
	Immunoglobulins (IgA, IgG, IgM, IgE and IgG subclasses 1–4)
Functional	Isohaemagglutinins
	Response to vaccines, e.g. diphtheria, Hib, polio

Phagocytes

Adhesion molecule expression	CD15s (LAD2), CD18 (LAD1)
Neutrophil function tests	Mobility and chemotaxis (rarely done)
	Phagocytosis – chemiluminescence
	Phagocyte enzyme analysis – cytochrome gp 92 phox, cytosolic proteins

TREATMENTS AVAILABLE

Infection treatment	Treatment of individual infections
	Prophylactic long-term antibiotics and antivirals
	Monoclonal antibodies against organism and target cell, e.g. B cells in EBV infections
Immune component replacement	Immunoglobulin infusions
Cure	Stem cell transplant
	Gene therapy, e.g. gamma chain deficient SCIDS and X-linked CGD

INHERITED IMMUNODEFICIENCIES

Classification of diseases in immunology is complex and changing; therefore, they may appear elsewhere classified slightly differently. It is best to concentrate on differentiating the individual diseases rather than their classification.

PREDOMINANTLY B CELL DISORDERS

X-linked agammaglobulinaemia (XLA, Bruton XLA)

X-linked recessive. Presents at 6 months–2 years.

Immune defect	Very low or absent B cells
	IgA, IgM, IgG, IgD, IgE *all* low
Underlying defect	Mutation in the Bruton tyrosine kinase (*btk)* gene at Xq22.3–22 causing absence of B cell's cytoplasmic tyrosine kinase
	Pre-B to B cell transformation is defective

Clinical features

- Recurrent bacterial infections after 6 months of age when maternal immunoglobulins have gone
- Unusual enterovirus infections (chronic meningoencephalitis)
- Tonsils, adenoids and lymph nodes small or absent

Management

Gamma-globulin (IVIG) infusions 3–4 weekly (IV or SC).

Common variable immunodeficiency (CVID)

| *Immune defect* | Abnormal B cell function (normal or reduced B cell numbers) |
| | Low IgA, IgG 6 IgM |

Abnormal T cell function in one-third (thus the disease could be considered a combined defect)

Underlying defect　　Unknown

Clinical features

Usually present later in life (in 2nd or 3rd decades).

Sinopulmonary infections	
Other infections	Gastrointestinal (giardia, campylobacter)
	Chronic enteroviral meningoencephalitis
Splenomegaly	(Diffuse lymphadenopathy may also occur)
GI tract	Follicular lymph node hyperplasia, malabsorption, weight loss, diarrhoea
Malignancies	Lymphomas, gastrointestinal malignancies
Autoimmune associations	Pernicious anaemia, haemolytic anaemia, thrombocytopenia, leucopenia

Management

Immunoglobulin replacement.

Selective IgA deficiency

Incidence 1:500 Caucasians, variable inheritance.

Associations	HLA-B8, DR3
	Autoimmune disease, e.g. RA, SLE, coeliac disease, thyroiditis
Immune defect	Low or absent IgA
	Sometimes IgG_2 and IgG_4 subclass deficiency also (20%)
Underlying defect	Impaired switching or maturational failure of IgA-producing lymphocytes

Clinical features

- Asymptomatic
- Respiratory infections (URTI, sinusitis, wheeze, polysaccharide infections)
- Chronic diarrhoea
- ↑ Type III hypersensitivity

Management

Specific therapy for infections. NB: Transfusion reactions more common.

Transient hypogammaglobulinaemia of infancy

Immune defect	Slow maturation of antibody production
	Low IgG 6 IgA before 6 months

Clinical features

- More common in preterm infants
- Recurrent respiratory tract infections in infancy
- Spontaneous improvement with age

Management

Usually none required.

IgG subclass deficiency

Immune defect	Low IgG subclasses (normal total levels of IgG)
	IgG$_2$ deficiency (most common type in children) often have low IgA levels
	IgG$_3$ most common in adults
Underlying defect	Defect of isotype differentiation

Clinical features

- Variable, usually mild
- Frequent infections
- Increased allergy
- Encapsulated bacterial infections if IgG$_2$ deficiency

Management

- Prophylactic antibiotics
- Intravenous immunoglobulin (occasionally)

Duncan syndrome (X-linked lymphoproliferative syndrome)

Immune defect	Inadequate immune response to EBV and other defects
Underlying defect	Unknown. Gene defect at Xq26

Clinical features

- Susceptibility to EBV infection
- Abnormal immune response leading to liver necrosis, aplastic crisis and lymphoproliferative disease
- If they survive primary infection, they develop hypogammaglobulinaemia and B lymphomas

Management

- Intravenous immunoglobulin and antibiotics
- Stem cell transplant

PREDOMINANTLY T CELL DISORDERS

22q11 Microdeletion syndrome (DiGeorge anomaly)

The autosomal dominant 22q11 microdeletion syndrome (DiGeorge anomaly) is caused by microdeletions of chromosome 22q, and includes the velocardiofacial (Shprintzen) syndrome.

Immune defect	One or more of:	Decreased numbers and function of T cells
		Reduced PHA
		Specific antibody deficiency
Underlying defect	4th branchial arch (3rd and 4th pharyngeal pouches) malformation	
	Microdeletions of chromosome 22q11	

Clinical features

The features result from fourth branchial arch development defect (3rd and 4th pharyngeal pouches).

Thymus	Aplasia or hypoplasia cellular immunity defect
Parathyroid	Hypoplasia/absence, hypoparathyroidism, Ca ↓, neonatal seizures, tetany, cataracts
Cardiac	Aortic arch anomalies (right-sided aortic arch, interrupted aortic arch, truncus arteriosus, VSD, PDA, TOF)

CNS	Learning difficulties
Growth	Short stature
Oesophagus	Atresia
Dysmorphism	Short palpebral fissures, low-set notched ears, long maxilla, micrognathia, bifid uvula, short philtrum, absent adenoids, cleft palate, prominent nose
Infections	Respiratory, diarrhoea, candida (severity varies, infections are not usually a presenting feature and immunodeficiency may correct over time)

Management

Thymus transplant and stem cell transplant if necessary.

Chronic mucocutaneous candidiasis

Immune defect	Impaired cell-mediated immunity to candida
	Negative skin tests to candida
Underlying defect	Unknown

Clinical features

Chronic candidiasis	Skin, nails and mucous membranes, not systemic infection
Others	Hypoparathyroidism, autoimmune disorders

Management

Antifungal therapy.

COMBINED IMMUNODEFICIENCIES

Severe combined immunodeficiency (SCID)

This comprises various syndromes, which have the following basic characteristics. The definition of SCID is based on the severity of the condition and presence of typical features. SCID is further distinguished on the basis of pathogenesis (where known). SCID must be differentiated from AIDS.

Immunological

Absence or impaired function of T and/or B cells from birth. There are two groups of SCID:

1. **T– B– SCID** (lack T and B lymphocytes) – RAG-1 or RAG-2 gene mutations
2. **T– B+ SCID** (lack T cells, normal number of B cells) – profound lymphopenia, hypogammaglobulinaemia, very small thymus

Clinical features

- Severe faltering growth
- Absent lymphoid tissue
- Diarrhoea
- Infections – pneumonia, otitis media, sepsis, cutaneous infections, opportunistic
- GvH symptoms – features similar to graft versus host disease in the neonatal period

Management

Death occurs < 2 years unless given stem cell transplant or gene therapy.

Causes

X-linked (50%)	T– B+
	Defective γc-chain of IL-2, 4, 7, 9 and 15
Autosomal recessive	T– B+
	Jak 3 mutation (intracellular kinase)
Omenn syndrome	T cell infiltration of tissues
	Hypereosinophilia, erythroderma, picture of GVHD
RAG-1/-2 deficiency	T– B–
	NK cells normal or ↑
	Mutations in RAG-1 or RAG-2 genes
	Autosomal recessive
Adenosine deaminase deficiency (ADA) (20%)	T– B–
	Autosomal recessive, chromosome 20q13
	Gene therapy currently being developed
Purine nucleoside phosphorylase (PNP) deficiency (4%)	T (reduced), B (less affected)
	Autosomal recessive, chromosome 14q13
	Neurological abnormalities (two-thirds)
	Autoimmune disease (one-third)
MHC class II deficiency	Failure of antigen presentation
	Heterogeneous condition
	CD4 lymphocytes particularly impaired

Wiskott–Aldrich syndrome

X-linked recessive (boys only).

Immune defect	Impaired cell-mediated immunity, *progressive* T lymphocyte ↓
	Impaired antibody production (normal initially, then IgM ↓)
	Isohaemagglutinins ↓
Underlying defect	Abnormal microvilli on T cells
	WASP gene on Xp11

Clinical features

Platelets	Small size, thrombocytopenic purpura over skin (normal megakaryocytes)
Eczema	Severe
Infections	Pneumonia, otitis media, meningitis
	HSV, VZV, PCP, encapsulated organisms, e.g. pneumococcus
Malignancies	Lymphoma
Autoimmune	JIA, haemolytic anaemia, vasculitis, glomerulonephritis

Management

These children will die < 2 years without stem cell transplant.

Ataxia telangiectasia

Autosomal recessive.

Immune defect	Impaired cell-mediated immunity (T cell numbers and function ↓)
	Impaired antibody production (IgA very low, IgE ↓, IgG_2 and IgG_4 ↓)
Underlying defect	Abnormal DNA repair especially chromosomes 7 and 14
	Mutations in *ATM* gene, chromosome 11q23.1

Additional	CEA ↑, α-FP ↑, fatty liver changes
	Cells have an extreme hypersensitivity to ionizing radiation (frequent somatic mutations)

Clinical features

Cerebellar ataxia	Progressive
Telangiectasia	Occulocutaneous, particularly on ear lobes and conjunctival sclera
Infections	Chronic sinopulmonary
Malignancy	Lymphomas, adenocarcinomas
Endocrine	Hypogonadism (ovaries or testes), glucose intolerance

Management

Supportive.

X-linked immunodeficiency with hyper IgM

Immune defect	Impaired antibody formation, low IgA and IgG
	IgM normal or ↑, absent germinal centres
	Recurrent neutropenia and thrombocytopenia
Underlying defect	Absent CD40 ligand on T cells (B cells need this to switch isotypes)

Clinical features

- Recurrent respiratory infection (URTI, LTRI, PCP)
- Autoimmune features may be present

Management

Gammaglobulin infusions.

Hyper IgE (Job syndrome)

Immune defect	Possible immune dysregulation of IgE
	Very high IgE (> 1000), impaired neutrophil locomotion
	T cell abnormalities
Underlying defect	Unknown

Clinical features

Eczema infections	Staphylococcal abscesses in lung, skin, joints

Management

1. Antibiotic prophylaxis (penicillin)
2. Gammaglobulin infusions if deficient
3. Drainage of abscesses

NEUTROPHIL DISORDERS

Chronic granulomatous disease (CGD)

Immune defect	Failure of superoxide production (therefore inability to kill)
Underlying defect	Defective cytochrome b558 (the enzymatic unit of NADPH oxidase) from a defect in one of its subunits. Absent gp91phox (X-linked, 66%). Absence of p22phox (autosomal recessive, 33%)

Clinical features

Infections	Recurrent abscesses of bone, lung, liver, lymph nodes, gastrointestinal tract
	Aspergillus infection
Granulomas	GIT, liver, spleen, skin, lung, bone
Other	Gingival hyperplasia, cervical lymphadenopathy, hepatosplenomegaly

Diagnosis

- NBT test (failure to reduce nitroblue tetrazolium)
- Biopsy granuloma
- Hypergammaglobulinaemia
- Radiology – liver/spleen CT scan, bone scan, CXR

Management

- Treat acute infection with antibiotics and neutrophil transfusions
- Long-term therapy with γ-interferon and prophylactic antibiotics
- Gene therapy for X-linked disease in development

Chediak–Higashi syndrome

Immune defect	Giant granules in all nucleated cells
	Neutropenia, granulocyte mobility and chemotaxis defects
	NK cell cytotoxicity defective
Underlying defect	Cytoskeletal microtubule defect
	Autosomal recessive

Clinical features

Infections	Recurrent, bacterial (skin, respiratory, abscesses)
Albinism	Partial occulocutaneous
	Photophobia, nystagmus
Neurological	CNS and peripheral nerve lesions

Accelerated phase of disease can occur with Epstein–Barr virus infection resembling familial lymphohistiocytosis (FLH), leading to pancytopenia, hepatosplenomegaly and death.

Diagnosis

- Neutrophil analysis (giant granules)
- Giant melanosomes in melanocytes
- Bleeding time prolonged due to platelet aggregation defects

Management

- Treatment of acute infections
- Stem cell transplant

Shwachman–Diamond syndrome (see p. 151)

Immune defect	Cyclical neutropenia, defective neutrophil mobility and chemotaxis
Underlying defect	Unknown
	Autosomal recessive

Clinical features

- Cyclical neutropenia
- Exocrine pancreatic failure (steatorrhoea)
- Metaphyseal dysostosis (short stature)
- Anaemia, thrombocytopenia (variable)

Management

Supportive, pancreatic exocrine supplements, GMCSF.

Leucocyte adhesion defects (LAD)

Immune defect	Abnormal leucocyte adhesion
	Peripheral neutrophils ↑
Underlying defect	Absence of CD18 (LAD1) resulting in LFA1, C3b or p150 deficiency
	Autosomal recessive

Clinical features

Infections	Skin, necrotic ulcers, periodontal infections
Fistulae	Intestinal or perianal

Management

- Aggressive use of antibiotics and antifungals
- BMT

COMPLEMENT DEFICIENCIES

Congenital deficiencies of almost all the complement components have been found, and of complement control proteins.

Two major patterns of infection exist:

1. Encapsulated bacteria – deficiencies of C2, C3, C4 and C1q (complement components); deficiencies of factor H or I (complement control proteins)
2. Neisserial infections – deficiencies of the lytic pathway (C5–9) (complement components)

Hereditary angioedema

This is due to C1 esterase inhibitor deficiency or defectiveness. Activation of C1 leads to uncontrolled C1 activity, breakdown of C2 and C4 and release of kinin (vasoactive peptide) from C2. The disease manifests as episodes of non-pitting oedema (with no itch, urticaria or redness) lasting 2–3 days. Laryngeal involvement may cause respiratory obstruction, and intestinal wall swelling can cause abdominal pain, vomiting and diarrhoea. Stress, surgery or exercise may trigger attacks. Treatment is with hydrocortisone ± adrenaline, FFP or purified inhibitor in acute attack. Danazol for long-term. Autosomal dominant acquired form exists.

ACQUIRED IMMUNODEFICIENCY

CAUSES

Immunoglobulin deficiency

- Lymphoproliferative disease, e.g. CLL
- Bone marrow aplasia, hypersplenism

- Protein loss: Protein-losing enteropathy
                  Burns
                  Nephrotic syndrome
                  Malnutrition states

Cell-mediated immunodeficiency

- Drugs, e.g. cyclosporin, cyclophosphamide, steroids, azathioprine, tacrolimus
- Lymphoproliferative disease, e.g. lymphoma
- Bone marrow aplasia, hypersplenism
- HIV infection

HIV AND AIDS

HIV (human immunodeficiency virus) is in the lentivirus group of retroviruses. Retroviruses contain the enzyme **reverse transcriptase**, which enables viral RNA to be incorporated into host cell DNA. There are two main types: HIV-1 (widespread) and HIV-2 (West Africa).

The cellular receptor for the virus is the CD4 molecule, which is found on T helper cells (Th1 subset), the cells most affected by the disease. The CD4 cell numbers decline and the host develops a profound immunodeficiency, encouraging opportunistic infections.

Transmission

Mode of transmission:

- Vertical transmission (mother to child, the majority of childhood HIV):   Prenatally
                                                                            Intrapartum
                                                                            Postnatally through breastfeeding

- Via mucous membranes during sexual intercourse (NB: sexual abuse)
- Blood transmission directly into the circulation, e.g. IV drug abusers

The overall vertical transmission rate estimates vary from 15% to 30% (see below).

Diagnosis

There are various techniques to detect HIV:

- Virus detection by PCR (rapid, sensitive and specific) or viral culture (slower)
- Viral p24 antigen – present shortly after infection until 8–10 weeks. Can reappear as disease becomes worse
- Detection of IgG antibody to envelop components (gp 120 and subunits). There is a window of < 3 months after infection before this becomes positive. These antibodies cross the placenta, therefore all infants of HIV-positive mothers possess them, whether they are infected or not. The antibody disappears by around 12–18 months if infant is not infected
- Detection of IgG antibody to p24, present early in infection only

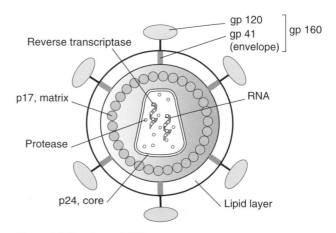

Figure 2.2 Structure of HIV

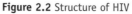

Repeat testing by PCR during the first few months should be done on all infants at risk to be sure of not missing an infected infant and to *confirm* a positive test.

Clinical manifestations

Infants are generally asymptomatic in the neonatal period. Two patterns of disease are seen:

1. Early-onset AIDS-defining symptoms (within a few months) (25%)
2. Late-onset AIDS-defining symptoms (around 8 years) (75%)

The disease develops more rapidly in children than in adults and opportunistic infections occur more frequently early in the disease. In addition to multiple infections, particular presentations in childhood include faltering growth, lymphocytic interstitial pneumonitis (LIP) and HIV encephalopathy. The disease criteria were revised in 1994, as below.

CDC 1994 classification for HIV disease in children < 13 years

This involves the four clinical categories listed below and three immunological categories based on the CD4 T lymphocyte counts at different ages.

Clinical categories	
Category N: Asymptomatic	No symptoms or only one of those in category A
Category A: Mildly symptomatic	$\geq$ 2 of the following symptoms: • Lymphadenopathy (>0.5 cm at >2 sites) • Hepatomegaly • Splenomegaly • Parotitis • Dermatitis • Recurrent or persistent URTIs (> 3 episodes/year)
Category B: Moderately symptomatic	Symptomatic conditions not listed in category C attributed to HIV infection There are many listed examples, including: • Anaemia < 8 g/dl or neutropenia < 1000/m^3 persisting >30 days Oropharyngeal candidiasis for > 2 months in a child > 6 months of age Chronic or recurrent diarrhoea • LIP • Herpes zoster, two episodes or > 1 dermatome
Category C: Severely symptomatic	Any condition listed in the 1987 surveillance case definition of AIDS except LIP. Examples include: • Oesophageal or pulmonary candidiasis multiple or recurrent serious bacterial infections (any combination of at least two culture-proven infections within a 2-year period, including septicaemia, pneumonia, meningitis) • *Pneumocystis jeuni* (formerly *carinii*) pneumonia • Progressive multifocal leucoencephalopathy • Kaposi sarcoma
From Centers for Disease Control 1994 classification system for HIV infection in children < 13 years old.	

Faltering growth

This may be apparent in the first few months of life. HIV with faltering growth is a differential diagnosis of SCID. It occurs due to a combination of factors:

- Reduced intake (appetite poor, HIV encephalopathy)
- Malabsorption (GI infections, HIV enteropathy)
- Increased metabolic requirements (recurrent infections)

Lymphocytic interstitial pneumonitis

This is a chronic lung disease of uncertain aetiology seen in 40–50% of vertically infected children.

Clinical features are variable. Patients may be asymptomatic, diagnosed on CXR or have features of respiratory distress including dyspnoea and hypoxia.

| CXR findings | Diffuse, interstitial reticulonodular infiltrate |
| | Hilar or mediastinal lymphadenopathy may be present |

Management is symptomatic only. Steroids may reduce oxygen dependency.

HIV encephalopathy

This is common in HIV-infected children. It presents as motor and language developmental delay, and an acquired microcephaly may occur. Brain imaging studies (CT/MRI) may demonstrate cortical atrophy, basal ganglia calcification, ventricular enlargement and white matter abnormalities.

Opportunistic infections

Protozoa

Pneumocystis jejuni (carinii) pneumonia (PCP)

Pnemocystis jejuni (formerly *carinii*) is an extracellular protozoan which causes opportunistic infection in immunocompromised individuals. It is an AIDS-defining illness. It often presents at 3 months of age in severely affected infants.

Clinical features:

- Hypoxia *often* more *severe* than expected from chest examination findings
- Persistent non-productive cough
- Dyspnoea
- High fever

Investigations:

CXR	Diffuse perihilar bilateral '*butterfly*' shadowing, ground glass appearance, cavities
	May be normal
Bronchoalveolar lavage	Immunofluorescence staining with monoclonal antibodies

Management:

| Pneumonia | High-dose co-trimoxazole (Septrin) IV/orally or pentamidine IV for 21 days |
| Prophylaxis | Low-dose co-trimoxazole orally or pentamidine nebulizers monthly |

Toxoplasmosis

Toxoplasma gondii	Cerebral abscesses, encephalitis (more common in adults)	
	Diagnosis	CT or MRI scan
		Positive IgG antibody to toxoplasmosis
	Treatment	Long-term pyrimethamine + sulphonamide

Cryptosporidiosis

Cryptosporidium parvum   Severe secretory diarrhoea, abdominal pain, bowel wall cysts, sclerosing cholangitis
                                          Diagnosis   Stool specimens (cysts), small bowel biopsy
                                          Treatment   Supportive, Paromamycin

Fungi

Candida

Candida albicans   Oropharyngeal (> 70% symptomatic children)
                        Oesophageal (dysphagia), vulvovaginal, disseminated (rare)
                        Treatment   Chronic antifungal therapy, e.g. fluconazole
                                               IV amphotericin B may be needed

Cryptococcus

Cryptococcus neoformans   Meningitis (atypical presentation), pneumonia
                             Diagnosis   CSF (India ink staining, antigen titres, culture)
                                               Serum (organism culture)
                             Treatment   Long-term fluconazole

Viruses

Many viruses can cause unusually severe disease in HIV-infected children. These include VZV (severe primary disease, recurrent zoster), RSV and adenovirus (severe pneumonitis), measles (pneumonitis and encephalitis), CMV and HSV (as below).

Cytomegalovirus (CMV)

Retinitis   Decreased acuity, floaters, orbital pain
               'Pizza-pie' appearance of haemorrhages and exudate on ophthalmoscopy
               Treatment with gancyclovir IV
Colitis   Bloody diarrhoea, fever, toxic dilatation, ulcers, hepatitis, sclerosing cholangitis
               Diagnosis on colonoscopy and biopsy ('owl's eye' cytoplasmic inclusion bodies)
               Treatment with gancyclovir IV
Other   Pneumonitis, hepatitis, pancreatitis, adrenal insufficiency

Herpes simplex virus (HSV)

HSV 1 and 2   Extensive oral and genital ulceration
                   Diagnosis   Clinical, virus isolation from ulcers, serology
                   Treatment   Acyclovir IV (NB: Resistance problems)

Bacteria

Recurrent serious bacterial infections are seen, as dysregulation of B cell function occurs in HIV. Of particular note is atypical mycobacterial infection, e.g. *Mycobacterium avium intracellulare*.

Tumours

Less common in children than adults.

Kaposi sarcoma

This is a tumour of vascular endothelial cells associated with HHV-8 and appears as purple lesions. It commonly involves skin, gut, lymphatics and lung. Treatment is with antiretrovirals, radiotherapy (if local) or chemotherapy (if disseminated).

Lymphoma

Non-Hodgkin B cell lymphoma, primary CNS lymphoma. Poor response to therapy unless it occurs when immuno-suppression is mild.

HIV therapy

A multidisciplinary team approach is used to manage the physical and emotional needs of these children and their families.

Currently Septrin prophylaxis is given until the child is shown to be HIV negative. If HIV positive, Septrin is continued until 12 months of age and then treatment is given according to the CD4 count and viral load. Combinations of drugs are used: the specific recommendations frequently change due to rapid therapeutic developments. Viral load and CD4 cell count are used as monitors of therapy.

Drug	Side-effect
Nucleoside analogues (reverse transcriptase inhibitors)	
Zidovudine (AZT, 3-azido-3-deoxythymidine)	Nausea, abdominal pain, headache, insomnia Bone marrow suppression, neutropenia, myopathy
Dideoxyinosine (DDI) and dideoxycitidine (DDC)	Gastrointestinal disturbance, pancreatitis, peripheral neuropathy
Non-nucleoside analogues (reverse transcriptase inhibitors) Nevirapine	
Protease inhibitors (prevent viral maturation) Indinavir	Gastrointestinal, headache, lethargy, rashes, elevation of bilirubin or liver transaminases, kidney stones

Reduction of vertical transmission

Pregnant women with HIV infection have a transmission risk (untreated) of approximately 15–30%. Measures to reduce transmission to < 5% include:

- Antiretroviral therapy during pregnancy and delivery
- Antiretroviral therapy during delivery only if unable to administer during pregnancy
- Elective Caesarean section
- Avoid invasive fetal procedures, e.g. fetal scalp electrodes and blood sampling
- Avoid breastfeeding (the WHO advises breastfeeding continue in developing countries to prevent malnutrition)
- Oral AZT to infant for the first 4–6 weeks

FURTHER READING

Primary Immunodeficiency Diseases, Report of a WHO Scientific Group *Clinical and Experimental Immunology* 1997 **109** (Suppl 1):1–28

Roitt IM, Brostoff J, Male D *Immunology,* 6th edn. Philadelphia: Mosby, 2001

3
Infectious diseases

- *Vaccination*
- *The febrile child*
- *The seriously unwell child*
- *Viral infections*

- *Bacterial infections*
- *Protozoal infections*
- *Fungal infections*
- *Helminthic infections*

VACCINATION

IMMUNIZATION SCHEDULE

Age	Vaccination
Birth	BCG (in at risk individuals)
2 months	DTP, polio, Hib, men C
3 months	DTP, polio, Hib, men C
4 months	DTP, polio, Hib, men C
Infancy	BCG (if in 'at-risk' group)
12 months	MMR, Hib
3–5 years	DTaP, polio, MMR
15 years	dT, polio

Key: D = diphtheria, d = low concentration diphtheria, P = pertussis, T = tetanus, MMR = measles, mumps, rubella, men C = meningococcal C conjugate, Hib = *Haemophilus influenzae* type b conjugate, aP = acellular pertussis, BCG = Bacille Calmette–Guerin

NB: Premature infants are scheduled for age since *birth (chronological age)*, irrespective of their prematurity.

VACCINES

Live attenuated vaccines	Killed organism vaccines	Subunit vaccines	Egg protein vaccines	Toxoid vaccines
Measles	Cholera	*Haemophilus influenzae* b	Measles	Diphtheria
Mumps	Pertussis		Influenza	Tetanus
Rubella	Typhoid	*Neisseria meningitides* (A,C,Y,W135)	Yellow fever	
Polio (oral, Sabin)	Polio (Salk)		Mumps	
Varicella zoster virus	Influenza	*Streptococcus pneumoniae* (7 valent, 23 valent)		
BCG	Rabies			
Yellow fever	Hepatitis B			
Cholera (live attenuated, oral) Typhoid (live, oral, attenuated)	Pertussis acellular			

NB: Polio Salk vaccine is a killed vaccine.

Contraindications to vaccination

All vaccines

1. Acute febrile illness – temporary contraindication. NB: Mild infection without fever or systemic upset is not a contraindication
2. Anaphylactic reaction to previous dose

Live vaccines

1. Immunosuppressed or on immunosuppressive treatment
2. On prednisolone (oral/rectal) 2 mg/kg/day for at least 1 week or 1 mg/kg/day for at least 1 month
3. Lower dose of prolonged steroids or in combination with immunosuppressives, to discuss with immunologist
4. Impaired cell-mediated immunity (antibody deficiency is a contraindication to oral polio vaccine)

HIV-positive children

These may receive all standard vaccines in the schedule except BCG. Inactivated polio vaccine may be used instead of live vaccine in symptomatic individuals.

Pertussis vaccine

In children with an *evolving* neurological problem, immunization is deferred until the condition is stable.

THE FEBRILE CHILD

The majority of children with a fever will have a self-limiting viral infection; however, it is important to distinguish and treat those children with a more serious cause.

Management of a febrile child includes a thorough history and examination to help elucidate the cause. There is no single clinical or laboratory finding that distinguishes viral from bacterial infection so it is necessary to develop an **impression** of the child as a whole and **frequently to reassess** the child.

Fevers can be divided into:

1. Fever with localizing signs
2. Fever without localizing signs

IMPORTANT POINTS IN THE HISTORY

*   Contact with infectious diseases
*   Travel
*   Contact with animals and insects
*   Dietary history, e.g. unpasturized milk consumption – listeria, brucellosis
*   Age (age-related infections)
*   Immunization status
*   Season
*   Immunocompromised state, e.g. chemotherapy patient, HIV patient, congenital immunodeficiency

IMPORTANT POINTS IN THE EXAMINATION

*   General clinical state and vital signs (see below)
*   Degree of fever
*   Rash
*   Lymphadenopathy, hepatosplenomegaly
*   Heart murmur
*   Localizing signs, e.g. tonsillar exudate, joint or bone tenderness
*   Features of immunodeficiency (see p. 26)

MANAGEMENT

Fever with localizing signs   Treat and investigate as appropriate for the condition

Fever without localizing signs
*   It is important not to miss a bacteraemic illness. Features suggestive of bacteraemia are outlined (see below); however, these are non-specific and none is diagnostic
*   Remember infections are **dynamic**. A child who has mild fever and looks well may be at the early stages of a septicaemic illness. **Regular review** (by family, primary or secondary health care workers) is imperative
*   Children who are clinically ill are investigated (with CRP and FBC; blood, throat and urine, stool $\pm$ CSF cultures) and then either commenced empirically on antibiotics, or observed with antibiotics only given if exact cause of illness is found, or sepsis is apparent
*   If a fever persists > a few days with no cause found, causes of prolonged fever should be looked for (see below). In particular, consider Kawasaki disease

Features suggestive of an unwell child

(Not necessarily a bacterial infection, but think of it in this context.)

NB: These features have low sensitivity and specificity.

Symptom/sign/test	Observation
Temperature	Markedly elevated (> 39°C) Hypothermia (neonates and impending severe sepsis)
Pulse rate	Tachycardia/bradycardia
Colour	Pale or mottled
Capillary refill time	Prolonged
Peripheries	Cool
Tone	Floppy
Responsiveness	Intermittent or unresponsive
WCC ESR, CRP elevated	$> 15 \times 10^9$/L or $< 2.5 \times 10^9$/L

Causes of prolonged fever

Viral infections	CMV, EBV, human herpes virus 6, HIV
Bacterial infections	TB, leptospirosis, brucellosis, spirochaetes, salmonella, bacterial endocarditis, osteomyelitis, abscesses
Other infections	Malaria, toxoplasmosis, chlamydia, rickettsia, fungal infections
Non-infectious causes	**Kawasaki disease**, collagen vascular disease, malignancies, drugs, inflammatory bowel disease, familial Mediterranean fever

THE SERIOUSLY UNWELL CHILD

SEPSIS

If a pathogen manages to break through the host's first line of defence and invades the blood stream, and if the host does not rapidly resolve the infection, bacterial proliferation can ensue and this results in a systemic host inflammatory response, which together with the virulent properties of the invading organism cause the features of sepsis.

In **septic shock** there is persistent hypotension despite adequate fluid resuscitation and/or hypoperfusion even after adequate inotrope or pressor support.

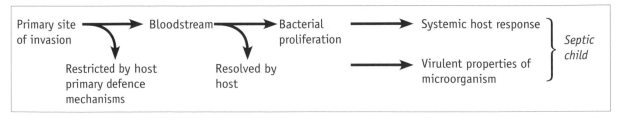

Figure 3.1 Pathway of sepsis

Main causes

Neonates (< 3 months age)	> 3 months of age children	Immunocompromised

Group B streptococcus
Escherichia coli
Other Gram-negative bacteria
Listeria monocytogenes
Staphylococcus aureus
	Streptococcus pneumoniae
	Neisseria meningitidis
	Haemophilus influenzae type b
	Staphylococcus aureus
	Group A streptococcus
	Salmonella spp.
		As for children and in addition:
		  Gram-negative organisms
		  Fungi
		  Opportunistic organisms

Clinical features

- The clinical features depend upon the organism, child's age and pre-existing health and duration of the illness
- Early bacteraemia can be difficult to assess. Therefore it is essential frequently to reassess the situation
- Non-specific early features: lethargy, irritability, hypotonia, poor feeding, mottled skin, nausea and vomiting
- Cardiovascular features: tachycardia/bradycardia, poor peripheral perfusion, prolonged capillary refill time, peripheral oedema, decreased urine output
- Other organs: respiratory, gastrointestinal, neurological derangement
- Rash: petechial, erythroderma, mucosal erythema and oedema (toxic shock syndrome, see p. 58)

Causes of petechial rash

Infections	Other
Meningococcal (sepsis, meningitis)	ITP
Haemophilus influenzae (sepsis, meningitis)	HSP (localized to buttocks, thighs, sockline)
Streptococcus pneumoniae (sepsis, meningitis)	Anaphylactoid purpura
Rickettsia, e.g. Rocky Mountain spotted fever	Leukaemia
Viral infection (EBV, CMV, atypical measles, enteroviruses)	DIC
Malaria	Vigorous coughing or vomiting ⎫ Localized to Attempted strangulation ⎬ head and neck

Management

Initially there is a small number of invading organisms, but these multiply (often logarithmically) resulting in rapid clinical deterioration. Therefore the most important management is *recognition of sepsis as early as possible* and initiation of antibiotics and supportive treatment. Frequent reassessment is therefore imperative.

Investigations	Source of infection:	Blood cultures Urine microscopy and culture Other samples, e.g. throat swab Lumbar puncture if suspected meningeal involvement
	Other indicators of infection: WCC, inflammatory markers	
	Other: FBC, coagulation profile, U&E, creatinine, glucose, LFTs, blood gas	
Treatment	Initial resuscitation as necessary Appropriate antibiotic therapy as soon as possible Supportive measures for septic shock Adjuvant therapy: new treatments administering antagonists of host-derived inflammatory mediators are being developed	

MENINGITIS

This is an acute infection with an inflammatory process involving the meninges, and may be bacterial, viral, fungal or other microbial.

Most common causes of bacterial meningitis

Neonates	2–3 months	3 months–5 years	> 5 years
Group B β-haemolytic streptococcus *Escherichia coli* *Listeria monocytogenes*	As for neonates *N. meningitidis*	*Neisseria meningitidis* (meningococcus) *Strep. pneumoniae* (pneumococcus) *Haemophilus influenzae type b* (uncommon since Hib vaccine)	Meningococcus Pneumococcus

Causes of viral meningitis

- Enteroviruses (> 80%, especially coxsackie and echovirus)
- Adenovirus
- Mumps
- EBV, CMV, VZV, HSV
- HIV

Clinical features

Sudden onset and rapid deterioration are seen in meningococcal meningitis.

Neonate	Non-specific features, lethargy, apnoea, poor feeding, temperature instability, respiratory distress, high-pitched cry, seizures, bulging fontanelle, shock, rash (occasionally)
Infant	Fever, lethargy, irritability, poor feeding, vomiting Bulging fontanelle, shock, seizures, coma, rash
Older child (*> 18 months*)	Fever, headache, drowsiness, shock, seizures (late), papilloedema (rare) Meningeal irritation: Headache, neck stiffness, photophobia **Kernig sign** (pain on lower leg extension, with hip flexed) **Brudzinski sign** (involuntary flexion of knees and hips with neck flexion)
Rash	Petechial rash seen classically in meningococcal infection (can also be seen in pneumococcal and *Haemophilus influenzae* infections)

Investigations

Blood	Glucose, blood gases, FBC, clotting profile, U&E, creatinine, CRP Bacterial cultures Bacterial PCR Viral (PCR) Viral serology, bacterial serology, e.g. *N. meningitidis*
CSF	Microscopy, culture, protein, glucose, bacterial antigens, viral and bacterial PCR
Throat and stool	M, C & S and viral culture
Urine	Rapid antigen tests
CXR	

Typical lumbar puncture findings

	Normal	Bacterial	Viral	TB
Appearance	Clear	Turbid	Clear	Viscous or clear
Lymphocytes/mm^3	< 5	< 50	10–100	100–300
Polymorphs/mm^3	Nil	> 200	Nil	0–200
Protein (g/L)	0.2–0.4	0.5–3 ↑	0.2–1.0 (N or ↑)	0.5–6.0 ↑↑
Glucose	> ½ serum	< ½ serum (↓)	> ½ serum (N)	< ⅓rd serum (↓↓)

NB: Neonates have different normal ranges, with higher white cell counts and CSF protein levels.

Contraindications to lumbar puncture

- ICP ↑ (focal or prolonged seizures, impaired consciousness, papilloedema, focal neurological signs)
- Cardiopulmonary compromise (sepsis)
- Local skin infection overlying LP site
- Coagulopathy

Management

Bacterial meningitis

Antibiotics	IV therapy to commence immediately. Do not delay for LP
	Choice depends on likely pathogen, generally third-generation cephalosporin, e.g. ceftriaxone, for 7–10 days
	Add ampicillin if < 3 months to cover listeria
	Rifampicin 2 days following treatment of meningococcal disease (if antibiotic other than ceftriaxone used)
Dexamethasone	Only of proven benefit in *H. influenzae* meningitis but generally administered in all bacterial meningitis
Supportive measures	Initial resuscitation with oxygen and IV fluids
	Monitoring of neurological status
	Intubation and ventilation if necessary and circulatory support (fluids, inotropes, CVP) as needed

Viral meningitis

Less severe infection, full recovery usual, enterovirus in the majority. Treat as bacterial if in doubt until culture results at 48 h. Aciclovir for HSV or VZV infection.

Complications

SIADH	Common complication, monitor plasma and urine electrolytes, and osmolality
Cerebral	Abscess, infarction, subdural effusion, hydrocephalus
Deafness	Due to VIIIth nerve vasculitis
Meningococcal disease	This may present as septicaemia (worse prognosis) or meningitis, with rapid deterioration
	Purpuric rash, may lead to necrotic areas
Haemophilus influenzae	Reduced incidence due to *H. influenzae* (Hib) vaccine. Subdurals common
Pneumococcal meningitis	High mortality (10%) and morbidity (30% neurological sequelae)

47

TB meningitis (see p. 66)

Unusual features	Chronic presentation, vague headache, anorexia, vomiting. Focal neurological signs, seizures, cortical blindness
Investigations	Mantoux or Heaf test (NB: May be negative)
	CXR (changes in 50%)
	CT brain (oedema, infarction, hydrocephalus, abscess, tuberculoma)
	CSF, gastric aspirate and early morning urine for microscopy, PCR and TB culture
Management	Commence on suspicion, 12 months of antituberculous therapy (rifampicin, isoniazid, pyrazinamide, ± ethambutol). Consider steroids

Partially treated bacterial meningitis

The picture may be confused, with culture-negative CSF but leucocytosis. Rapid antigen tests ± PCR may be useful. If concerned, treat as bacterial.

Prevention for contacts

Contacts	Meningococcal *H. influenzae*: all close contacts given 2 days oral rifampicin and 4 days oral rifampicin if there is an unvaccinated child < 4 years in household
Vaccination	Hib vaccine all children
	Meningococcal vaccine currently available to groups A, C, Y and W135 only

Prognosis

- Mortality of bacterial meningitis 5–10% with treatment
- Neurological impairment in survivors > 10%

ENCEPHALITIS

An inflammation of the brain parenchyma, which may be due to:

- Direct viral invasion
- Secondary to post-infectious due to immune response or slow virus infection, e.g. SSPE

Viral encephalitis and meningitis are caused by the same organisms and form a continuum.

Viral encephalitis

Cause	Specific features
HSV 1 and 2	Temporal lobe abnormalities on EEG and MRI 70% mortality untreated Aciclovir treatment
VZV	Aciclovir treatment. Post-infectious cerebellar ataxia
Mumps	VIIIth nerve damage, with deafness
Enteroviruses Measles Rubella HIV-I Rabies	Echovirus, coxsackie virus

Clinical features

- Insidious onset compared to bacterial meningitis
- Fever, headache, lethargy, behavioural change, meningeal irritation (uncommon in young infants), decreased consciousness, seizures
- Focal neurology, features of ICP ↑
- Neurological sequelae common (cognitive and motor deficits, epilepsy, behavioural changes)

Investigations

Samples	As for bacterial meningitis
	In particular, blood serology (including viral, mycoplasma raised specific IgM, or increase in IgG in paired sera), viral cultures (blood, urine, stool, throat and CSF) and PCR for specific pathogens
Imaging	MRI
Other	EEG

Management

- Supportive care (shock, ICP ↑ treatment)
- Antiviral agents (intravenous)
- Treat with antibiotics as for bacterial meningitis until viral aetiology confirmed/bacterial cultures negative

VIRAL INFECTIONS

DNA VIRUSES

Family	Virus	Disease
Adenoviridae	Adenovirus	Croup, pharyngitis, mesenteric adenitis
Herpesviridae	HSV (HHV1)	HSV-1 and -2 infections
	VZV (HHV2)	Chicken pox, shingles
	CMV (HHV3)	CMV infection
	EBV (HHV4)	Infectious mononucleosis
	HHV6 ⎫ HHV7 ⎭	Roseola infantum (exanthum subitum, sixth disease)
	HHV 8	Kaposi sarcoma
Hepadnaviridae	HBV	Hepatitis (see p. 191)
Papovaviridae	Human papillomavirus	Warts (see p. 296)
Parvoviridae	Parvovirus B19	Fifth disease (erythema infectiosum, slapped cheek syndrome)
Poxviridae	Variola virus	Smallpox
	Orf	Orf (hard skin lesions, from sheep)
	Molluscum contagiosum	Molluscum contagiosum (see p. 295)

Herpes simplex virus (HSV)

Transmission	Direct contact
Incubation	2–15 days

Two types of HSV exist:

HSV-1   Transmitted mainly via saliva and the cause of most childhood infections

HSV-2   Transmitted mainly via genital secretions or via vaginal delivery and the primary cause of genital herpes. Dormancy in sacral ganglia

(NB: The two forms of HSV infections overlap.)

Primary infection causes a severe vesicular rash wherever the primary inoculation was:

- **Mouth infection (gingivostomatitis**). The most common primary infection. If severe, swallowing is painful and NG or intravenous fluids may be required. Fever for 2–3 days, then ulceration, healing in 1 week. Peak age 1–3 years. Dormancy in trigeminal ganglia
- **Skin infection**, e.g. **herpetic Whitlow** (infection on finger)
- **Eye infection (keratoconjunctivitis)** can result in corneal scarring. Ophthalmological review is important

Recurrent disease is triggered by stress, illness, sun exposure. Local recurrence generating from dormancy:

- **Herpes labialis (cold sore)** – the most common site
- Herpes genitalis

Serious HSV infection	
CNS infection	Encephalitis (temporal lobe damage, 70% mortality untreated) Meningitis
Eczema herpeticum	Widespread infection seen in children with atopic eczema
Immunocompromised child	Severe infection, may become disseminated
Neonatal infection	From maternal genital tract active lesions during delivery; high morbidity and mortality.

Diagnosis

Usually clinical.

Vesicle fluid	Electron microscopy (EM), immunofluorescence, viral culture
Blood	Serology
CSF	PCR

Treatment

Aciclovir	IV in severe disease (neonates, immunocompromised, eczema herpeticum, encephalitis, ophthalmic disease) Oral treatment considered in some cases Topical to cold sores Eye drops (ocular infection)

Varicella zoster virus (VZV)

This produces two diseases.

Varicella (chicken pox)

Transmission	Airborne or contact
Incubation	14–21 days, infectious 48 h pre-rash to 5 days after onset of rash
Clinical features	Mild prodromal illness with fever 2–3 days (not in young children) Peak age 2–8 years Rash: face, scalp and trunk, spreads *centrifugally* Macules → papules → vesicles → pustules → crusts. *All stages are seen at once* on the skin

Complications	Superinfection of the skin – crusts, pustules, prolonged fever. May develop toxic shock syndrome (*Staphylococcus aureus* or *Streptococcus pyogenes*) Encephalitis – acute truncal cerebellar ataxia (*post*-infectious). Recovery good Purpura fulminans – a vasculitis in skin and subcutaneous tissues Pneumonia – common in adults (30%), CXR dramatic Other – Sepsis, thrombocytopenia, DIC, hepatitis, Reye syndrome, arthritis, pancreatitis, nephritis, stroke Immunocompromised – severe disseminated haemorrhagic disease, high mortality
Congenital infection	This can produce severe malformations, with limb deformities

Zoster (shingles)

This occurs from reactivation of dormant VZV, from the dorsal root or cranial ganglia. Triggered by immunocompromise, though commonly seen in normal children. Lesions identical to varicella, itchy and slightly painful in children, and usually restricted to < 3 dermatomes. Infection of the geniculate ganglion causes ear pinna vesicles and facial nerve palsy (= Ramsay–Hunt syndrome).

Diagnosis

Clinical diagnosis	Vesicle fluid – electron microscopy, immunofluorescence, viral culture (difficult)
Serology	CSF – PCR

Treatment

Chicken pox	No treatment required in uncomplicated cases IV aciclovir if complications or immunocompromised
Shingles	Aciclovir (oral or IV, dependent on severity and site)
Neonatal	Maternal infection 5 days predelivery to 2 days post: give ZIG to infant. If infant develops vesicles, treat with IV aciclovir

Prophylaxis

Zoster immunoglobulin (ZIG), i.e. passive immunization is given to:

1. Immunocompromised children exposed to VZV, e.g. stem cell transplant patients, congenital immunodeficiency, on immunosuppressives or high dose steroids in previous 3 months
2. Neonates (as above)

VZV vaccine exists but is currently not routinely used in the UK.

Cytomegalovirus (CMV)

Transmission	Close contact (saliva, breast milk, genital secretions) Transplacental Blood (NB: An important pathogen in organ transplant)

Most children are infected when toddlers, and half of adults have positive serology (IgG to CMV).

Clinical features

Healthy individuals	Asymptomatic (usually) Similar clinical picture to EBV (but tonsillitis less obvious)
Immunocompromised	Severe infection including encephalitis, retinitis, pneumonitis, gastrointestinal infection, atypical lymphocytes, hepatitis
Congenital infection	See p. 449

Investigations

Serology	Primary infection (IgM), latent infection (IgG)
Urine	For CMV DEAFF (signifies active replication)
CMV PCR	On blood and other secretions
Blood count	Lymphocytosis with atypical lymphocytes. Sometimes neutropenia
Tissues	Intranuclear 'owl's eye' inclusions on microscopy, direct immunofluorescence, viral culture

Treatment

None in healthy individuals. Ganciclovir, foscarnet or cidofovir IV if immunocompromised.

Epstein-Barr virus (EBV)

This produces infectious mononucleosis (glandular fever). The virus infects the B lymphocytes.

Transmission	Aerosol, saliva
Incubation	20–30 days

Clinical features

- Often asymptomatic in young children. Classical picture in adolescents
- Fever, headache, tonsillopharyngitis, palatal petechiae, generalized lymphadenopathy
- Maculopapular rash. Bright red rash in 90% if ampicillin given
- Splenomegaly (tender), hepatitis, hepatomegaly
- Arthropathy
- Thrombocytopenia, haemolytic anaemia, atypical lymphocytes, mononuclear cells
- May produce depression and malaise for months

Complications

- Meningitis, encephalitis
- Myocarditis
- Myelitis, Guillain–Barré syndrome
- Mesenteric adenitis
- Splenic rupture

Burkitt lymphoma, nasopharyngeal carcinoma and lymphoproliferative disease in the immunocompromised are thought to be caused by EBV infection (see p. 52).

Diagnosis

- Atypical lymphocytes in the blood
- Monospot test positive (heterophile antibodies to horse RBCs, unreliable < 5 years due to false negatives)
- Positive Paul–Bunnell reaction positive (IgM antibodies that agglutinate sheep RBCs. Non-specific. False positives: leukaemia, non-Hodgkin lymphoma, hepatitis)
- EBV IgM may be detected (75–90% by end of third week)
- EBV VCA (EBV viral capsid antigen) ⎫
- EBV NA (EBV nuclear antigen) ⎬ Antigens for serology
- EBV PCR ⎭

Treatment

Not usually required except in the rare cases of lymphoproliferation where monoclonal antibodies to the B cell antigen CD20 are used.

Roseola infantum (exanthem subitum, HHV6)

Almost all children are infected with this during infancy. Roseola infantum is the cause of approximately one-third of febrile convulsions in children < 2 years of age.

Transmission	Droplet
Incubation	9–10 days

Clinical features

- High fever and malaise
- Cervical lymphadenopathy
- Few days later red macular rash over face, trunk and arms 1–2 days
- Red papules on the palate
- Febrile convulsions
- Sudden improvement after the rash
- Rarely: meningitis, encephalitis, hepatitis
- One-third of children asymptomatic

There is no specific treatment

Parvovirus B19

This virus attacks the erythroid precursors, and leads to transient arrest of erythropoiesis.

Transmission	Respiratory route, blood, vertical transmission
Incubation	Variable

Clinical features

It produces various clinical features:

1. **Slapped cheek disease (erythema infectiosum, Fifth disease):**
   Incubation 4–21 days
   Seen in school-age children, most commonly in spring
   Fever, malaise, myalgia
   Then after 1 week: very red cheeks, macular erythema over trunk and limbs with central clearing of the lesions, resulting in a **lacy pattern** which may recur over weeks
2. **Asymptomatic infection** – common
3. **Arthropathy** – usually transient, older children may develop arthritis
4. **Immunocompromised** – chronic infection with anaemia
5. **Transient aplastic crisis** – occurs in children in states of chronic haemolysis, e.g. sickle cell disease, thalassaemia, spherocytosis
6. **Congenital infection** – severe anaemia with hydrops fetalis.

RNA VIRUSES

Family	Virus species	Disease
Picornaviridae	Polio virus	Poliomyelitis (see p. 364)
	Coxsackie A virus (A1–A24)	Herpangina, hand, foot and mouth (HFM) disease, encephalitis
	Coxsackie B virus (B1–B6)	Myocarditis (B5), Bornholm disease, HFM disease
	Echovirus (types 1–33)	Herpangina, encephalitis, myocarditis (type 6)
	Enterovirus (types 68–72)	HFM disease, encephalitis
	Rhinovirus (many)	Common cold
	HAV	Hepatitis (see p. 191)
Reoviridae	Reovirus (many)	URTI, diarrhoea
	Rotavirus (many)	Diarrhoea
Togaviridae	Rubella virus	Rubella
	Alphaviruses	Ross River fever, etc
Flaviviridae	HCV	Hepatitis (see p. 194)
		Yellow fever, dengue fever, Japanese encephalitis
Orthomyxoviridae	Influenza virus A,B,C	A – pandemic, epidemics
		B – small outbreaks
Paramyxoviridae	Parainfluenza virus	Common cold, croup
	Measles virus	Measles
	Mumps virus	Mumps
	Respiratory syncytial virus	Bronchiolitis (see p. 129)
Rhabdoviridae	Rabies virus	Rabies
Retroviridae	Human immunodeficiency virus	HIV and AIDS (see p. 36)
Calciviridae	Hepatitis E virus	Hepatitis
Arenavirus	Lassa virus	Lassa fever

NB: Poliovirus, coxsackie A and B, echovirus and enterovirus are all in the genus Enteroviruses.

Hand, foot and mouth disease

Organisms   Coxsackie A (A16) and B, enterovirus (71)
Transmission   Faecal–oral, droplet, direct contact

Clinical features

- Mild disease lasting a week, mostly in pre-school children
- Fever with vesicles in the oropharynx, palms and soles
- Maculopapular rash also on palms, soles and buttocks
- In X-linked agammaglobulinaemia (XLA) enteroviruses can cause extensive cerebral infections

Rubella (German measles)

Transmission   Droplet, winter and spring
Incubation   14–21 days. Infectious <7 days from onset of rash

Clinical features

< 5 years	Usually asymptomatic
> 5 years	Prodrome of conjunctivitis, low grade fever, cervical lymphadenopathy (suboccipital and postauricular)
	Forcheimer spots (palatal petechiae)
	Splenomegaly
	< 7 days fine pink maculopapular rash on face, then body, lasting 3–5 days

Complications

- Arthritis (small joints)
- Myocarditis
- Thrombocytopenia
- Encephalitis
- Congenital rubella syndrome (see p. 451)

Diagnosis

Viral culture	Throat swab, urine
Serology	Rubella-specific IgM levels and rising antibody titre (acute and convalescent samples)

Management

- No treatment usually necessary
- Vaccination (contraindicated during pregnancy)

Measles

A potentially serious illness, whose incidence is rising again as the MMR vaccine uptake is poor. A vaccine coverage of > 90% is required to prevent epidemics.

Transmission	Droplet (coughing, sneezing)
Incubation	7–14 days
	Infectious from pre-eruptive stage until 1 week after onset of rash

Clinical features

Pre-eruptive stage	Unwell, high fever, conjunctivitis, cough, coryza
	Koplik spots (pathognomonic small white spots on labial mucosa and gums around 2nd molar). 2–3 days later:
Eruptive stage	Fine red maculopapular rash behind ears and on face, progressing to whole body
	NB: EEG abnormalities seen in 50%

Complications

- Common in malnourished children with vitamin A deficiency (developing countries)
- Otitis media
- Secondary bacterial pneumonia bronchitis
- Hepatitis, myocarditis, diarrhoea
- Post-measles blindness secondary to keratitis (seen in developing countries)
- Encephalomyelitis (post-infectious)
- Subacute sclerosing pan-encephalitis (SSPE) (a rare progressive dementia occurring several years after measles infection in < 1:100 000 cases) This is not caused by vaccine strains (see p. 358)

Investigations

Viral isolation	Immunofluorescence (CSF, serum, nasal secretions)
Viral culture	Throat swab
Serology	Serum, CSF, saliva (anti-measles IgM)

Treatment

- Symptomatic only
- Human pooled immunoglobulin and ribavirin can be given < 6 days of exposure (immunocompromised, < 3 years)
- MMR immunization

Mumps

Transmission	Droplet, direct contact, winter and spring
Incubation	14–21 days, infectious for 6 days pre–9 days post parotid swelling appears

Clinical features

- Prodrome of fever, anorexia, headache, earache. Usually asymptomatic
- Painful salivary gland swelling – bilateral (usually) or unilateral, parotid 60%, parotid and submandibular 10%
- Trismus may occur

Complications

- Meningeal signs (10%), encephalitis (1:5000), transient hearing loss
- Epididymo-orchitis (20% after puberty), pancreatitis, oophoritis, myocarditis, arthritis, mastitis, hepatitis

Investigations

Viral isolation/culture	Urine, saliva, throat swab, CSF (meningism)
Serology	Rise in antibody titre ('S' antigen early and 'V' antigen later, for life).

Rabies

Transmission	Saliva (animal bite)
Incubation	1–3 months (average 10 days)

The rabies virus enters through the bite wound, replicates in local muscle, travels up the peripheral nerves to the brain and replicates further. Then it travels via autonomic nerves to the salivary glands, lungs, kidneys, etc.

Clinical features

Initial	Pain at site of wound, fever, headache
Furious rabies	Anxiety, hallucinations, hyperexcitability with visual and auditory stimuli
	Hydrophobia (50%), aerophobia (*pathognomonic*)
	Sympathetic overactivity, cardiac arrhythmias, convulsions
	Death < 10–14 days
Dumb rabies	Symmetrical ascending paralysis with areflexia

Diagnosis

Rabies antigen	Salivary secretion, corneal impressions or skin sections (using fluorescent antibodies)
Postmortem	Negri bodies in cerebellum and hippocampus

Treatment

1. Clean the wound
2. Local antiserum (rabies immunoglobulin) around wound

3. Postexposure vaccine, human diploid cell strain vaccine (HDCSV) IM on days 0, 3, 7, 14 and 28
4. Symptomatic treatment with quiet, dark environment, sedation and analgesia

Prophylaxis

Rabies vaccine HDCSV IM two or three doses.

BACTERIAL INFECTIONS

GRAM-POSITIVE AND -NEGATIVE COCCI

Group	Organism		Disease
Gram-positive cocci			
Staphylococci	Coagulase positive	*Staph. aureus*	25% population carriers
	Coagulase negative	*Staph. epidermidis*	
		Staph. saprophyticus	
Streptococci	Group A β-haemolytic strep. (GAS) (*Strep. pyogenes*)		Most (95%) infections (15–20% children have asymptomatic nasal carriage of GAS)
	Group B β-haemolytic strep. (GBS)		Neonatal sepsis
	Strep. pneumoniae (non-β-haemolytic streptococci)		Pneumonia, meningitis Otitis media
	α-haemolytic strep. (*Strep. viridans*)		Infective endocarditis
Gram-negative cocci			
Neisseria	*N. meningitidis*		Meningitis, septicaemia (see p. 46)
	N. gonorrhoea		Gonorrhoea

STAPHYLOCOCCAL INFECTIONS

Staphylococci are part of the normal flora of skin, upper respiratory tract and gastrointestinal tract.

Infections due to bacterial invasion		Toxin mediated
Skin	Impetigo (see p. 294), cellulitis	Bullous impetigo, SSSS (see p. 294)
		Staphylococcal scarlet fever
General	Septicaemia	Toxic shock syndrome (TSS)
Gut	Enterocolitis	Food poisoning (onset 6 hours from ingestion)
Bones	Septic arthritis (p. 495), osteomyelitis	
Eyes	Orbital cellulitis, preseptal cellulitis (see p. 383)	
Lungs	Pneumonia, lung abscess (see p. 134)	
CNS	Meningitis (see p. 46)	
Cardiac	Acute endocarditis (see p. 108)	

Toxic shock syndrome

This severe infection is due to exotoxins, e.g. toxic shock syndrome toxin-1 (TSST-1) usually from *Staph. aureus*. The focus of infection is usually minor, e.g. a boil. There is an association with tampon use.

Diagnostic features

- Fever ≥ 38.9°C
- Conjunctivitis
- Patchy then diffuse tender pale red rash followed by desquamation
- Hypotension
- Vomiting and diarrhoea
- Toxic effects in other systems (≥ 3 required for diagnosis): myalgia, renal impairment, thrombocytopenia, drowsiness, mucous membrane involvement

Anti-TSST-1 antibodies are positive. Management is mostly supportive, with IV antibiotics, cardiovascular support, IPPV and renal dialysis as necessary. IVIG may be considered.

Streptococcal TSS is similar and often due to a deep-seated streptococcal infection.

STREPTOCOCCAL INFECTIONS

Infections due to bacterial invasion		Toxin mediated	Post-infectious
Skin	Impetigo, bullous impetigo Cellulitis, erysipelas	Scarlet fever Streptococcal scalded skin syndrome	Erythema nodosum
Respiratory	Otitis media Tonsillitis, pneumonia Mastoiditis, sinusitis		
Bone	Osteomyelitis (usually Staph.)		Arthritis
CNS	Meningitis	(In neonates)	PANDAS (see below) Sydenham chorea
General	Septicaemia	Streptococcal TSS	
Cardiac	Infective endocarditis		Rheumatic fever
Renal			Glomerulonephritis

Scarlet fever

This is due to a strain of Group A β-haemolytic streptococci producing an **erythrogenic exotoxin** in individuals with no neutralizing antibodies. The entry site is usually the pharynx (after tonsillitis).

Transmission	Contact, droplets
Incubation	2–4 days post-streptococcal pharyngitis

Clinical features

- Fever, headache, sore throat, rigors, vomiting, anorexia
- 'White strawberry tongue' (white coating, red papillae), then
- 'Strawberry tongue' (bright red)

- Flushed cheeks with circumoral pallor. Erythematous, coarse rash (feels like sandpaper) commencing on the neck, spreading to the rest of the body (face, palms and soles usually involved), desquamation after 5 days
- School-age children

Diagnosis

- Throat swab (positive culture)
- ASOT (antistreptolysin O toxin) and anti-DNAse B present

Management

Oral penicillin for 10 days (erythromycin if penicillin allergic).

PANDAS (paediatric autoimmune neuropsychiatric disorders associated with streptococcal infections)

- Onset or symptom exacerbation of obsessive–compulsive disorder and/or tic disorders following Group A β-haemolytic streptococcal infection (scarlet fever or streptococcal sore throat)
- Symptoms episodic

GRAM-POSITIVE AND -NEGATIVE BACILLI

Bacteria		Disease
Gram-positive bacilli		
Corynebacteria	C. diphtheriae	Diphtheria
Listeria	L. monocytogenes	Meningitis, sepsis
Clostridium	C. tetani	Tetanus
	C. botulinum	Botulism
	C. perfringens	Gas gangrene
	C. difficile	Pseudomembranous colitis
Bacillus	B. anthracis	Anthrax
	B. cereus	Food poisoning, wound sepsis
Gram-negative bacilli		
Brucella	B. abortus	Brucellosis
	B. melitensis, B. suis	
Bordatella	B. pertussis	Whooping cough
	B. parapertussis	(see p. 135)
Bartonella	B. henselae	Cat scratch disease
Haemophilus	H. influenzae type b	Meningitis, epiglottitis
	Non-capsulated	Otitis media, pneumonia
	H. influenzae	
Legionella	L. pneumophilia	Legionnaire disease
Pseudomonas	P. aeruginosa	Opportunistic infections (usually)
	P. cepacia	End-stage cystic fibrosis
		continued

Bacteria		Disease
Vibrio	*V. cholerae*	Cholera
Escherichia coli		Gastroenteritis
Salmonella	*S. enteritidis*	Enterocolitis, food poisoning
	S. typhi	Typhoid/paratyphoid fever
	S. paratyphi	Osteomyelitis
Shigella	*Sh. boydii*	Gastroenteritis
		Gastritis (see p. 151)
Yersinia	*Y. enterocolitica*	Enterocolitis
	Y. pseudotuberculosis	Mesenteric adenitis
Klebsiella	*K. pneumoniae*	
Campylobacter	*C. coli, C. jejuni*	Gastroenteritis
	Helicobacter pylori	Gastritis (see p. 151)

DIPHTHERIA

Organisms   *Corynebacterium diphtheriae*, types mitis (mild disease), intermedius and gravis

Exposure of the bacteria to bacteriophage – results in toxin production and disease. The toxin has:

- Subunit A – produces clinical disease
- Subunit B – transports the toxin to target receptors

Transmission   Droplets, fomites
Incubation   2–7 days

Clinical features

Local	Thick grey membrane over tonsils, progressing to husky voice, dyspnoea and respiratory obstruction
Systemic	Fever, tachycardia, irritability
	'Bull-neck' from lymphadenopathy
Other	Day 10 acute myocarditis (usually fatal)
	Myocarditis weeks later
	Neurological, e.g. palatal paralysis, cranial nerve palsies, peripheral neuropathy. Recovery usual
Cutaneous diphtheria	(Cutaneous ulcers with covering membrane) seen in burns patients

Diagnosis

Clinical diagnosis and organism culture.

Management

- Antitoxin IV (NB: Only neutralizes unfixed toxin, anaphylaxis risk)
- Antibiotics IV, e.g. penicillin
- Supportive therapy as needed

LISTERIOSIS

Listeriosis (due to *Listeria monocytogenes*) can be severe in pregnant mothers, neonates and immunocompromised individuals.

Transmission	Ingestion of unpasturized soft cheese, pâté, raw vegetables and chicken
Diseases seen	Neonates – pneumonia, meningitis, septicaemia (see p. 46)
	Pregnancy – miscarriage
	Immunocompromised – meningitis, septicaemia

Diagnosis

Blood or CSF culture.

Treatment

Antibiotics, e.g. ampicillin and gentamicin.

TETANUS

Clostridium tetani produces disease via tetanospasmin (neurotoxin).

Transmission	Direct contact onto open wound
Incubation	4–21 days

Clinical features

Generalized tetanus	Malaise, trismus, *risus sardonicus* (fixed smile) within 42–72 h spasms, opisthotonus, autonomic dysfunction
Localized tetanus	Wound site pain and stiffness
Cephalic tetanus	This occurs from entry via the middle ear, mortality nearly 100%
Tetanus neonatorum	Features as for generalized disease, entry via umbilical stump, mortality nearly 100%

Diagnosis

Clinical.

Management

- Wound debridement, IV penicillin, antitetanus immunoglobulin IM
- Control of spasms, e.g. diazepam and systemic support as necessary

Tetanus immunization recommendations

Immunization status	Clean wound	Tetanus prone wound
3 dose course given	Nil	Nil or adsorbed vaccine dose or reinforcing dose < 10 years
Course or reinforcing dose > 10 years	Reinforcing dose of adsorbed vaccine	Human antitetanus immunoglobulin + reinforcing dose adsorbed vaccine
Not immunized or status uncertain	Full 3 course dose of absorbed vaccine	Human antitetanus immunoglobulin + full 3 dose course of adsorbed vaccine

Tetanus prone wound
1. Wound or burn > 6 h prior to surgery
2. Wound or burn of: Puncture type
                 Significant degree of devitalized tissue
                 Soil or manure contact
                 Sepsis present

GRAM-NEGATIVE BACILLI

Cat scratch disease

Common worldwide infection due to *Bartonella henselae*.

Transmission:	Scratch or contact from cat (especially kitten), sometimes a dog
	50% no history of scratch obtained
	September–February mostly
Incubation:	3–30 days

Clinical features

- Inoculation pustule/papule (lasts days–months)
- Conjunctivitis
- Regional lymphadenopathy (2–4 months)
- Well child (50%)
- Malaise, low-grade fever (50%)
- Other symptoms unusual (maculopapular rash, splenomegaly, hepatitis, thrombocytopenia, encephalopathy with convulsions)

Diagnosis

- History and primary inoculation site found
- Serology for *B. henselae*

Treatment

- Spontaneous recovery common
- Azithromicin effective for severe disease

Brucellosis

Brucella endotoxin produces disease symptoms.

Organism	*Brucella melitensis*
Transmission	Ingestion of raw milk (cows, goats, camels)
	Also abraded skin, respiratory tract and genital tract entry
Incubation	1–3 weeks

Clinical features

Acute brucellosis	Fever, headache, malaise, night sweats
	Hepatomegaly, lymphadenopathy, splenomegaly (if severe), arthritis (33%, large joints, oligoarticular), endocarditis, osteomyelitis, epididymitis, meningoencephalitis
Chronic brucellosis	Tiredness, episodes of fever, depression, splenomegaly

Diagnosis

- Blood cultures (50% positive during acute phase)
- Serological tests (titre rise over 4 weeks, raised IgG)

Treatment

Cotrimoxazole high dose.

Typhoid fever

Organism	*Salmonella typhi*
Transmission	Ingestion food contaminated from faeces (humans only reservoir)
	Common in Asia, Africa, S. America
Incubation	10–14 days

Clinical features

Week 1	Fever, malaise, sore throat, headache, abdominal pain, confused
	Toxic child with *relative bradycardia*
Week 2	'Rose spots' (pink macules) on chest and upper abdomen
	Splenomegaly (75%), toxic, confused, hepatomegaly (30%)
Week 3	Complications: seizures, pneumonia, myocarditis, gastrointestinal haemorrhage and perforation, meningitis, peripheral neuropathy, haemolytic anaemia, glomerulonephritis, renal failure, osteomyelitis
Week 4	Recovery

Diagnosis

- Blood cultures (80% positive during week 1, 30% during week 3)
- Stool cultures (more positives after 2nd week)
- Urine cultures (positive with bacteraemia)
- Widal test (high titre of O antigens)
- Anaemia and leucopenia

Treatment

This depends on age and clinical severity. If unwell, IV antibiotics are given, e.g. cephalosporin or oral ciprofloxacin if appropriate.

Carrier state – chronic carriers excrete salmonella for > 1 year (gallbladder often the focus) and may be treated with 4 weeks of antibiotic and, if ineffective, cholecystectomy.

Paratyphoid fever is a similar, milder illness caused by *S. paratyphi* A, B or C. Treatment is co-trimoxazole for 2 weeks.

OTHER BACTERIA

Group	Bacteria	Disease
Mycobacterium	*M. tuberculosis*	TB (see p. 64)
	M. leprae	Leprosy
Mycoplasma	*M. pneumoniae*	Pneumonia in children and adolescents
Spirochaetes	*Treponema pallidum*	Syphilis, bejel, yaws, pinta
	Leptospira interrogans	Leptospirosis
	Borrelia burgdorferi	Lyme disease
Rickettsiae	*R. prowasekii*	Epidemic typhus
	R. typhi, *R. conorii*	Endemic, tick and scrub typhus
	R. rickettsii	Rocky mountain spotted fever
	Coxiella burnetii	Q fever
Chlamydiae	*C. trachomatis*	Trachoma, urethritis, cervicitis
	C. psittaci	Psittacosis
	C. pneumoniae	Pneumonia (see p. 134)

Mycoplasma

Mycoplasma pneumoniae is unusual in that it is the smallest organism that can survive outside a host cell and has no cell wall. The most common condition it causes is a bronchopneumonia in school-age children and adolescents.

Transmission	Droplet
Incubation	10–14 days

Clinical features

Bronchopneumonia	Gradual onset mild URTI, then persistent cough, fever, malaise, headache, wheeze
	Young school-age children. Resolves within 3–4 weeks.
Other features	Skin rashes (maculopapular erythematous, vesicular) common
	Vomiting, diarrhoea, arthralgia, myalgia (common)
	Bullous myringitis, haemolytic anaemia, Stevens–Johnson syndrome
	Hepatitis, pancreatitis, splenomegaly
	Aseptic meningitis, encephalitis, cerebellar ataxia, Guillain–Barré syndrome

Investigations

Blood	Serology (specific IgM antibody)
	Cold agglutinins (in 50%)
CXR	Diffuse patchy shadowing, often looks unexpectedly severe

Treatment

Erythromycin 2 weeks.

Tuberculosis

Infective agent   Usually *Mycobacterium tuberculosis* (an acid- and alcohol-fast bacillus).

- TB is on the increase in the UK, particularly London as a result of the widespread migration of people from Asia and Africa
- The clinical features depend greatly on the **host reaction**. If there is a good immune response the infection is locally contained and can become dormant. Small numbers of organisms may spread via the bloodstream and infect other organs. If there is a poor immune response the infection becomes overwhelming and disseminated
- In children, tuberculosis is usually a **primary infection** (rarely becoming disseminated), whereas in adults it is usually a **reactivation** of previous pulmonary infection
- The amount of TB organisms in primary TB in children is *very small*
- The lung manifestations are mostly due to a marked **delayed hypersensitivity reaction**
- Children are usually infected from an adult with active pulmonary TB
- Children with primary TB are generally *not* infectious

Clinical features

Primary infection

Asymptomatic pulmonary TB infection

- A **primary complex** develops: a small local lung parenchymal area of TB infection and regional lymph node involvement
- This is asymptomatic

- On CXR the lymph nodes are usually visible but not the TB focus
- The Mantoux/Heaf test may become positive (in which case anti-TB medication should be given)
- It becomes dormant and goes fibrotic. The lung focus may calcify over a couple of years and may then be visible on the CXR
- NB: This can reactivate later in life and develop into highly infectious 'open' pulmonary TB, and should therefore be treated

Symptomatic primary pulmonary TB

- Enlargement of the primary complex (in around 50% of children), i.e. local lung reaction + regional lymph nodes, visible on CXR (the lymph nodes but not the lung TB focus)
- Child becomes **symptomatic** after 4–8 weeks when the immune system responds: wheeze, cough, dyspnoea, fever, anorexia, weight loss
- Local pulmonary complications can occur from:
  Obstruction of a bronchus (due to lymph nodes) – cough, localized wheeze
  Rupture into a bronchus – bronchopneumonia, bronchitis
  Rupture into pleural cavity – pleural effusion
- This is treated with anti-TB medication
- It may become dormant (and may reactivate later) going fibrotic, and calcifying over a couple of years when the lung focus is visible on the CXR
- Small numbers of bacilli may escape into the bloodstream and lodge in other sites where they can cause abscesses or spontaneously become dormant, e.g. the kidney
- Sometimes this primary infection is not contained by the immune system and spreads (see below)
- NB: It is the **immune response** mounted by the child that is primarily responsible for the lung manifestations. Only a few organisms may be present, but release of organisms with rupture causes a marked hypersensitivity reaction, as delayed hypersensitivity to TB has developed by this time (4–8 weeks post-infection)

Primary TB infection at sites other than the lung	
The primary TB infection is usually the lung, but may be in other organs (and sometimes in multiple sites):	
Skin	Primary inoculation TB
Superficial lymph nodes	Tender lymphadenopathy in neck (from the mouth)
Gut	Mesenteric lymphadenopathy, abdominal pain, fever and weight loss

Massive TB spread (acute miliary TB)

- TB will rarely enter the bloodstream (from the primary infection – lung or other, or from reactivation of dormant TB)
- This can result in a few tubercles that can lodge in other organs, e.g. kidney, and spontaneously become dormant, or form a local abscess
- Or it can result in disseminated TB, which has a high mortality if untreated
- Disseminated infection is more likely in children < 4 years, with malnutrition and immunosuppression

Features of disseminated TB:

Acute miliary TB	Acutely unwell, fever, weight loss, hepatosplenomegaly, lymphadenopathy, widespread internal organ infection including: • **TB pericarditis** – a constrictive pericarditis • **Renal TB** • **Bones and joints** – osteomyelitis, infective arthritis 'Miliary' picture on CXR, i.e. scattered white dots throughout the lung fields

65

TB meningitis   A slow, insidious onset of meningitis
                    Night sweats, weight loss, malaise
                    Symptoms of meningeal irritation occur later

Skin manifestations of TB	
Primary TB infection	Inoculation TB developing at skin site of inoculation
Lupus vulgaris	Red plaque(s), usually on head and neck
Metastatic TB abscess	Subcutanoues TB abscess from endogenous spread
Scrofuloderma	TB lymphadenitis which ulcerates. Often on neck from endogenous spread
Acute miliary TB	Scattered macules and papules may occur
Erythema nodosum (see p. 298)	A hypersensitivity reaction

Late reactivation

Dormant TB (post-asymptomatic or symptomatic) can reactivate any time, usually during intercurrent illness or immunosuppression, causing post primary TB. This can be:

- Disseminated TB (as above)
- Open 'pulmonary' TB which is very infectious. This generally occurs in adults, with an approximate life-long risk of 5–10%

Diagnosis

TB is an elusive disease. There are two main forms of investigation:

1. **Direct detection of bacilli** (microscopy, PCR)
2. Assessment of **host immunity**

Ideally all TB would be diagnosed by visualization of the bacteria; however, this is rarely the case. More frequently diagnosis is made through a combination of radiological findings and evidence of host immunity to the organism.

Immunological tests

The immunological test is the **Mantoux test.**

- A test of delayed hypersensitivity to tuberculin using an intradermal injection of purified protein derivative (PPD) of tuberculin on the forearm
- The presence of induration is measured at 48–72 h
- A positive Mantoux is > 10 mm induration (indicating active infection)
- Interpretation is however variable depending on the individual estimated risk of TB

Other immunological investigations are being developed such as interferon-γ release from T cells in response to myco-bacterial antigens.

Direct detection of organisms

Places to look for TB organisms		
Early morning urine		
Sputum	Early morning gastric aspirate	Samples for PCR, microscopy (Ziehl–Neilson stain) and culture (4–8 weeks)
	Bronchoscopy washings	
	Coughed up sputum (older child)	
Biopsies	(Of lymph nodes, pleura, skin, gut, tuberculoma)	

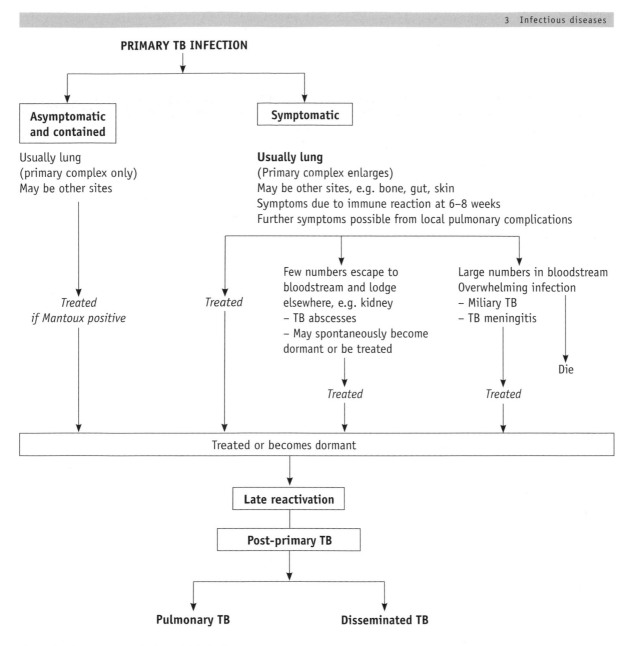

Figure 3.2 Management of primary TB infection

Management

1. Mantoux positive but no other evidence of disease: isoniazid or rifampicin + pyrazinamide for 3–6 months (two agents given if concern about multiresistance)
2. Evidence of infection in addition to a positive Mantoux test:
   For pulmonary disease – 6 months combination therapy
   For disseminated disease – 12 months therapy
   Combination therapy is used with various combinations of isoniazid, rifampicin, pyrazinamide and ethambutol

Prevention

- Vaccination with the **BCG** (Bacille Calmette–Guérin, a live attenuated strain) gives up to 75% protection.
- This is now recommended for neonates in high-risk groups, i.e. most infants in London, and Asian and African populations, and at 10–14 years to tuberculin test-negative children

Antituberculous drugs	
Drug	**Features and side-effects**
Isoniazid	Increased effects in slow acetylators Skin rashes and hepatoxicity (rare in children) Psychosis rarely occurs (due to pyridoxine deficiency)
Rifampicin	Liver enzyme inducer Pink/orange secretions, 4–8 h Skin rashes, gastrointestinal upset and hepatotoxicity (rare)
Pyrazinamide	Skin rashes, gastrointestinal upset and hepatotoxicity
Ethambutol	Ocular effects (colour-blindness, blurred vision, scotoma) Ophthalmological opinion with visual acuity assessment must be done prior to commencing. Caution in < 7–8 years as young children not capable of reporting visual disturbances

Leprosy

Organism	*Mycobacterium leprae*. Acid and alcohol – fast, weekly Gram-positive bacilli
Transmission	Uncertain
Incubation	Months–years
	Found in Asia, Africa, the USA and Russia. The clinical disease is dependent on the immune status of the individual.

Clinical features

Tuberculoid leprosy (TL)	Good immune response mounted A single hypopigmented skin lesion with decreased sensation, central atrophy and a thickened, tender nerve
Lepromatous leprosy (LL)	Poor cell-mediated immunity Many florid skin lesions All internal organs may be involved Nasal snuffles, saddle nose deformity, **leonine facies**, hoarse voice, fingers disappear, peripheral neuropathy
Intermediate forms	Borderline leprosy, indeterminate leprosy, neuritic leprosy (nerve lesion only)

Investigations

Clinical diagnosis

Organism isolation	Acid-fast bacilli found in skin or nasal mucosa smears NB: Organism cannot be cultured in artificial media
Culture	In mouse foot pad
Lepromin test	This is a measure of **host resistance** to disease. Dead bacilli are injected intradermally

Treatment

Multidrug regimens, e.g. dapsone, rifampicin and clofazimine, for at least 2 years.

Syphilis

Organism   *Treponema pallidum*
Transmission Sexual contact, transplacentally (congenital syphilis, see p. 452)
Incubation   10–90 days

Clinical features

Early stages	Primary (3 weeks)	Painless hard chancre, regional lymphadenopathy
	Secondary (4–10 weeks)	Fever, malaise, sore throat, arthralgia, myalgia
		Maculopapular, itchy rash, mucosal ulcers
		Condylomata lata (perianal plaque warts)
Late stages	Tertiary (years)	Gummas (granulomatous ulcers) in bones, liver, testes
		CNS disease (meningovascular involvement, general paralysis of the insane, tabes dorsalis)
		Cardiac disease (aortitis, aortic regurgitation)

Diagnosis

Dark ground microscopy	From chancres or mucous ulcers
Serology	VDRL (Venereal Disease Reference Laboratory):
	• Positive 3 weeks of infection, negative 6 months after treatment
	• False positive: EBV, hepatitis, mycoplasma, malignancy, autoimmune disease
	TPHA (*T. pallidum* haemagglutination assay). Specific for treponema, remains positive
	FTA–ABS (fluorescent treponema antibodies). Specific for treponema

Treatment

This is dependent on the stage. Penicillin is given via the IM route (long-acting) for some stages or IV route, e.g. for CNS disease.

Lyme disease

Organism   *Borellia burgdorferi*
Transmission Ixodid ticks on deer (or sheep, cattle, dogs or squirrels), Europe, the USA, Australia, Asia
Incubation   7–30 days

Clinical features

Within days	**Erythema chronicum migrans** (painless, red annular rash slowly enlarging) from site of tick bite
	Headache, conjunctivitis, malaise, fever, arthralgia, myalgia, lymphadenopathy
Weeks to months later	CNS 15% (meningoencephalitis, cranial and peripheral nerve palsies, especially VIIth nerve palsy)
	Cardiac 10% (myocarditis, heart block)
	Recurrent arthritis (oligoarticular, episodic, often the knee with erosion of bone and cartilage)
	Other (myelitis, hepatitis, hepatosplenomegaly)

Diagnosis

This is a clinical diagnosis.

Organism isolation	Serum, CSF, skin biopsy (difficult)
Serology	IgM antibodies in CSF and serum may be positive after 3–6 weeks

Treatment

For early general symptoms, oral antibiotics (amoxicillin or erythromycin if < 9 years, doxycycline if > 9 years). If CNS or articular involvement, give ceftriaxone.

Typhus

Organism   Rikettsiae (small bacteria that multiply intracellularly and cause a **vasculitis**)
Transmission   Human lice (epidemic), rat flea (endemic) in tropical areas
Incubation   1–3 weeks

Clinical features

Epidemic typhus:

Week 1   Profound malaise, high fever, severe headache, orbital pain, conjunctivitis. Measles-type rash on day 5, *becoming purpuric*
Week 2   Meningoencephalitis, myocarditis, pneumonia, splenomegaly, gangrene of peripheries, renal failure; death may occur
Week 3   Slow recovery

NB: Recurrence years later = Brill–Zinsser disease (from lymph node storage).

Endemic typhus – similar but milder disease

Diagnosis

Serology.

Treatment

Oral tetracycline.

Rocky Mountain spotted fever

Organism   *Rikettsia rikettsii*
Transmission   Tick on dogs and rodents in America
Incubation   1–2 weeks

Clinical features   As for epidemic typhus. NB: Crusted papule at bite site
Diagnosis   Serology
Treatment   Tetracycline

PROTOZOAL INFECTIONS

Group	Organism	Vector/reservoir	Disease
Plasmodium	P. falciparum, P. malariae, P. vivax, P. ovale	Mosquito	Malaria
Leishmania	L. donovani, L. mexicana, L. braziliensis	Sandfly	Leishmaniasis
Trypanosoma brucei	T. b. gambiense, T. b. rhodesiense	Tsetse fly	Trypanosomiasis
Toxoplasma	T. gondii	Cats, sheep, pigs	Toxoplasmosis
Entamoeba	E. histolytica	Water	Amoebiasis
Giardia	G. lamblia	Humans	Giardiasis
Cryptosporidium	C. parvum	Cattle	Cryptosporidiosis
Trichomonas	T. vaginalis	Humans	Trichomoniasis

Malaria

Malaria is found in all countries between latitude 40 N and 30 S, and there are four species: *Plasmodium vivax*, *P. ovale*, *P. malariae* and *P. falciparum*.

Transmission	Anopheles mosquitos	
Incubation	18 days–6 weeks	*Pl. malariae*
	10–14 days	All others

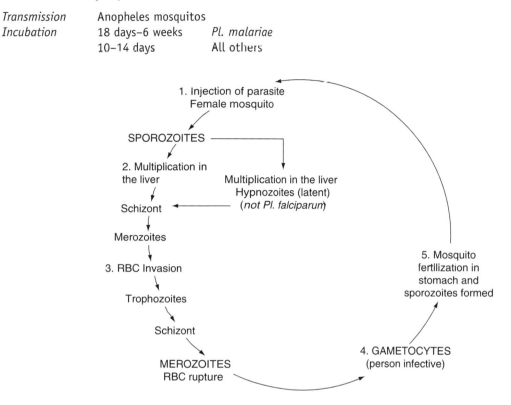

Figure 3.3 Malaria parasite lifecycle

Clinical features

General

Intermittent fevers	Due to schizont rupture:
	• **Cold stage** (½–1 h, vasoconstriction, rapid temperature rise, patient feels cold)
	• **Hot stage** (2–6 h, patient feels hot, delirium)
	• **Sweating stage** (profuse sweating, patient sleeps)
Other	Anaemia, splenomegaly, hepatomegaly
P. vivax and *P. ovale*	Mild disease, young RBCs and reticulocytes only affected. NB: Relapses and difficult to eradicate due to **latent phase**
P. malariae	Mild, chronic course, growth retardation, massive splenomegaly, old RBCs only affected. **Nephrotic syndrome** may occur
P. falciparum	Most severe form, all RBCs affected and become sticky to endothelium, causing vascular occlusion and ischaemic organ damage (brain, kidneys, liver, gastrointestinal tract)
	Worse if high parasitaemia (> 2%)
	Complications:
	• Cerebral malaria, fits, hyperpyrexia
	• Acute renal failure (Blackwater fever)

- Shock, metabolic acidosis, DIC, jaundice
- Severe anaemia
- Hypoglycaemia, splenic rupture

Diagnosis

Thin and thick peripheral blood smears (parasites seen with staining). Three negative smears on three successive days required to declare malaria-free. NB: Consider malaria in any febrile child returning from an endemic area.

Treatment

Acute attack	Disease-type specific oral medication given and because resistance is increasing, up-to-date therapy advice should be obtained from the malaria reference laboratory
	In severe disease (< 2% RBCs) IV quinine infusion and intensive care as necessary
	If infective species unknown or mixed, initial treatment as for *Falciparum malariae*
Eradication (for *P. vivax* and *P. ovale*)	Primaquine for 2–3 weeks after acute treatment (NB: Not if G6PD deficiency present)

Prevention

Prophylaxis	Drugs taken 2 weeks prior to entering malaria area and for 6 weeks after return. Resistance affects choice of drugs, so up-to-date advice should be obtained
	Drugs used (sometimes in combination) are: chloroquine (weekly), proguanil (daily), maloprim (weekly), mefloquine (weekly), doxycycline (daily, not if < 12 years old)
Natural protection	This is present in people with: Duffy-negative blood group (*P. vivax*), HbS and *(partial)* G6PD, thalassaemia, PK deficiency (*P. falciparum*)

Amoebiasis

Organism	*Entamoeba histolytica*
Transmission	Faecal–oral (cysts transferred). Tropics and sub-tropics

Clinical features

In the intestine, trophozoites emerge from the cysts and multiply in the colon producing symptoms:

Amoebic colitis	Colonic mucosa invaded, ulcers, bloody diarrhoea, amoebic granulomas (10%). Acute amoebic dysentery may occur
Hepatitis	Travel of trophozoites via portal vein
	Amoebic *'anchovy sauce'* liver abscesses, high mortality
Asymptomatic cyst carrier	

Diagnosis

'Hot' stools	Trophozoites and cysts seen
Serology	Amoebic fluorescent antibody titre (FAT) positive in symptomatic disease
Liver USS	Abscess
Liver function	Alkaline phosphatase – (in liver abscess)

Treatment

Metronidazole orally. Drainage of liver abscesses.

Giardiasis

Organism	*Giardia lamblia*
Transmission	Faecal–oral, spreads easily in nurseries and institutions

Clinical features

Asymptomatic carrier
Gastroenteritis | Abdominal pain, watery diarrhoea, vomiting
If prolonged: malabsorption, steatorrhoea, weight loss, growth retardation

Diagnosis

Isolation | 'Hot' stool (trophozoites and cysts) (20% pick up rate only)

Treatment

Metronidazole orally for 5–7 days (20% resistance rate).

Toxoplasmosis

Organism | *Toxoplasma gondii* (intracellular protozoan)
Transmission | Faecal–oral from cat faeces, sheep, pigs or goats

Clinical features

This may present as:

1. Lymphadenopathy
2. Acute febrile illness with lymphadenopathy
3. Immunocompromised – headache, neck stiffness (ICP $\uparrow$), intracerebral lesions, acute febrile illness, hepatosplenomegaly, chorioretinitis, sore throat
4. Congenital infection – classical triad of choreoretinitis, hydrocephalus and cerebral calcification (see p. 449)

Diagnosis

Serology – rising antibody titre, IgM.

Treatment

None if mild disease. Pyrimethamine and sulphadiazine in severe disease and pregnancy.

FUNGAL INFECTIONS

Fungus	Disease
Histoplasma capsulatum	Histoplasmosis
Aspergillus fumigatus	Aspergillosis
Cryptococcus neoformans	Cryptococcosis
Coccidioides immitis	Coccidioidomycosis
Blastomyces dermatitidis	Blastomycosis
Candida albicans	Candidiasis (systemic, oral, perianal)
Dermatophytoses	Tinea (see p. 296)

HELMINTHIC INFECTIONS

Group	Organism	Disease
Nematodes (round worms)	*Ascaris lumbricoides* (roundworm)	Intestinal infection
	Trichuris trichuria (whipworm)	Intestinal infection
	Enterobius vermicularis (thread worm)	Intestinal infection
	Strongyloides stercoralis	Strongyloidiasis
	Ankylostoma duodenale }	Hookworm infection and
	Necator americanus (hookworms) }	cutaneous lava migrans
	Toxocara canis and *cati*	Toxocariasis
	Wucheria bancrofti	Filariasis, elephantiasis
	Loa loa	Loiasis
	Onchocerca volvulus	Onchocerciasis, elephantiasis
	Brugia malayi	Filariasis, elephantiasis
	Dracunculus medinensis (guinea worm)	Dracunculiasis
Trematodes (flukes)	*Schistosoma*	Schistosomiasis (bilharzia)
	Fasciola hepaticus	Fascioliasis
	Clonorchis sinensis	Clonorchiasis
Cestodes (tapeworms)	*Taenia saginata* (beef tapeworm)	Intestinal infection
	Taenia solium (pork tapeworm)	Intestinal infection
	Echinococcus	Hydatid disease

INTESTINAL NEMATODE INFECTIONS

Organism	Clinical features	Diagnosis	Treatment
Roundworm *Ascaris lumbricoides* Worldwide	Asymptomatic Abdominal pain and distension Ileo-caecal valve obstruction, appendicitis, bile duct obstruction Pneumonitis, pulmonary ascariasis, eosinophilia and dyspnoea (Loeffler syndrome)	Ova in stool	Mebendazole or piperazine
Threadworm *Enterobius vermicularis* Worldwide	Asymptomatic Pruritis ani, worse at night (the female lays her eggs perianally)	Sticky tape test	Mebendazole or piperazine
Whipworm *Trichuris trichuria* Worldwide	Asymptomatic Intestinal ulcers, blood and mucus loss, rectal prolapse, appendicitis	Ova in stool	Mebendazole

continued

Organism	Clinical features	Diagnosis	Treatment
Hookworm *Ankylostoma duodenale* (Europe, Middle East, N. Africa) *Necator americanus* Temperate, sub-tropical and tropical areas	Local irritation Intestinal ulcer-like symptoms Anaemia (0.2 ml blood loss/day) Mild pulmonary symptoms	Ova in stool	Mebendazole
Strongyloidiasis *Strongyloides stercoralis* Worldwide	Local reaction Cough, pneumonitis Abdominal pain, diarrhoea, malabsorption, steatorrhoea (in heavy infection) Disseminated infection if immunocompromised	Larvae in stool or duodenal aspirates	Thiabendazole or albendazole
Toxicariasis (visceral larva migrans) *Toxocara canis* (puppies) *Toxocara cati*	Clinical diagnosis Young children Lungs – asthma, eosinophilia Urticaria, pica, anaemia, fever Hepatosplenomegaly Faltering growth	Thiabendazole Serology may be positive	

FURTHER READING

Department of Health *Immunisation Against Infectious Disease, Manual on Immunisation Practices in the UK*, HMSO, London, 1997

Feigin RD, Cherry JD *Textbook of Pediatric Infectious Diseases*, 5th edn. Philadelphia: WB Saunders, Philadelphia, 2003

Isaacs D, Moxon RE *A Practical Approach to Paediatric Infectious Diseases*. Edinburgh: Churchill Livingstone, 1996

Long SS, Pickering LK, Prober CG *Principles and Practice of Pediatric Infectious Diseases*, 3rd edn. Philadelphia: WB Saunders, 2007

4
Cardiology

- *Physiology*
- *The ECG*
- *Cardiac positions*
- *Innocent murmurs*
- *Heart failure*
- *Eisenmenger reaction*
- *Teratogens and maternal disorders associated with CHD*
- *Inherited conditions associated with CHD*

- *Structural congenital heart disease*
- *Duct-dependent circulations*
- *Arrhythmias*
- *Rheumatic fever*
- *Infective endocarditis*
- *Myocarditis*
- *Cardiomyopathy*
- *Pericarditis*

PHYSIOLOGY

FETAL CIRCULATION

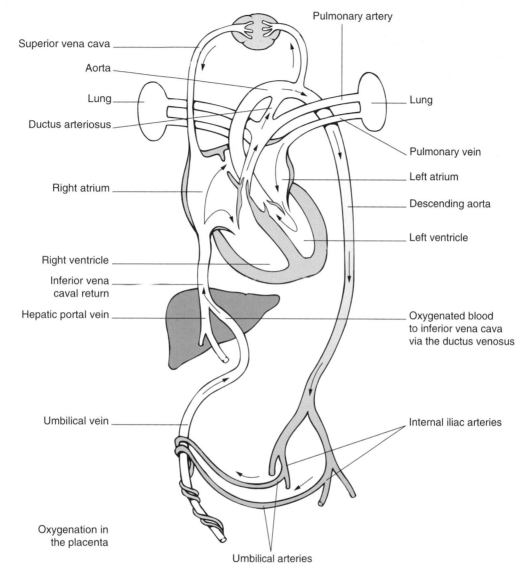

Figure 4.1 Fetal circulation

CARDIAC CYCLE

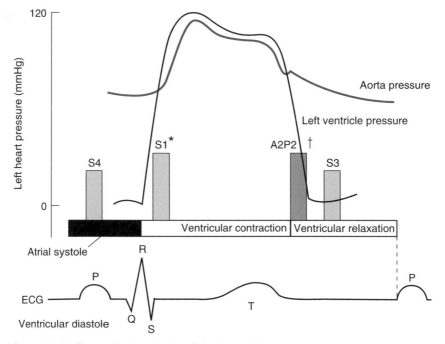

Figure 4.2 Cardiac cycle: * = ejection click; † = opening snap

HEART SOUNDS

First heart sound (S1)

Loud **S1** seen with: High cardiac output state, e.g.:   Anxiety
     Exercise
     Fever
     Thin chest
     Thyrotoxicosis
     Vasodilatation
     Mitral stenosis

Soft **S1** seen with: Obesity
     Emphysema
     Impaired left ventricular function

Second heart sound (A2 P2)

Soft **P2** (Fig. 4.3B)   Stenotic pulmonary valve, e.g. Fallot
Loud **P2** (Fig. 4.3C)   Pulmonary hypertension
Normal splitting (Fig. 4.3D)   Children
     Young adults
Wide mobile splitting (Fig. 4.3E)   Pulmonary stenosis
     Pulmonary hypertension
     RBBB

Reversed splitting (Fig. 4.3F)   Aortic stenosis
                                     LBBB
                                     HOCM
Wide fixed splitting (Fig. 4.3G)   ASD

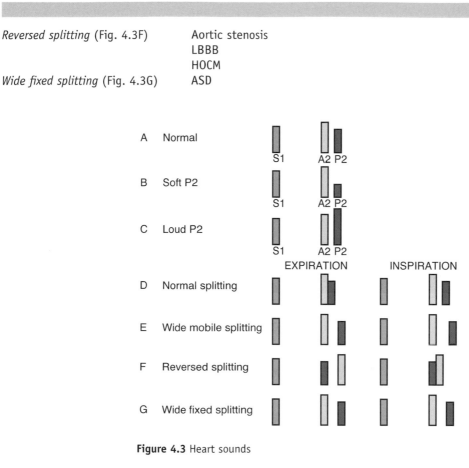

Figure 4.3 Heart sounds

Third heart sound (S3)

Due to rapid ventricular filling.

Causes

- Normal (in children, athletes and pregnancy)
- Increased left ventricular stroke volume (aortic regurgitation, mitral regurgitation)
- Restrictive ventricular filling (constrictive pericarditis, restrictive cardiomyopathy)
- Ischaemic heart disease

Fourth heart sound (S4)

Due to forceful atrial contraction.

Causes

- HOCM
- Long-standing hypertension
- Ischaemic heart disease

JUGULAR VENOUS PULSE (JVP)

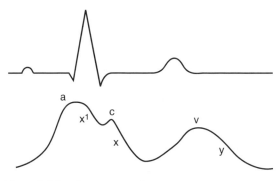

a = atrial systole
x^1 = atrium begins to relax
c = onset of ventricular contraction
v = atrial filling in ventricular systole
x = atrial relaxation commencing
y = tricuspid valve opens and
     ventricle relaxes

Figure 4.4 Jugular venous pulse

Changes in the JVP

	Seen in	Cause
Giant a waves (large a waves)	Pulmonary hypertension Pulmonary stenosis Tricuspid stenosis	↑ Resistance to ventricular filling
Cannon a waves (very large a waves)	Complete heart block VT	Atrial contraction against closed tricuspid valve
Large v waves	Tricuspid regurgitation	
Steep y descent	Constrictive pericarditis Tricuspid regurgitation	

NORMAL VITAL SIGNS – AGE RELATED

Age	HR	RR	SBP	DBP
< 1 year	120–160	30–60	60–95	35–69
1–3	90–140	24–40	95–105	50–65
3–5	75–110	18–30	95–110	50–65
8–12	75–100	18–30	90–110	57–71
12–16	60–90	12–16	112–130	60–80
Ref: Duke J, Rosenberg SG *Anesthesia Secrets*, Hanley & Belfus, Mosby, 1996.				

CARDIAC CATHETERIZATION DATA

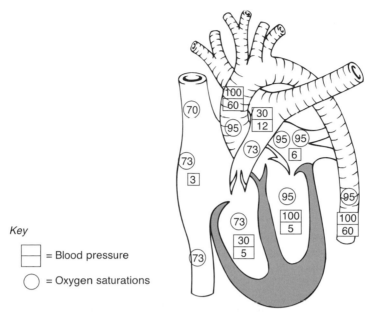

Key

☐ = Blood pressure

◯ = Oxygen saturations

Figure 4.5 Cardiac catheterization data

CXR SILHOUETTE

Right sided aortic arch	Big heart
Fallot tetralogy	Heart failure
Truncus arteriosus	Significant left-to-right shunts
Pulmonary atresia	HOCM/DCM
Congenital vascular ring	Pericardial effusion
	Ebstein anomaly

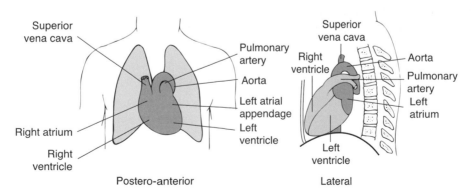

Figure 4.6 CXR silhouette

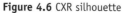

CARDIAC SCARS

Scar	Cause	Left brachial pulse
Left thoracotomy (only)	PDA ligation	N
	Blalock–Taussig shunt	↓ or N
	Coarctation repair (left subclavian flap)	↓ or N
	Pulmonary artery banding	N
	Non-cardiac	N
Right thoracotomy (only)	Right Blalock–Taussig shunt	N
	Non-cardiac	N
Median sternotomy	Any correction	N

THE ECG

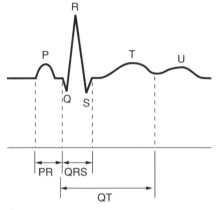

Figure 4.7 ECG

	Birth–1 year	1–10 years	10–15 years	> 15 years
PR interval (s)	0.08–0.15 (**0.10**)	0.08–0.15 (**0.12**)	0.09–0.18 (**0.14**)	0.10–0.22 (**0.16**)
QRS duration (s)	0.03–0.07 (**0.05**)	0.04–0.08 (**0.06**)	0.04–0.09 (**0.07**)	0.06–0.1 (**< 0.1**)
Maximum QTc (s)	0.45	0.44	0.44	0.44

RATE

The heart rate varies with age (outlined above). It is calculated by noting the number of large squares between QRS complexes:

1 large square = 300/min
2 large squares = 150/min
3 large squares = 100/min
4 large squares = 75/min
5 large squares = 60/min

NB. 5 large squares = 1 s, 1 large square = 0.2 s

AXIS

The cardiac axis is the average direction of spread of the depolarization wave through the ventricles (as seen from the front) and it changes from right and anterior in infants to left and posterior in adults.

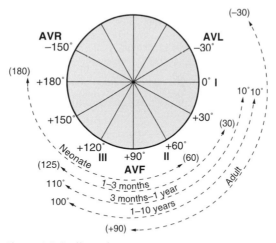

Figure 4.8 Cardiac axis

The axis can be derived by noting the direction of the QRS complexes in leads I, II and III. It can also be estimated by observing the direction in leads I and AVF (though this is less accurate).

The axis may be normal, left axis deviation (LAD) or right axis deviation (RAD). A superior axis is seen when the S wave > R wave in AVF.

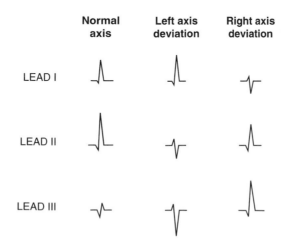

Figure 4.9 Calculating the cardiac axis

Axis deviation		
RAD	**LAD**	**Superior axis**
Normal in children	Primum ASD	Primum ASD
RVH	LVH	AVSD
RBBB	LBBB	Tricuspid atresia
Secundum ASD	AVSD	Noonan syndrome Double inlet left ventricle Familial Myocarditis

HEART BLOCK

FIRST DEGREE BLOCK

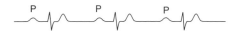

SECOND DEGREE BLOCK

1. Mobitz type I (Wenkebach)

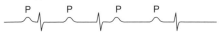

The PR interval gradually increases until it does not conduct to the ventricles

2. Mobitz type II

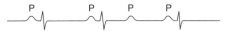

The P waves that do not conduct to the ventricles are *not* preceded by a gradual PR prolongation

3. 2:1 AV block

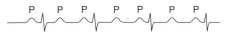

THIRD DEGREE (COMPLETE) BLOCK

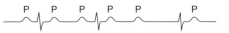

No relation between P waves and QRS complexes

Figure 4.10 Heart block

BUNDLE BRANCH BLOCK

Right bundle branch block (RBBB) (Fig. 4.11a)

The left ventricle and septum are activated normally and the right ventricle has a slower conduction spreading from left to right. ECG features include:

- QRS complex is prolonged
- An RSR pattern in the right precordial leads

Left bundle branch block (LBBB) (Fig. 4.11b)

The septum depolarizes from right to left and the left ventricle relies on late transmission of the activation wave. ECG features include:

- QRS complex prolonged
- Lead V1 negative and V5–V6 mostly positive with an M pattern

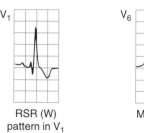
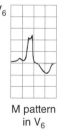

A. RBBB B. LBBB

V_1 V_6

RSR (W) pattern in V_1 M pattern in V_6

Figure 4.11 (a) Right bundle branch block. (b) Left bundle branch block

NB: With complete LBBB or RBBB, ventricular hypertrophy and ischaemia changes *cannot* be interpreted from the ECG.

VENTRICULAR HYPERTROPHY

Left ventricular hypertrophy (LVH) (Fig. 4.12a)

This is difficult to predict accurately from the ECG and so it is best to have a combination of criteria, which include:

- R wave amplitude in V5–V6 higher than the 98th centile for age (NB: voltage criteria for LVH are not very exact)
- S wave in V1
- Lateral t wave inversion (strain pattern, in V5–V6 and II, III and AVF)
- LAD

A. LVH

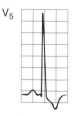

V_5 V_6

(a) In V_5 or V_6 there is a tall R wave (>25 mm in adults)

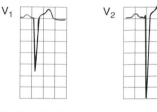
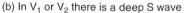

V_1 V_2

(b) In V_1 or V_2 there is a deep S wave

B. RVH

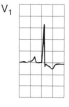

V_1

(a) In V_1 the height of the R wave is > the depth of the S wave

V_6

(b) In V_6 there is a deep S wave

Figure 4.12 (a) Left ventricular hypertrophy. (b) Right ventricular hypertrophy

Right ventricular hypertrophy (RVH) (Fig. 4.12b)

ECG features include:

- R wave amplitude in V1 > 98th centile for age
- Abnormal T wave direction in V1 (NB: the T wave direction changes with age: it is upright in newborns, negative > 7 days of age, then becomes positive again in adolescents and adults)
- S wave depth in V6 is lower than the 98th centile for age
- In marked RVH the R wave is big and the T wave inverted (a strain pattern)

EFFECTS OF HYPER- AND HYPO-KALAEMIA ON THE ECG

K⁺ ↑	K⁺ ↑
Peaked T waves	Flat T waves
Wide QRS complexes	QRS axis rotates
Long PR interval	Long PR interval
Flat P waves	Long QT interval – *torsades de pointes*
Bradycardia/asystole	U waves ST depression

K⁺ ↓   K⁺ ↓

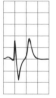

Figure 4.13 Effects of hyper- and hypo-kalaemia on the ECG

CARDIAC POSTIONS

The classification of the normal and abnormal cardiac positions involves looking at the **visceroatrial situs** and the **apex** of the heart.

VISCEROATRIAL SITUS

Situs solitus   Viscera normal, lungs normal, atria normal
Situs inversus   Viscera reversed, lungs reversed, atria reversed
Situs ambiguous (isomerism)   Asplenia syndrome (right isomerism)
                          No spleen, central liver, two right lungs
                          Polysplenia syndrome (left isomerism)
                          Multiple small spleens, no intrahepatic portion of IVC
                          Bilateral left lungs

NB: Isomerism (right worse than left) is usually associated with severe congenital heart disease.

APEX OF THE HEART

Laevocardia   Normal (apex points to the left)
Dextrocardia   Apex points to the right

The following combinations are associated with severe congenital heart disease:

- Situs solitus + dextrocardia
- Situs inversus + laevocardia

ECG in dextrocardia

The P waves are negative in lead I and reflect the position of the atria. The chest leads V1–V6 show right ventricular complexes.

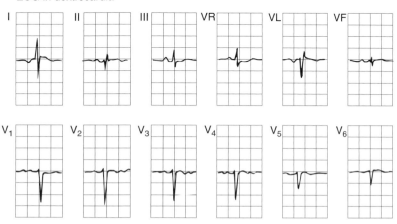

Figure 4.14 ECG in dextrocardia

INNOCENT MURMURS

These are heard in 30% of children. There are two types:

Ejection murmur   Due to turbulent flow in the outflow tracts from the heart
                    A buzzing or blowing quality in the 2nd–4th left intercostal space
Venous hum   Due to turbulent flow in the head and neck veins
                    A continuous low-pitched rumble heard beneath the clavicles
                    Disappears with compression of ipsilateral jugular veins or on lying down

Specific features

- Soft
- Change with altered patient position
- More pronounced if child tachycardic
- Child asymptomatic
- Normal examination: Normal heart sounds
                         No thrill or radiation
                         Normal pulses
- Normal CXR and ECG

HEART FAILURE

Symptoms	Signs
Sweating	Tachypnoea, intercostal and subcostal recession
Poor feeding	Tachycardia
Faltering growth	Cardiomegaly
Shortness of breath (SOB)	Hepatomegaly
Recurrent chest infections	Gallop rhythm/murmur/muffled heart sounds
Abdominal pain (big liver)	Central cyanosis
Collapse/shock	Cool peripheries (NB. Lungs often sound clear in children/neonates)

CXR

Prominent pulmonary markings and cardiomegaly. NB: An important exception is with infradiaphragmatic TAPVD where the heart size is normal and therefore this can appear like primary lung disease.

Management

Sit patient up
Give oxygen
Diuretics — E.g. frusemide (with potassium supplements), spironolactone (reduce preload and afterload)
Inotropes — For acute heart failure use IV dobutamine (peripherally) or dopamine (centrally)
If less severe, oral digoxin may be used
Vasodilators — E.g. captopril and hydralazine (reduce afterload)
Intubation and ventilation — If necessary

EISENMENGER REACTION

This is when persistently increased pulmonary blood flow leads to increased pulmonary artery vascular resistance, pulmonary hypertension and, eventually, reversal of a previous left-to-right shunt. When this is due specifically to a VSD, it is called **Eisenmenger syndrome.**

The Eisenmenger reaction is becoming rarer as the diagnosis of CHD improves and there is earlier management.

Causes

VSD, AVSD, PDA, ASD (rare) and any other condition with a communication between PA and the aorta.

Clinical features

- Progressively worsening cyanosis, malaise, dsypnoea and haemoptysis
- Right ventricular heave
- Loud P2

ECG

- RVH
- P wave tall and spiked

CXR

- Prominent pulmonary artery with peripheral tapering of pulmonary vessels
- Cardiomegaly
- May be normal

Management

Medical   Symptomatic treatment (oxygen, calcium channel blockers)
Surgical   Heart–lung transplant or bilateral lung transplant with repair of the cardiac defect

Causes of peripheral pulmonary stenosis	
Williams syndrome	Supravalvular AS, hypercalcaemia, mental retardation, elfin facies
Congenital rubella syndrome	Myocarditis, PDA, microphthalmia, cataracts, deafness
Alagille syndrome	Progressive bile duct destruction, TOF, butterfly vertebrae, nephritis, facial features, posterior embryotoxon (see p. 186)
CHD	ASD,VSD, PDA,TOF, supravalvular AS

TERATOGENS AND MATERNAL DISORDERS ASSOCIATED WITH CHD

	Cardiac lesion
Drugs	
Sodium valproate	Coarctation of aorta, hypoplastic left heart, AS, interrupted aortic arch, secundum ASD, pulmonary atresia with no VSD, VSD
Lithium	Ebstein anomaly
Alcohol	ASD, VSD, TOF, coarctation of aorta
Phenytoin	AS, PS, coarctation of aorta, PDA
Maternal disorders	
Rubella	PDA, peripheral pulmonary stenosis
SLE, Sjögren	Complete heart block
Diabetes	All types of CHD increase

INHERITED CONDITIONS ASSOCIATED WITH CHD

Condition	Cardiac lesion
Down syndrome	AVSD, VSD, PDA, ASD, aberrant subclavian artery
Edwards syndrome	VSD, ASD, PDA, coarctation of aorta
Patau syndrome	VSD, PDA, ASD, coarctation of aorta
Turner syndrome	Bicuspid aortic valve, coarctation of aorta, AS
Chromosome 22 microdeletion	Aortic arch anomalies, truncus arteriosus, PDA, TOF
Holt–Oram	Secundum ASD, VSD
Marfan syndrome	Dissecting aortic aneurysm, AR, mitral valve prolapse
Neurofibromatosis	PS, coarctation of aorta
Noonan syndrome	PS, hypertrophic cardiomyopathy, AVSD, coarctation of aorta
Williams syndrome	Supravalvular aortic stenosis, PS, peripheral pulmonary stenosis, VSD, ASD
Tuberous sclerosis	Cardiac rhabdomyoma
Ehlers–Danlos	Mitral valve prolapse, tricuspid valve prolapse, dilated aortic root
Hunter syndrome	AR, MR
Pompe disease	Hypertrophic cardiomyopathy
CHARGE syndrome	TOF, PDA, double outlet right ventricle, VSD, ASD, right-sided aortic arch

STRUCTURAL CONGENITAL HEART DISEASE

The incidence of structural congenital heart disease is 8 in 1000. Recurrence risk is 3% if one child affected, 10% if two children affected and 25% if three children affected.

It can be divided into **acyanotic** conditions and **cyanotic** conditions. If CHD is suspected the child should be investigated with a CXR and ECG initially, then an echocardiogram with Doppler ultrasound to outline the defect(s). Cardiac catheterization may be used for presurgical evaluation, evaluation of pulmonary vascular resistance, to monitor progress after surgical intervention and as a therapeutic tool in interventional cardiac catheterization, e.g. balloon dilatation, embolization and closure of intracardiac defects.

ACYANOTIC CONGENITAL HEART DISEASE

Ventricular septal defect (VSD)

This comprises 32% of CHD, being the most common form. There are several types of VSD that may be classified as:

- Inlet
- Muscular
- Perimembranous
- Outlet
- Doubly committed

The symptoms and signs depend on the size of the hole and any other cardiac defects present. Large ones and outlet VSDs are less likely to close spontaneously.

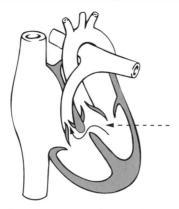
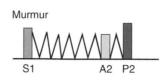

Figure 4.15 Ventricular septal defect

Clinical features

- Asymptomatic murmur
- Features of cardiac failure
- Recurrent chest infections
- Endocarditis
- Cyanosis (Eisenmenger syndrome) may develop at 10–20 years (only in untreated large VSDs)

Signs

Murmur   Loud pansystolic murmur
Lower left sternal edge (LSE)
Parasternal thrill
± Mid-diastolic apical murmur (due to increased mitral flow) if large defect (smaller holes may have shorter, louder murmurs)

Heart sounds   Loud P2 if pulmonary hypertension

ECG

Normal or LVH (RVH if pulmonary hypertension).

CXR

- Cardiomegaly and increased pulmonary vascular markings
- May be normal

NB: Important findings in **pulmonary hypertension**:

- RVH on the ECG
- Loud P2

Management

Treat cardiac failure if present: oxygen, sitting up, diuretics (frusemide, spironolactone, ACE inhibitors, thiazides), digoxin.

Surgical repair is required in < 10% as most will close spontaneously during the first few years of life. Repair is needed if:

- Severe symptoms with failure to thrive
- Pulmonary hypertension develops
- Aortic regurgitation develops
- Persistent significant shunting > 10 years of age

Atrial septal defect (ASD)

There are two types of ASD: **ostium secundum** and **ostium primum**.

Ostium secundum

This is the most common form of ASD and involves a defect(s) in the atrial septum. The defects may be single or multiple.

Associations	Holt–Oram syndrome
Clinical features	Asymptomatic (commonly)
	Heart failure (rare until adult life)
	Atrial arrhythmias (onset at 30–40 years)
Signs	*Murmur*:
	• Ejection systolic
	• Upper LSE (due to increased RV outflow)
	• ± Mid-diastolic tricuspid flow murmur at the lower LSE (due to increased tricuspid flow)
	Heart sounds: fixed wide splitting of the second heart sound
ECG	RAD
	Partial RBBB (in 90%) } NB: All right
	RVH
CXR	Cardiomegaly, large pulmonary artery, straight left heart border and increased pulmonary vascular markings
Management	Elective surgical or transcatheter device closure performed at 3–5 years (earlier if necessary) if child is symptomatic. Small defects will usually close spontaneously

Ostium secundum atrial septum defect

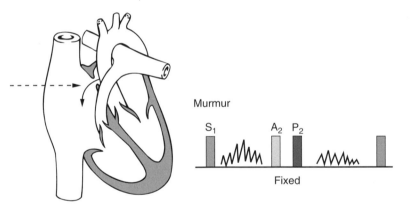

Murmur

S_1 A_2 P_2

Fixed

Figure 4.16 Atrial septal defect

Ostium primum

Here there is failure of development of the septum primum (which divides the mitral and tricuspid valves) and usually also a cleft in the anterior leaflet of the mitral valve.

Associations	Down syndrome and Ellis–van Crevald syndrome
Clinical features	Many asymptomatic (if small defect)
	Heart failure and recurrent pneumonias (severity depending on A-V valve regurgitation)
Signs	As for ostium secundum with a mitral regurgitation murmur (apical, pansystolic)

ECG	LAD or superior axis
	Partial RBBB
	RVH
Management	Surgical repair is always required

Atrioventicular septal defect (AVSD)

Association – common in Down syndrome

Atrioventricular septal defect (also known as A-V canal defect or endocardial cushion defect) is a severe form of CHD where there is a contiguous atrial and ventricular septal defect and defects of the mitral and tricuspid valves. (There are variable degrees of severity of AVSD.)

Clinical features

Usually severe with early development of heart failure, recurrent pneumonias, faltering growth and pulmonary hypertension due to the large left-to-right shunt across both the atria and the ventricles. Some right-to-left shunting may also occur.

ECG

LAD or superior axis and biventricular hypertrophy.

CXR

Large heart with pulmonary plethora

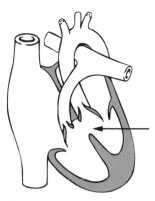

Atrioventricular defect

Figure 4.17 Atrioventricular septal defect

Management

Repair is usually needed within 6 months to prevent the development of pulmonary hypertension.

Patent ductus arteriosus (PDA)

Associations	Sick premature neonates
	Maternal warfarin and phenytoin therapy
	Congenital rubella
	Commoner in girls

Clinical features and signs

Preterm infants	Systolic murmur at the left sternal edge
	Collapsing pulse (visible brachial artery)
	Heart failure
Older children	Continuous murmur beneath the left clavicle, '**machinery murmur**' (continuous because the PA pressure is always lower than the aortic pressure) Collapsing pulse, '**waterhammer pulse**' (systolic pressure = twice the diastolic pressure). If severe there is heart failure and eventually pulmonary hypertension

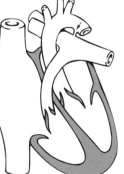

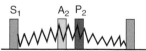

Murmur

S_1 A_2 P_2

Figure 4.18 Patent ductus arteriosus

ECG

- Usually normal
- May show LVH (or RVH if pulmonary hypertension)
- Indistinguishable from VSD

CXR

- Increased pulmonary vascular markings
- May be normal

Management

Neonate	Fluid restrict
	Indomethacin if < 34 weeks' gestation and within 3 weeks of birth (check renal function, platelets and predisposition to NEC)
	Surgical ligation if failure of medical management
Older child	Transcatheter device occlusion or surgical ligation

NB: PDA must be closed even if asymptomatic because of the risk of endocarditis.

Pulmonary stenosis (PS)

Associations	Noonan syndrome
	Maternal warfarin therapy

Clinical features

- Usually asymptomatic
- Right heart failure
- Arrhythmias (later in life)

NB: In neonates critical pulmonary stenosis presents as a duct-dependent circulation with cyanosis.

Signs

Murmur	Ejection systolic
	Upper left intercostal space
	No carotid radiation
	No carotid thrill
	Right ventricular heave
Heart sounds	Ejection click
	If severe: delayed P2 and soft P2

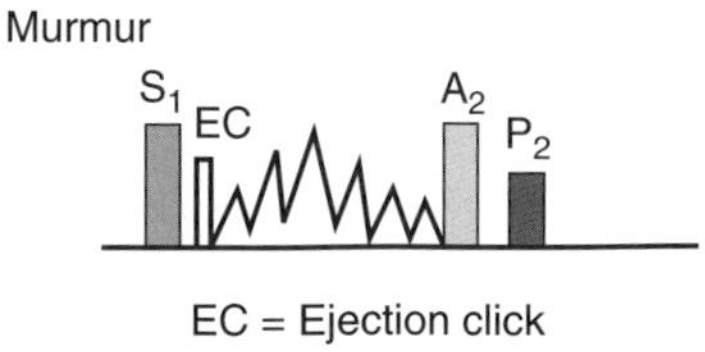

EC = Ejection click

Figure 4.19 Pulmonary stenosis

ECG

RVH.

CXR

Post-stenotic dilatation of the pulmonary artery.

Management

If the pressure gradient across the pulmonary valve is > 50 mmHg, found on Doppler scan, e.g. right ventricular pressure 70, pulmonary artery pressure 20, or there is severe pulmonary valve thickening, then transvenous balloon dilatation may be necessary. Surgical valvotomy is performed if balloon dilatation is unsuccessful.

In critical neonatal PS, emergency balloon valvuloplasty or surgical valvotomy is performed.

Aortic stenosis (AS)

This is usually anatomically a bicuspid aortic valve.

Associations	Aortic incompetence
	Coarctation of the aorta
	Mitral stenosis

Williams syndrome is *supravalvular* aortic stenosis with hypercalcaemia, elfin facies, mental retardation (see p. 12).

Clinical features

Neonate	Severe heart failure
	Duct-dependent circulation
Older child	Asymptomatic murmur
	Thrill on the chest
	Decreased exercise tolerance
	Chest pain, syncope
	Endocarditis
	Sudden death

Signs

Murmur	Ejection systolic
	Aortic area
	Radiation to the neck
	Carotid thrill
Heart sounds	Paradoxical splitting of second heart sound and soft A2
	Apical ejection click (due to opening of deformed aortic valve)
Slow rising plateau pulse	

ECG

LVH.

Murmur

S_1 EC A_2 P_2

Figure 4.20 Aortic stenosis

CXR

Post-stenotic aortic dilatation.

Management

Neonate	Valvotomy (balloon or surgical), then valve replacement later on
Older child	If symptomatic or resting pressure gradient across aortic valve >50 mmHg, then valvotomy (balloon or surgical) is required

Coarctation of the aorta

The descending aorta is constricted at any point between the transverse arch and the iliac bifurcation, but usually *just distal to the left subclavian artery*. Male > female 2:1.

Associations	Bicuspid aortic valve (40%)
	Mitral valve anomaly (10%)
	VSD
	Turner syndrome
	Berry aneurysm

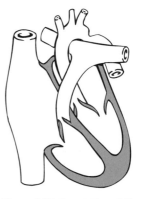

Figure 4.21 Coarctation of the aorta

Clinical features

This may present early or late.

Early   Circulatory collapse in the first week (duct-dependent circulation)
Late   Asymptomatic murmur discovered
           Hypertension (in the upper limbs only), weak pulses in legs
           Heart failure
           Subarachnoid haemorrhage (Berry aneurysm or SBE)

Signs

- Femoral pulses weak or absent (± left radial pulse)
- Four-limb blood pressure measurements show BP higher in right arm (± left arm) than legs
- Radiofemoral delay may be observed in older children
- Murmur: Ejection systolic
              Between the shoulder blades

ECG

- RVH in neonates (because the right ventricle is systemic in the fetus)
- LVH in older children

CXR

- May be normal
- Cardiomegaly with increased pulmonary vascular markings
- Rib notching (due to collaterals developing beneath the ribs) > 8 years of age

Management

Unstable neonates to be stabilized as for duct-dependent circulation (PGE_2, ventilation and inotropes as necessary). Surgical repair with an end-to-end repair or a left subclavian flap procedure. A left thoracotomy is used. The left subclavian flap procedure leaves the child with an absent left radial pulse. Recoarctation rate is approximately 5%. Mortality < 2%.

Balloon dilatation has been used successfully in older children.

Interrupted aortic arch

This is a form of severe coarctation where there is complete interruption of the aorta.

Associations   VSD
                  Chromosome 22 microdeletion (these can also have truncus arteriosus)

Clinical features

These present as neonates with features of a duct-dependent circulation.

Management

Complete correction is required within days of birth. The operative mortality is around 20%.

CYANOTIC CONGENITAL HEART DISEASE

In cyanotic CHD there is central cyanosis, manifested as a blue-coloured tongue, which occurs when capillary deoxygenated haemoglobin is > 3 g/dl (100 ml) of blood. It can be difficult to detect clinically in the presence of anaemia.

Causes of central cyanosis

- Lung disease
- Cardiac disease
- Persistent pulmonary hypertension of the newborn (PPHN)
- Methaemoglobinaemia

Cyanotic congenital heart disease results from:

1. Right-to-left shunting with decreased pulmonary blood flow, e.g. TOF, TA, PA, Ebstein anomaly, or
2. Abnormal blood mixing with normal or increased pulmonary blood flow, e.g. TGA, TAPVD, double inlet ventricle, hypoplastic left heart

Complications

- Metabolic acidosis (occurs when PaO_2 < 40 mmHg). Treated with sodium bicarbonate
- Increased affinity for oxygen (because the oxyhaemoglobin dissociation curve shifts to the left)
- Polycythaemia, which may lead to thrombosis, embolism, haemorrhage and abscess formation
- Necrotizing enterocolitis

Nitrogen washout test

This test is used to distinguish cardiac from respiratory causes of central cyanosis. The baby is given > 90% oxygen to breath for 10 min.

- If the PaO_2 rises to > 100 mmHg (14 kPa) the cause is respiratory or a central disorder
- If there is no change in the PaO_2 or a small rise but it remains < 100 mmHg (14 kPa) the cause is cardiac or it is PPHN

Prostaglandin (PGE2)

This is a relatively specific ductal smooth muscle relaxant. It is used as an emergency measure in duct-dependent circulations. It is given as an intravenous infusion.

The common side-effects are: hypotension, fever, apnoea (dose related) and jitteriness.

Methaemoglobinaemia

Iron in haemoglobin is usually in the ferrous form (for both oxygenated and deoxygenated Hb). In methaemoglobin (MetHb) iron is in the ferric form, non-functional and brown in colour. Normally methaemoglobin accounts for < 2% of total body haemoglobin.

Causes

- Congenital – autosomal recessive enzyme deficiencies
- Nitrites
- Nitrobenzine
- Aniline dyes

Clinical features

- Cyanosis with normal or only slightly reduced oxygen saturations
- Cardiac and respiratory distress on exertion

Investigations

- Nitrogen washout test (PaO_2 rises)

- Shaken blood turns brown
- Oxygen saturations are 80–100%
- Spectrophotometry of blood reveals MetHb

Management options

1. Reducing agents (IV) – methylene blue or ascorbic acid
2. Exchange transfusion
3. Reducing agents (orally) – methylene blue or ascorbic acid

Tetralogy of Fallot (TOF)

This is the most common congenital cyanotic heart condition. The cyanosis results from right-to-left shunting.

Associations   Down syndrome
22q microdeletion (DiGeorge) syndrome
CHARGE syndrome
VACTERL syndrome

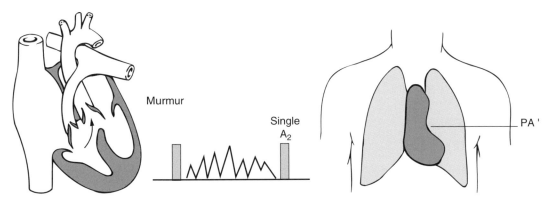

Figure 4.22 Tetralogy of Fallot

Anatomical features

- Malaligned VSD
- RV outflow obstruction (valvular + infundibular stenosis)
- Overriding aorta
- RV hypertrophy

Clinical presentations

- Cyanosis present in the first few days of life (rare)
- Murmur detected in first 2–3 months of life
- **Hypercyanotic spells** (late infancy) due to **infundibular spasm:**
  Occur in the morning and on crying
  Cyanosis or pallor
  Acidosis
  Child assumes squatting position (increases pulmonary blood flow by increasing systemic vascular resistance)
  Murmur becomes inaudible (due to *no* flow through pulmonary valve)

Management

1. Put child in knee–chest position and hold them over one shoulder with their knees bent, and reassure them (increases systemic vascular resistance and therefore pulmonary flow)
2. IV fluids
3. Morphine
4. Propranolol IV (decreases infundibular spasm and peripheral resistance)
5. Bicarbonate, then as necessary: IPPV (paralysed, therefore decreased oxygen demand)
   Noradrenaline (increases systemic vascular resistance and so increases pulmonary flow)
   Emergency surgery

Complications

Cerebral thrombosis, endocarditis, heart failure, myocardial infarction, brain abscess.

Signs

Murmur	Ejection systolic
	Upper left sternal edge (due to flow through pulmonary artery)
Heart sounds	Single second heart sound
Cyanosis	
Clubbing	

ECG

- RAD
- RVH

CXR

- Small boot-shaped heart: 'coeur en sabot'
- Prominent pulmonary artery bay
- Right-sided aortic arch (30%)
- Pulmonary oligaemia

Management

1. Palliative early surgery in the first few months of life if symptomatic with a modified Blalock–Taussig shunt (side-to-side anastomosis of subclavian artery to pulmonary artery)
2. Corrective surgery at 4–12 months of age (patch closure of the VSD and relief of the obstruction of the RVOT by removing muscle bundles, pulmonary valvotomy or outflow tract patch). Mortality of total correction is approximately 2%. Long-term problems are those of pulmonary regurgitation

NB: In a classical Blalock–Taussig shunt the subclavian artery is anastomosed to the pulmonary artery (child is left with an absent right radial pulse).

Tricuspid atresia

Clinical features

- Cyanosis usually present at birth and increases with age as pulmonary flow decreases
- Systolic murmur at LSE
- Single second heart sound

ECG

- Superior axis or LAD
- Tall P wave in V2

NB: Severe cyanosis + superior axis – can only be TA.

CXR

Small heart with pulmonary oligaemia.

Management

1. Initial palliation with a Blalock–Taussig shunt if too little pulmonary flow, or pulmonary band if too much pulmonary artery flow

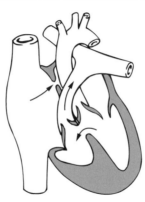

1. *Absence of tricuspid valve*
2. *ASD*
3. *VSD*
4. *Small, non-functional right ventricle*

Figure 4.23 Tricuspid atresia

2. Definitive palliation (usually at 2–5 years) with the Fontan procedure (SVC and IVC connected to pulmonary artery). Long-term problems are due to a single effective ventricle and concern of atrial arrhythmias developing

Double inlet ventricle

Here both atria empty into a single ventricle. The ventricle may be left, right or indeterminate. Both the aorta and the pulmonary artery arise from this ventricle.

Clinical features

The degree of cyanosis depends on the pulmonary blood flow:

If pulmonary flow is high   Relatively pink with severe heart failure and eventually Eisenmenger reaction

If pulmonary flow is low   Severe cyanosis and no heart failure

CXR

Cardiomegaly with either pulmonary plethora or oligaemia.

Management

1. Initial palliation with pulmonary artery banding (if no stenosis) or aortopulmonary shunt (if stenosis)
2. Then a bidirectional Glenn shunt (SVC to PA) at 4–12 months.
3. A modified Fontan procedure is performed for later surgical management at 1.5–3 years

Ebstein anomaly

- Abnormal tricuspid valve, leaflets adherent to ventricle wall (anterior cusp most normal)
- Distally displaced TV
- Atrialization of right ventricle
- ASD
- Functional pulmonary atresia
- WPW syndrome type B

Clinical features

- Cyanosis
- Failure to thrive
- SVT, extrasystoles
- May be asymptomatic, especially if mild anatomical abnormalities

Signs

- Soft, long systolic murmur (due to tricuspid regurgitation)
- Diastolic murmurs, extra heart sounds

ECG

- RBBB, RAD
- WPW (negative deflection of δ wave)
- Tall P waves, long PR interval

CXR

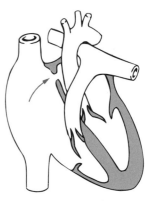

Figure 4.24 Ebstein anomaly

- Massive 'box cardiomegaly' and pulmonary oligaemia
- May be normal

Management

Neonate	Consider pulmonary vasodilatation (with O_2, prostacyclin or nitric oxide); if unsuccessful, the duct is opened using PGE_2
Older child	Control of SVTs and cardiac failure medically
	Tricuspid repair or replacement with closure of the ASD and ablation of the WPW pathway (this procedure is delayed as long as possible)

Hypoplastic left heart

This involves underdevelopment of the left side of the heart:

- Small left ventricle
- Small mitral valve
- Aortic valve atresia
- Small ascending aorta

Clinical features

Duct-dependent systemic circulation on closure of the ductus arteriosus in the first week of life, i.e. cyanosis, collapse, acidosis and impalpable peripheral pulses.

Management

Norwood procedure – a series of surgical procedures to rebuild the aorta and use the right ventricle as a systemic ventricle.

Pulmonary atresia

This may be:

1. Complete atresia of the pulmonary valve ± VSD with a PDA or collateral vessels and variable pulmonary arteries
2. Complete atresia of the pulmonary valve, no VSD, a PDA, hypoplastic right heart and good pulmonary arteries supplied by the duct. This type is totally duct dependent

Clinical features and signs

- Early neonatal cyanosis (duct-dependent circulation)
- No murmurs at the front, continuous murmur at the back (from collaterals in those with a VSD)
- Single second heart sound

ECG

RAH + RVH.

CXR

- Prominent right atrium (both types)
- Those with a VSD: right-sided aortic arch (30%) and 'coeur en sabot' finding
- Pulmonary oligaemia

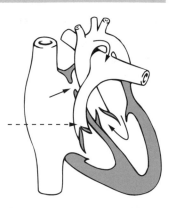

Figure 4.25 Pulmonary atresia

Management

- Emergency neonatal treatment with PGE$_2$ if duct dependent
- Pulmonary valvotomy or outflow patch ± a Blalock–Taussig-type shunt as a neonate
- Formation of a systemic–pulmonary connection when older
- Fontan operation in those with hypoplastic right heart

Total anomalous pulmonary venous drainage (TAPVD)

All the pulmonary veins drain into the right atrium instead of the left atrium. There are three types:

1. **Supracardiac** – drainage of pulmonary veins to SVC
2. **Cardiac** – drainage to right atrium and coronary sinus
3. **Infracardiac** – drainage below the diaphragm to the IVC, ductus venosus and portal vein. This type is always associated with obstruction to pulmonary venous return

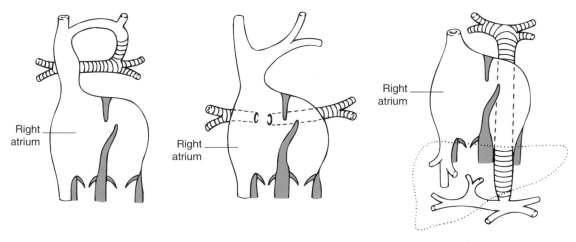

Supracardiac   Cardiac   Infracardiac

Figure 4.26 Total anomalous pulmonary venous drainage

102

There is mixing of blood between right and left sides at the:

- Patent foramen ovale
- Ductus arteriosus
- ASD

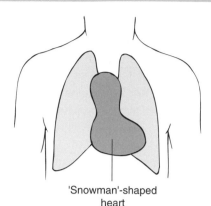

'Snowman'-shaped
heart

Figure 4.27 'Snowman'-shaped heart

Clinical features and signs

There are two presentations.

If obstruction present (type 3)	Severe cyanosis as a neonate
	Respiratory distress
	Hepatomegaly
	No murmurs
No obstruction (types 1 and 2)	Mild cyanosis
	Cardiac failure
	Recurrent chest infections
	Pulmonary hypertension

ECG

Normal or RVH.

CXR

1. Infracardiac – small heart and hazy lung fields
2. Supracardiac – big supracardiac shadow (classic 'snowman' appearance)

Management

1. If obstructive type, emergency prostaglandin infusion in neonates, then urgent cardiac surgery
2. Elective surgical correction in infancy (pulmonary venous trunk connected to left atrium)

Transposition of the great arteries (TGA)

Association   Maternal diabetes

There are *two parallel* circulations. Survival is due to mixing of blood at the:

- Ductus arteriosus
- Foramen ovale
- ASD
- VSD

Clinical features and signs

- Cyanosis within hours (on closure of DA and FO)
- Acidosis
- Mild tachycardia
- No murmur (there may be a systolic murmur from increased pulmonary flow)
- Single second heart sound

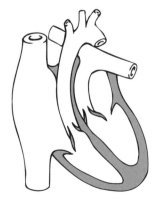

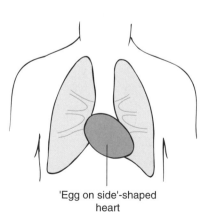

'Egg on side'-shaped
heart

Figure 4.28 Transposition of the great arteries

103

ECG

Normal.

CXR

- 'Egg on side' appearance of heart
- Increased pulmonary markings

Management

1. Emergency neonatal prostaglandin (PGE$_2$) infusion
2. Atrial balloon septostomy (Rashkind)
3. Corrective surgery with anatomical correction (aterial switch procedure) within a few weeks of birth

DUCT-DEPENDENT CIRCULATIONS

These are circulations that depend on the ductus arteriosus to maintain pulmonary or systemic blood flow, and deterioration occurs when the duct closes in the first week.

Causes of collapse in first week (duct-dependent systemic blood flow)	Causes of cyanosis in first week (duct-dependent pulmonary blood flow)
• Coarctation of the aorta • Hypoplastic left heart • Critical aortic stenosis • Interrupted aortic arch	• Transposition of the great arteries • Pulmonary atresia with a VSD • Critical pulmonary stenosis • Pulmonary atresia with no VSD • Tetralogy of Fallot • Tricuspid atresia • TAPVD with obstruction • Ebstein anomaly

ARRHYTHMIAS

SUPRAVENTRICULAR TACHYCARDIA (SVT)

This is the commonest arrhythmia in children. It is a re-entry tachycardia causing premature reactivation of the atria. In neonates the rate is > 220 bpm, and in older children > 180 bpm.

Wolff–Parkinson–White syndrome (WPW)

A congenital condition caused by an abnormal connection between the atria and the ventricle (an accessory pathway). The features are:

- δ Wave
- Short PR interval
- Wide QRS complexes

There are two types:

Type a   Activation of the left ventricle via the accessory pathway (most common)

Type b   Activation of the right ventricle via the accessory pathway (occurs in Ebstein anomaly)

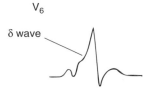

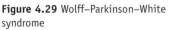

Figure 4.29 Wolff–Parkinson–White syndrome

The tachycardia may be stopped by IV adenosine, oral digoxin or oral flecainide. Flecainide reduces the recurrence risk of tachycardias.

Clinical presentation of SVT

Older child   Palpitations, dizziness, chest pain, collapse
Infant   Poor cardiac output, cardiac failure
In utero   Fetal tachyarrhthymia which can cause IUD or hydrops fetalis

Investigation

- ECG (particularly of the tachycardia, recording the response to adenosine if possible)
- It is helpful to do an echocardiogram to exclude structural CHD

Management

1. Vagal stimulation:
   Diving reflex: Babies   Immerse head and face in basin of ice-cold water for 5 seconds
                     Older child: Place polythene bag full of ice-cold water on face for 15 seconds
   Unilateral carotid sinus massage (older children only)
2. Adenosine – treatment of choice, given by rapid IV bolus
3. Synchronized DC cardioversion (1–2 J/kg). Anaesthetize or sedate the child (first line if child severely ill, otherwise use if drugs fail)
4. Other drugs that may be used are: Amioderone
                                        Flecainide – IV over 15 min
                                        Digoxin – oral or IV (slow acting)

Maintenance therapy to prevent recurrence may be required and this can be achieved with either flecainide, propranolol, digoxin or amiodarone. NB: Stop maintenance when > 1 year of age as 90% will have no further attacks.

Adenosine

Adenosine is an endogenous purine nucleotide. The half-life is very short (3–6 s). It acts to block A-V conduction. The side-effects are common and unpleasant.

- Dyspnoea, flushing, nausea
- Chest pain (this is not angina, though feels the same)
- Bradycardia (therefore do not use in the presence of sinus node disease)
- Heart block
- Atrial and ventricular premature beats
- If inhaled, bronchoconstriction (therefore do not use in asthmatics)

The antidote is aminophylline.

VENTRICULAR TACHYCARDIA (VT)

This is the occurrence of three or more ventricular beats in a row at a rate of at least 120/min.

Causes

- Metabolic – calcium, magnesium, potassium imbalances
- Long QT syndrome
- HOCM
- Infantile VT
- Postcardiac surgery

Management

- Adenosine to make the diagnosis if necessary
- DC cardioversion
- IV lignocaine or IV amiodarone

NB: It can be hard to distinguish VT from SVT (see below). If unsure whether it is VT or SVT, always treat as VT.

VT	SVT
Wide complexes	Narrow complexes
Irregular complexes	Usually regular
A-V dissociation	A-V association
Intermittent P waves seen	Regular P waves (if seen)
Fusion and capture beats	
Fusion beat – early beat with abnormal QRS	
Capture beat – early beat with normal QRS	

CONGENITAL COMPLETE HEART BLOCK

This is associated with:

- Maternal connective tissue disease – SLE and Sjögren syndrome (maternal anti-Rho antibodies cause atrophy and fibrosis of the AV node)
- Structural CHD (in 15% of cases):   AVSD
                                        Congenitally corrected TGA

Clinical presentation and management

- *In utero*: fetal bradycardia, hydrops fetalis or fetal death
- Neonatal bradycardia and heart failure
- Investigations include a 24-h ECG (as it may be intermittent)
- Treatment with the placement of a pacemaker is necessary if symptomatic or if the daytime pulse rate is < 60/min in an infant or < 50/min in an older child

PROLONGED QT SYNDROME (TORSADES DE POINTES)

Torsades de pointes is an arrhythmia usually of short duration. The ECG has a prolonged QT between the tachycardias. The arrhythmia usually spontaneously reverts to sinus rhythm; however, it can convert to VF and result in sudden death.

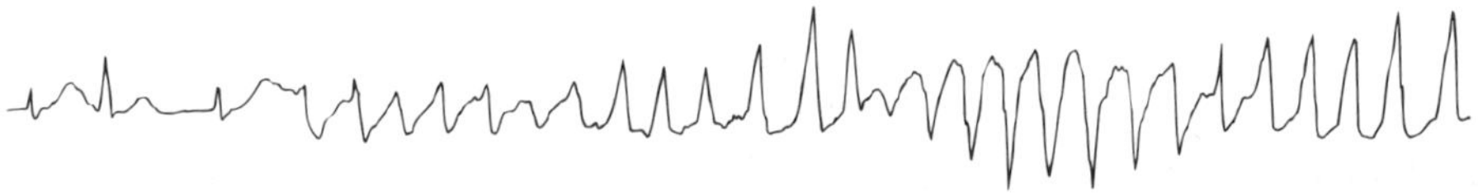

Figure 4.30 *Torsades de pointes*

Causes of prolonged QT interval

Congenital	**Jervell–Lang–Neilson**:
	• Autosomal recessive
	• Long QT plus congenital deafness. Suffer repeat drop attacks
	• Triggering factors: fear, excitement, exercise
	• May be misdiagnosed as epilepsy
	Romano–Ward:
	• Autosomal dominant
	• Isolated prolonged QT. Prognosis better than Jervell–Lang–Neilson
Acquired	Electrolyte disturbances – hypercalcaemia, hypomagnesaemia
	Drugs – amiodarone, quinidine, sotalol, MAOIs, tricyclics, erythromycin
	Poisoning – organophosphates
	Low-protein diets
	Anorexia nervosa
	Any cause of a bradycardia – myxoedema, complete heart block, head injury

Management

Congenital	β-blockers (mortality reduced from around 80% to 6%)
	Other antiarrhythmic drugs
	Left stellate ganglionectomy
	Implantable defibrillator if future treatment required
Acquired	Isoprenaline IV (this is contraindicated in congenital types)
	Pacing wire if associated heart block

RHEUMATIC FEVER

This is an inflammatory disease occurring in response to **Group A β-haemolytic streptococcal (GAS)** infection. It is now rare in the UK due to antibiotics. A streptococcal infection (usually sore throat or scarlet fever) is followed 2–6 weeks later by a polyarthritis, fever and malaise, and cardiac symptoms (the exact symptoms depending on the organs involved). The diagnosis is made on the basis of the Duckett Jones criteria. Two major criteria or one major and two minor criteria are needed to make the diagnosis.

Major criteria		Minor criteria
1. **Carditis**	Endocarditis (murmur) Myocarditis (heart failure) Pericarditis (pericardial rub, pericardial effusions)	1. **Fever** 2. **Arthralgia** 3. **Long PR interval** 4. **Raised ESR or CRP**
2. **Polyarthritis**	Medium joints, 'flitting'	5. **Leucocytosis** 6. **Previous rheumatic fever**
3. **Sydenham chorea**	'St Vitus dance' (involuntary movements) lasts 3–6 months	
4. **Erythema marginatum**	Pale red rings and segments of rings in recurrent crops lasting hours–days	
5. **Subcutaneous nodules**	Extensor surfaces Hard, painless, pea-like	

Investigations

- Evidence of recent streptococcal infection (ASOT raised, blood cultures, throat cultures, serology, recent scarlet fever)
- Investigation of symptoms and signs (FBC, U&E, creatinine), acute phase proteins, ECG, CXR, echocardiogram)

Management

- Bed rest (when active fever, carditis or arthritis is present)
- High-dose aspirin
- Steroids
- Treat heart failure
- Benzathine penicillin intramuscularly or oral penicillin course
- Then *lifelong* penicillin prophylaxis (monthly IM or daily oral penicillin)

Long-term complications

Mitral stenosis ± aortic stenosis.

INFECTIVE ENDOCARDITIS

This is infection of the endocardium, which occurs particularly with congenital heart disease (especially cyanotic) and on previously damaged or prosthetic valves. A high-velocity flow is needed to damage the endocardium. It can be acute (rare) or subacute (SBE).

Infecting organisms

- α-Haemolytic streptococcus (*Strep. viridans*) (50% of SBE)
- *Staphylococcus aureus* (50% of acute endocarditis, occurs with central lines and postcardiac surgery)
- *Enterococcus faecalis*
- *Staphylococcus epidermidis* (central lines, postcardiac surgery)
- *Candida albicans* (central lines, immunosuppressed)
- Aspergillus, brucella, histoplasma, *Coxiella burnetii* (Q fever) (all rare)

Clinical features

These may be subtle, therefore *always think of SBE* in a patient with a known cardiac defect who is unwell.

- Sustained fever, night sweats, malaise
- Development of *new* cardiac murmur
- Persistence of fever after acute illness (in the acute form)
- Splenomegaly and splenic rub
- Small vascular lesions: **Splinter haemorrhages**
   Roth spots (retinal haemorrhages)
   Janeway lesions (erythematous macules on thenar and hypothenar eminences)
   Osler's nodes (hard, painful embolic swellings on toes, fingers, soles and palms)
- Major embolic phenomena – cerebral, coronary, pulmonary and peripheral arterial
- Renal lesions – haematuria, focal glomerulosclerosis, renal failure
- Clubbing
- Arthritis of major joints

Investigations

Blood tests   Serial blood cultures (at least three sets, more if negative)
   FBC (anaemia almost invariably)

ESR and CRP (↑), immunoglobulins
C3 (low due to immune complex formation)
Serology (chlamydia, candida, coxiella and brucella) if culture negative

Urine Microscopic haematuria and proteinuria
CXR and ECG
Echocardiogram Looking for vegetations

Management

1. 4–6 weeks of antibiotic therapy with suitable antibiotic (initially IV for 2 weeks)
2. Antibiotic prophylaxis in the future for procedures
3. Surgery (if extensive valve damage, cardiac failure, vegetations or embolization)

NB: 'At-risk' individuals should receive prophylactic antibiotics for certain procedures.

MYOCARDITIS

This is an inflammation of the heart, with necrosis and fibrosis, causing serious weakening of the heart muscle with cardiac and respiratory failure. May become chronic.

Causes

Infectious Viral (*most common cause in children*) – coxsackie B, adenovirus
Bacterial – diphtheria, rikettsia
Fungal
Parasitic
Toxic E.g. pneumonia, sepsis, drugs
Connective tissue
disease
Idiopathic

Clinical features

- Cardiac failure – tachycardia, weak pulses, respiratory distress
- Arrhythmias
- Sudden death
- Asymptomatic (in adolescents)

Investigations

CXR Gross cardiomegaly, pulmonary plethora
ECG Arrhythmias
Bloods Cardiac enzymes (CK ↑, LDH ↑, troponin ↑)
Viral serology (specific IgM ↑), PCR
Echocardiography Poor ventricular function, large heart, pericardial effusion

Management

Most cases of mild inflammation will resolve spontaneously but in a proportion irreversible devastating damage is done to the heart.

Supportive Cardiac failure, arrhythmias management, ECMO may be necessary
Cardiac transplant If refractory heart failure

CARDIOMYOPATHY

DILATED CARDIOMYOPATHY (DCM)

This is a disease involving dysfunction of the cardiomyocytes, resulting in dilatation and impaired function of the left ± right ventricle. Most cases are idiopathic.

Associations

Genetic diseases	Familial, mitochondrial abnormalities, Friedreich ataxia, carnitine deficiency, muscular dystrophy, Fabrey disease, Refsum disease, Pompe disease
Infections	Post-viral myocarditis, e.g. coxsackie, echovirus, sepsis, diphtheria, rheumatic fever, HIV, trypanosomiasis (Chagas disease)
Nutrition	Selenium deficiency, e.g. TPN, short bowel syndrome, Keshan disease, thiamine, or calcium deficiency, iron overload, severe chronic anaemia
Toxins	E.g. doxorubicin, cyclophosphamide, adriamycin

Clinical features

- Heart failure (tachycardia, cardiomegaly, raised JVP, third and fourth heart sounds present)
- Arrhythmias
- Embolism

Investigations

CXR	Cardiomegaly and pulmonary plethora
ECG	LVH, non-specific T wave abnormalities
Echocardiogram	Large baggy heart (poorly contracting with atrial and ventricular dilatation) Reduced ejection fraction, mitral and tricuspid regurgitation
Cardiac biopsy (rarely)	Fibrosis, myocardiocyte hypertrophy and white cell infiltration (often unhelpful)
Other	If indicated to detect the cause: metabolic screen, nutritional bloods and genetic screening

Treatment

1. Treatment of cardiac failure and arrhythmias, and anticoagulants (aspirin or warfarin)
2. Cardiac transplant if needed

HYPERTROPHIC CARDIOMYOPATHY

This is characterized by hypertrophy of the interventricular septum and left ventricular wall, in the absence of a cardiac or systemic cause. Left ventricular outflow tract obstruction may be present.

Associations/causes

- Maternal IDDM (transient)
- Premature infants receiving steroids for lung disease (transient)
- Neurofibromatosis, mucopolysaccharidoses
- Autosomal dominant in some cases

In some of the familial cases mutations have been found in chromosome 14, cardiac β-myosin heavy chain (β-MCG) defect.

Clinical features

- Syncope, angina
- Arrhythmias (AF and VF)

- Sudden death (60–70%)
- Family history of sudden death

Signs

- Murmur: Ejection systolic (due to left ventricular outflow obstruction) mid-diastolic
              ± pan-systolic (mitral regurgitation)
- Fourth heart sound (palpable = double apex beat)
- Left ventricular failure

Investigations

Echocardiogram
24-h ECG   VT or VF (treat with amiodarone first line)
                             AF (dangerous as they are dependent on atrial contraction)
ECG   Long Q waves (due to thick interventricular septum)
                             LVH, non-specific T wave changes
Electron microscopy (EM)   'Myocardial disarray'
CXR   Cardiomegaly, prominent left ventricle

Treatment

1. Amiodarone
2. β-blockers
3. Cardiac pacing (causes an LBBB)
4. Surgical resection of the septum if significant LV outflow obstruction

PERICARDITIS

ACUTE PERICARDITIS

This is inflammation of the pericardium.

Causes

- Coxsackie virus
- Staphylococcus, *Haemophilus influenzae,* TB
- Rheumatic fever, malignancy, e.g. Hodgkin disease

Symptoms

Chest pain   Substernal, sharp, radiating to the neck
               Worse on lying flat and respiration
               Better on sitting forward

Signs

- Pericardial friction rub
- Fever

Investigations

- ECG: ST elevation, concave upwards
            T inversion
- Cardiac enzymes elevated (if associated myocarditis)

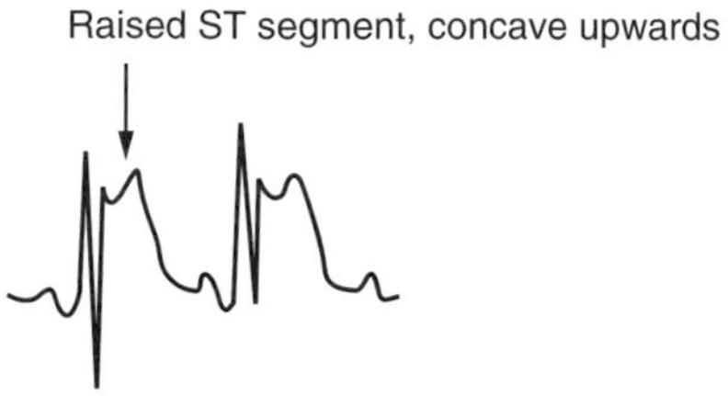

Raised ST segment, concave upwards

Figure 4.31 ECG in pericarditis

111

Treatment

- Anti-inflammatory drugs
- Drainage if indicated (always in post-viral pericarditis)

PERICARDIAL EFFUSION

All cases of acute pericarditis eventually develop a pericardial effusion.

Clinical features (if significant)

- Decreased cardiac output, impalpable apex beat
- Soft heart sounds, friction rub (quiet)
- Pulsus paradoxicus (BP decreases on inspiration)
- Kusmaul's sign (neck veins distend on inspiration)
- Raised JVP with Friedreich's sign (steep y descent)

Investigations

ECG	Small voltages
CXR	Large, globular heart
Echocardiogram	Diagnostic

Treatment

Pericardiocentesis with pericardial window formation if indicated.

CONSTRICTIVE PERICARDITIS

Causes

- TB
- Acute pericarditis
- Haemopericardium

Clinical features

- Cardiac failure – dyspnoea, sweatiness, hepatosplenomegaly
- Decreased ventricular filling – pulsus paradoxus, Kusmaul's sign, Friedreich's sign
- Atrial fibrillation (30%)
- Pericardial knock (loud third heart sound)

Investigations

CXR	Small heart with calcification
ECG	Low voltage QRS complexes and T wave inversion
Echocardiogram	Thick pericardium

Treatment

Surgery (**pericardiectomy** – removal of pericardium).

FURTHER READING

Archer N, Burch M *Paediatric Cardiology – An Introduction*. London: Chapman & Hall, 1998

Emmanouilides GC, Allen HD, Reimenschneider TA, Gutgesell HP, eds *Clinical Synopsis of Moss and Adams' Heart Disease in Infants, Children and Adolescents.* Baltimore: Williams & Wilkins, Baltimore, 1998

Park MD, Guntheroth WG *How to Read Pediatric ECGs*, 4th edn. Philadelphia: Mosby, 2006

Trusler GA, Freedom RM, Mawson JB, Yoo S, eds *Congenital Heart Disease: Textbook of Angiocardiography*. New York: Futura Publishing Company, 1997

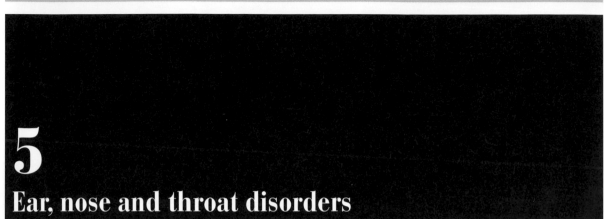

5

Ear, nose and throat disorders

- *Ears*
- *Nose*

- *Throat*

EARS

HEARING TESTS

Age	Test	Use
Birth onwards	Otoacoustic emission (OAE) Brain stem-evoked potential (BSER) 'gold standard'	Neonatal screening When OAEs fail
9–24 months	Distraction testing/behavioural audiometry (baby turns towards sounds made)	Establish thresholds
15 months–2½ years	Cooperative testing (whisper instructions with hand covering mouth)	Hearing assessment
2 years–3 years	Performance testing (condition, e.g. balls into a bucket)	Hearing assessment
2 years–4 years	Speech discrimination tests (similar words, e.g. man, lamb)	Hearing assessment
From birth	Impedance audiometry – tympanometry	For conductive loss
> 3 years approx	Pure tone audiometry	Hearing assessment

Causes for concern regarding hearing in newborns

- Family history of deafness
- Craniofacial malformations
- Birthweight < 1500 g
- Neonatal meningitis
- Severe perinatal asphyxia
- Potentially toxic levels of ototoxic drugs

- Neonatal jaundice requiring exchange transfusion
- Congenital infection, e.g. rubella, CMV, toxoplasmosis
- Parental concern

Tuning fork hearing tests

These tests may be used on older children to distinguish sensorineural hearing loss from conductive hearing loss. Beware – they are not always reliable.

Rinne test   Tuning fork held in front of the ear (air conduction) and then firmly on the mastoid process (bone conduction):

- Rinne positive = heard louder in front of the ear – normal or sensorineural hearing loss
- Rinne negative = heard louder on the mastoid process – conductive hearing loss

Weber test   Tuning fork held on the forehead in the midline. A conductive loss in one ear results in the sound being referred to that ear and heard as a louder sound

Possible test results

Interpretation	Right ear	Left ear
Normal or mild bilateral sensorineural loss	Rinne+ Weber central	Rinne +
Left conductive or mixed loss	Rinne + Weber referred to the left	Rinne +
Left severe sensorineural loss	Rinne + Weber referred to the right	Rinne −
Bilateral conductive or mixed loss	Rinne − Weber central	Rinne −

HEARING LOSS

Mild hearing loss   25–35 dB
Moderate hearing loss 40–60 dB
Severe hearing loss   60–90 Db
Profound hearing loss > 90 dB

	Conductive deafness	Sensorineural deafness
Site of lesion	Middle ear defects, e.g. Eustachian tube blockage	Cochlear or central neural damage
Incidence	Common in children	Uncommon
Cause	Glue ear is the commonest diagnosis	Usually congenital or neonatal
Presentation	Poor school performance and behavioural problems	Developmental delay
Severity	Usually mild or moderate	Entire spectrum from mild to profound
Management	Watchful waiting Medical or surgical therapy	Hearing aids Cochlear implants (if profound)

Audiograms

Hearing loss may be conductive (common in children) or sensorineural (uncommon).

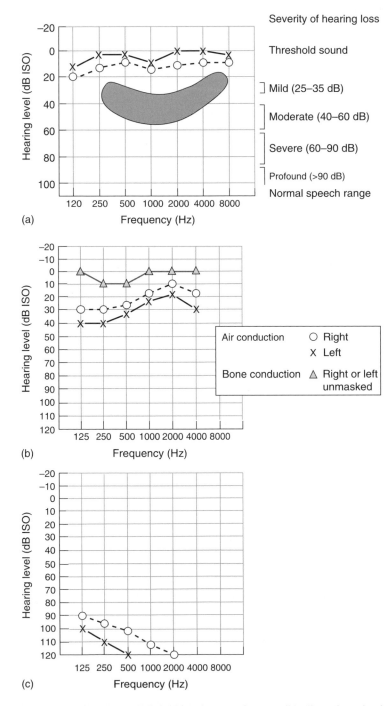

Figure 5.1 Audiograms. (a) Normal hearing speech range. (b) Bilateral conductive hearing loss. (c) Bilateral profound sensorineural hearing loss

EAR CONDITIONS

Acute otitis media (AOM)

This is infection of the middle ear.

Causes

Viral	RSV, rhinovirus
Bacterial	*Streptococcus pneumoniae, Haemophilus influenzae, Moxarella catarrhalis,* Group A β-haemolytic streptococcus, *Streptococcus pyogenes*

Frequently a bacterial infection will follow an initial viral infection.

Clinical features

- Earache (not in 20%)
- Fever
- URTI
- Hearing loss

Signs

Injected tympanic membrane (TM), bulging TM, loss of light reflex, perforated TM, discharge. Middle ear effusion post-infection in most children for 2–3 weeks.

Management

1. Analgesia and antipyretics for 24 h; if no improvement, commence oral antibiotics
2. Oral antibiotics
3. Myringotomy and drainage very rarely required

Glue ear (otitis media with effusion)

Glue ear occurs after acute otitis media when fluid persists for > 8 weeks without signs of inflammation. Incidence and prevalence are high but the majority of effusions resolve spontaneously. The initial infection may not be noticed.

Associations	Down syndrome, cleft palate and other craniofacial abnormalities
	IgG subclass deficiency, food allergies

Clinical features

- Conductive hearing loss, earache
- Speech and learning difficulties, behavioural difficulties

Signs

- Retracted TM, loss of light reflex, bubbles and fluid levels on the TM
- There may be a normal-looking drum
- Rinne test negative (if > 5 years)
- Tympanometry usually shows a flat (type B) response
- Pure tone audiometry shows a conductive hearing loss

Management

1. Initial observation for spontaneous resolution, 'watchful waiting' for 3 months
2. Trial of antibiotics may benefit a few children, e.g. 6 weeks of low dose co-amoxiclav

3. Grommet insertion
4. Adenoidectomy may be combined with grommets (leads to higher resolution rates)

Chronic otitis media (COM)

This is chronic disease of the middle ear, and is subdivided into different conditions depending on where the perforation lies and whether it is active.

COM classification (synonym)	Otoscopic abnormalities
Healed COM **Healed perforation** **(with or without tympanosclerosis)**	Thinning and/or local or generalized opacification of the pars tensa without perforation or retraction
Inactive mucosal COM (dry **perforation**) 'Safe' perforation	Permanent perforation of the para tensa but the middle ear mucosa is not inflamed
Active mucosal COM (**discharging perforation**) 'Safe' perforation	Permanent defect of the pars tensa with an inflamed middle ear mucosa which produces mucopus that may discharge
Inactive squamous epithelial (**retraction**) 'Unsafe' perforation	COM retraction of the pars flaccida or pars tensa (usually posterior-superior), which has the potential to become active with retained debris
Active squamous epithelial **Cholesteatoma** 'Unsafe' perforation	Retraction of the pars flaccida or tensa that has retained squamous epithelial debris and is associated with inflammation and the production of pus, often from the adjacent mucosa

Perforation of the central tympanic membrane is a '**safe**' perforation, and may be active, i.e. discharging, or inactive when the only sign is the perforation. There is conductive deafness and in long-standing cases a coexistent sensory loss. This can heal spontaneously leaving tympanosclerosis.

Perforation of the margin of the tympanic membrane (squamous epithelia) or pars tensa that has retained squamous epithelia is an 'unsafe' perforation, and become an active cholesteatoma.

Cholesteatoma

A potentially serious condition in which squamous epithelial debris, granulation tissue and pus develop in the middle ear and progress to damage neighbouring structures. Treatment is nearly always surgical.

Complications

Extracranial   VIIth nerve palsy, suppurative labyrinthitis, perimastoid abscess
Intracranial   Extradural, subdural and intracerebral abscess, meningitis, sigmoid sinus thrombosis and
hydrocephalus

Otitis externa

This is relatively uncommon in children. It comprises an infected, oedematous external auditory canal and usually presents as a discharging ear which then becomes painful (unlike otitis media which is initially painful and then may discharge). Treatment is with aural toilet and topical antibiotics given as eardrops or impregnated onto a wick.

Acute mastoiditis

Clinical features

This is a serious condition, usually following AOM which presents with similar symptoms plus swelling and tenderness in the postauricular region.

Investigations

Blood tests	FBC (neutrophilia), blood cultures
CT scan	(If diagnosis uncertain) Opacification of the mastoid air cell system with breakdown of bony septa

Treatment

Admit immediately for IV antibiotics and analgesia. Surgical exploration and mastoidectomy are performed in cases that fail to resolve with medical therapy or are advanced in presentation.

Complications

The concern with this condition is the development of **brain abscess**, **meningitis** or **venous sinus thrombosis**.

NOSE

Rhinitis

This is divided into allergic rhinitis (where known allergens trigger the symptoms) and non-allergic rhinitis. The symptoms are very similar.

Clinical features

- Persistently runny nose, clear discharge, occasionally becoming purulent
- Sneezing and itchy nose
- Nasal obstruction
- Mouth breather, hyponasal speech
- Family history of atopy

Signs and investigations

- Nasal mucosa pale and purple (normally pink)
- Serum IgE ($\uparrow$) and RAST tests may be done (allergic rhinitis)
- Postnasal space X-ray if concern about enlarged adenoids

Differential diagnosis

- Adenoidal hypertrophy
- Foreign body (unilateral)

Management

- Allergen avoidance
- Topical steroids (nasal drops or spray)
- Decongestants for short-term (< 1 week) usage for acute exacerbations, e.g. ephedrine, xylometazoline
- Antihistamines (nasal or systemic)
- Mast cell stabilizers, e.g. disodium chromoglycate
- Check for nasal foreign body (if unilateral discharge)

Epistaxis

This is a common problem in childhood, usually involving bleeding from Little's area of the nasal septum (the bit they pick!). Immediate management involves applying pressure to the soft part of the nose; vasoconstrictors such as xylometazoline (paediatric otrivine) will usually arrest bleeding if this fails.

Very rarely epistaxis is persistent: a nasal pack can be inserted (with admission) if this fails. If recurrent nose bleeds are occurring, underlying defects of coagulation, hypertension and neoplasms should be excluded. Cauterization of Little's area can be carried out if necessary.

Common cold (nasopharyngitis)

Causes

Rhinoviruses, coronaviruses, RSV.

Clinical features

- Snuffles, nasal discharge, sneezing
- Mouth breathing, headache, fever, malaise, anorexia, sore throat

Management

- Rest, oral fluids, simple analgesics
- For infants, saline nasal drops help clear the nose

Sinusitis

Sinusitis is rare in children. Infection of the sinuses in children usually involves the ethmoid and maxillary sinuses as the frontal sinuses are not fully developed. The serious complication of **subperiosteal abscess** or **orbital cellulitis** may be the presentation.

Clinical features

- Purulent nasal discharge, fever, local tenderness and pain
- Postnasal drip and chronic cough in chronic sinusitis

Investigations

Blood tests	FBC and blood cultures (if acutely unwell)
Sinus CT	Opaque maxillary sinuses (or X-ray – less frequently requested)

Management

- Broad-spectrum antibiotics (IV if acutely unwell)
- Nasal decongestion, e.g. xylometazoline
- Intranasal steroid drops
- Steam inhalations

If orbital cellulitis is present, an ophthalmologist must be involved to assess and help make the differentiation between pre- and post-septal cellulitis, and an ENT surgeon should also be involved. A CT of the sinuses will show sinus involvement as well as intraorbital complications necessitating surgical intervention.

Progression of orbital cellulitis:

- Pre-septal
- Post-septal
- Subperiosteal abscess

- Orbital abscess
- Cavernous sinus thrombosis

Danger signs indicating need for surgery
• Decreased acuity • Impaired globe mobility • Decreased colour vision • Proptosis

THROAT

STRIDOR

Stridor is a harsh sound caused by upper airway obstruction. Associated hoarse voice or cry, barking cough, tracheal tug or sternal recession, dyspnoea, tachycardia, tachypnoea, cyanosis (if severe) and agitation progressing to drowsiness may be seen.

- **Inspiratory stridor** is caused by extrathoracic obstruction
- **Expiratory stridor** is caused by intrathoracic obstruction
- Stridor arising from the subglottis and cervical trachea is often **biphasic**

Causes

Intraluminal
- Foreign body
- Tumour (including haemangioma)
- Papilloma
- Diphtheria

Intramural
- Infection (croup, epiglottitis, diphtheria, bacterial croup)
- Angioneurotic oedema
- Hypocalcaemia
- Haemangioma
- Laryngomalacia
- Subglottic stenosis
- Laryngeal web
- Tracheomalacia
- Vocal cord paralysis or prolapse

Extramural
- Goitre
- Cystic hygroma
- Haemangioma
- Mediastinal tumour
- Retropharyngeal abscess

LARYNGOMALACIA (FLOPPY LARYNX)

- A common condition in neonates where soft laryngeal cartilage collapses on inspiration or an elongated epiglottis flops into the larynx resulting in stridor
- Stridor worse on crying, agitation or lying supine
- Diagnosis clinical or by direct laryngoscopy
- Develops in first few days of life and usually resolves by 1 year (occasionally 2 years)
- Gastro-oesophageal-laryngo-respiratory reflux (GOLR) may prolong or exacerbate it

CROUP (ACUTE LARYNGOTRACHEOBRONCHITIS)

This is the commonest cause of acute stridor in children. It is a viral condition caused by parainfluenza virus, respiratory syncytial virus (RSV) or rhinovirus. The child's already small airway is narrowed by secretions and oedema.

Clinical presentation

- Usual age 1–2 years
- Stridor, mild fever, hoarse voice, barking cough and little constitutional disturbance. Worse in evening and overnight. Sometimes viral croup can deteriorate into a much more severe condition

Management

1. Calm atmosphere with avoidance of unnecessary blood tests, direct airway vision and neck X-rays which may frighten the child, making the condition worse
2. Humidified oxygen as necessary (keep oxygen saturations > 92%)
3. Steroids as nebulizer (budesonide 1 mg 12 hourly) or oral dexamethasone 12 hourly
4. Racemic epinephrine (adrenaline) nebulizer 1 ml 1/1000 if necessary (NB: Rebound increased stridor common 30–45 min later)
5. Intubation and IPPV are needed in approximately 1% of children and tracheostomy very rarely

Indications for IPPV

- Drowsiness due to hypoxia
- Tiring
- Rapid deterioration

Recurrent (spasmodic) croup

- Recurrent episodes of sudden onset at night of inspiratory stridor and croupy cough
- Most common in infants 1–3 years old
- Responds to inhaled steroids in acute phase
- Thought to be related to bronchial hyper-reactivity/reflux (GORL)

Bacterial tracheitis (pseudomembranous croup)

An uncommon condition usually caused by *Staphylococcus aureus*. The child is unwell for 2–3 days and is usually severely unwell on presentation. Soft hoarse voice, quiet cough and soft stridor. Intubation with IPPV for several days is usually required together with antibiotic therapy.

ACUTE EPIGLOTITIS

This is an infection usually caused by *Haemophilus influenzae* type b. It presents between 1 and 7 years (peak 2–3 years). It has become much less common since the introduction of the Hib vaccine.

Clinical presentation

- Toxic child
- Drooling, no cough, stridor, high fever and a short history (usually < 6 h)
- Muffled voice, pain in throat

Management

- Immediate involvement of senior ENT surgeon and anaesthetist
- Transfer to intensive care or high-dependency setting with intubation equipment and anaesthetist, paediatrician and ENT surgeon

- Intubation with IPPV for 1–3 days electively or in response to hypoxia
- Antibiotic therapy, e.g. cefuroxime, IV for 5 days
- Rifampicin prophylaxis for contacts

Differences between viral croup and epiglotitis		
	Viral croup	**Epiglotitis**
General state	Mildly unwell	Very unwell, toxic
Fever	Low grade	High
Length of history	Few days	Few hours
Drooling	No	Yes
Cough	Barking	No cough
Voice	Hoarse	Muffled
Incidence	Common	Rare
Age	1–3 years	2–7 years

PHARYNGITIS

This is a common infection usually caused by a virus (adenovirus or para-influenza virus) or, more rarely, a bacteria (*Group A streptococcus*).

Clinical features

- Sore throat, nasal congestion, fever
- Oropharyngeal inflammation (red throat)

Treatment

Symptomatic treatment with antipyretics and plenty of fluids, and antibiotics if bacterial infection is suspected.

Differential diagnoses

- Infectious mononucleosis, measles, scarlet fever, diphtheria, chronic adenoiditis, HIV
- Presentation of acute leukaemia or lymphoma

ACUTE TONSILITIS

Clinical features

- Sore throat, fever, malaise, bad breath
- Red tonsils sometimes with pus
- Cervical lymphadenopathy

Investigations

- Throat swab
- FBC and Monospot test

It can be difficult to distinguish bacterial (usually *Streptococcus pneumoniae*) from viral tonsillitis.

Management

- Analgesics, antipyretics and plenty of fluids
- Antibiotics may be required (penicillin V as first-line management – usually streptococcal if bacterial)

Complications

- Quinsy (peritonsillar abscess) – surgical drainage required
- Post-streptococcal complications (see p. 58)
- Obstructive sleep apnoea syndrome

Tonsillectomy indications
At least six attacks of tonsillitis per year for 2 years
Three attacks per year over a number of years for the older child
Obstructive sleep apnoea syndrome is a strong indication

OBSTRUCTIVE SLEEP APNOEA SYNDROME

This is upper airway obstruction with periods of desaturation. It is usually due to adenotonsillar hypertrophy. Children with certain craniofacial abnormalities are more at risk. Children with sickle cell disease are particularly affected due to a lower resting oxygen saturation and propensity to precipitate a sickle crisis. There is a spectrum of disease from mild and intermittent, e.g. with a URTI, to marked desaturation.

Clinical features

During sleeping	Snoring with apnoeas of > 10 s as the child struggles for breath
	Mouth breathing
	Frequent awakenings
	Unusual sleeping postures
Daytime	Sleepiness, morning headaches
	Learning problems and behavioural change

Complications

In extreme cases prolonged periods of hypoxia and hypercapnoea can cause ventricular hypertrophy, hypertension, polycythaemia and eventually cor pulmonale.

Investigations

- ENT examination
- X-ray postnasal space
- Sleep studies if diagnosis is in doubt or child at high risk. In practice not all children require sleep studies

Treatment

Adenotonsillectomy is usually curative.

CLEFT LIP AND PALATE

Incidence 1:1000 babies, polygenic inheritance. Subsequent pregnancy risk 5%.

Associations

- Older mothers
- Syndromes, e.g. Patau syndrome
- Drugs, e.g. maternal anticonvulsant therapy, alcohol

They may be unilateral or bilateral and isolated or combined.

Problems

- Inability to feed
- Choking episodes
- Otitis media with effusion
- Speech problems

Management

A multidisciplinary approach involving plastic surgeons, ENT surgeons, geneticists, paediatricians, speech therapists, audiologists, orthodontists. Special feeding teats, speech therapy.

Surgical repair   Lip may be repaired early (first week of life), though some surgeons prefer to wait until infant is 3 months old
Palate usually repaired at several months of age

Pierre–Robin sequence

A sequence of:

- Midline cleft of soft palate
- Micrognathia
- Glossoptosis (posterior displacement of the tongue)

These result in difficulty with feeding and upper airway obstruction.

Management includes:

- Nasopharyngeal airway
- Special feeding teat
- Surgical repair of palate (mandible grows)

6

Respiratory disorders

- *Physiology*
- *Congenital malformations*
- *Causes of wheeze*
- *Bronchiolitis*
- *Inhalation of a foreign body*
- *Aspiration (acute and recurrent)*
- *Asthma*
- *Viral-induced wheeze*

- *Causes of chronic cough*
- *Infection*
- *Cystic fibrosis*
- *Bronchiectasis*
- *Immotile cilia syndrome*
- α_1-*Antitrypsin deficiency*
- *Pulmonary fibrosis*
- *Sarcoidosis*

PHYSIOLOGY

LUNG FUNCTION TESTS

Peak respiratory flow rate (PEFR)

The PEFR is a useful and very simple lung function test. It varies with height, sex, age and ethnic group. It also varies during the day, being lowest in the early morning, and with exercise, being low shortly after moderate exercise. It is used to assess asthma severity by comparing a child's PEFR to normal corrected PEFR and to the individual child's normal PEFR.

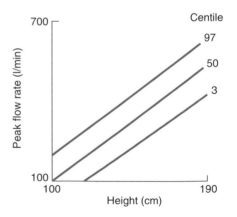

Figure 6.1 Peak flow readings

Spirometry

Spirometry provides timed measurements of expired volumes from the lung. It enables obstructive and restrictive lung conditions to be differentiated.

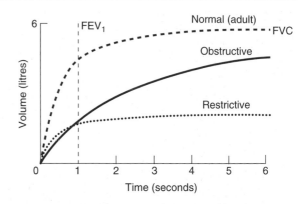

Figure 6.2 Spirometry

Obstructive lesions	Restrictive lesions
Low FEV$_1$:FVC ratio, RV ↓, FVC ↓, TLC ↑	FVC ↓, TLC ↓, FEV$_1$:FVC ratio ↑ or N
Asthma	Cystic fibrosis (both)
Bronchiolitis/bronchitis	Sarcoidosis
Emphysema (α_1-antitrypsin)	Myaesthenia gravis
Cystic fibrosis (both)	Fibrosing alveolitis
	Scoliosis

Lung volumes

Methods of measuring the lung volumes:

- Helium dilution
- Nitrogen washout
- Whole-body plethysmography

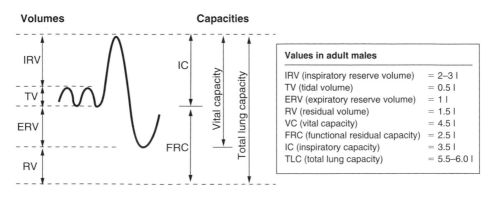

Values in adult males

IRV (inspiratory reserve volume)	= 2–3 l
TV (tidal volume)	= 0.5 l
ERV (expiratory reserve volume)	= 1 l
RV (residual volume)	= 1.5 l
VC (vital capacity)	= 4.5 l
FRC (functional residual capacity)	= 2.5 l
IC (inspiratory capacity)	= 3.5 l
TLC (total lung capacity)	= 5.5–6.0 l

Figure 6.3 Lung volumes and capacities

Transfer factor

This measures the rate at which a gas will transfer from the alveoli into the blood. It is a function of both the membrane-diffusing capacity and pulmonary vascular components, which together reflect the alveolar-capillary unit function. Carbon monoxide is used to measure this. Normal diffusing capacity (Dco) is 25–30 ml/min/mmHg.

Decreased Dco	Increased Dco
Anaemia	Polycythaemia
Cystic fibrosis	Pulmonary haemorrhage
Interstitial lung disease: • Pneumonia • Pulmonary fibrosis	Heart failure Left-to-right shunt Hyperkinetic states
Pulmonary vascular disease: • Pulmonary emboli • Pulmonary hypertension	Exercise Asthma

Flow–volume curves

These are constructed from spirometric data and are used to locate the site of an airway obstruction.

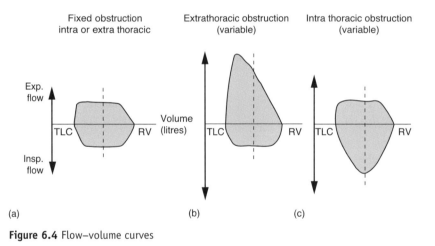

Figure 6.4 Flow–volume curves

CONGENITAL MALFORMATIONS

- Laryngomalacia (see p. 121)
- Tracheo-oesophageal fistula (see p. 479)
- Congenital lobar emphysema
- Bronchogenic cyst. These are usually asymptomatic at birth and present when secondarily infected or they enlarge in size and compromise an adjacent airway. There is an air–fluid level on CXR and treatment is with surgical excision
- Cystic adenomatoid malformation (CAM lung). This is the second most common congenital lung malformation after congenital lobar emphysema. A single lobe of one lung is enlarged and cystic, and usually causes mediastinal shift with compression of the other lung. It presents with neonatal respiratory distress, a pneumothorax or recurrent respiratory infections. It may be seen on CXR and CT scan of the thorax. Management is surgical

CAUSES OF WHEEZE

Common	Rare

Infection:
• Bronchiolitis
• Viral-induced wheeze (<1 year of age)
• Whooping cough
• Pneumonia
Asthma (> 1 year of age)
Recurrent aspiration
Foreign body inhalation
	Cystic fibrosis
	Immunodeficiency
	Congenital lobar emphysema
	External compression of airway:
	  • Congenital vascular ring
	  • Mediastinal mass (glands, tumours, cysts)
	Heart failure
	Fibrosing alveolitis
	Cow's milk protein intolerance (aspiration)

BRONCHIOLITIS

This is a common condition usually presenting between 1 and 9 months. It is due to the respiratory syncytial virus (RSV) in 80% of cases, and otherwise to adenovirus types 3, 7 and 21, para-influenza virus, rhinovirus or influenza viruses.

Clinical features

- Coryza, cough, dyspnoea, tachypnoea, wheeze
- Worsening for first 5 days then resolution over next 2 weeks
- Feeding difficulties (secondary to breathing difficulties), poor intake, vomiting
- Apnoea in small babies
- Secondary bacterial chest infection can develop

Signs

- Tachypnoea, tachycardia, intercostal, subcostal and suprasternal recession
- Inspiratory crackles, wheeze
- Low grade fever, and if severe cyanosis

Investigations

Nasopharyngeal aspirate (NPA)	Immunofluorescence test for RSV antibodies
CXR	(Only if severe or bacterial superinfection suspected) Hyperinflation (horizontal ribs and flattened diaphragm) Patchy atelectasis (often RUL), peribronchial thickening
Blood tests	Paired antibody titres (for RSV) Viral culture

Treatment

- Oxygen via nasal prongs or head box
- IV fluids as necessary with NG feeding in recovery phase
- CPAP or intubation with IPPV if deterioration with exhaustion or persistent apnoeas
- Bronchodilators advocated in some centres, these cause short-term improvement in a minority and must be monitored for efficacy
- Antibiotic therapy if secondary bacterial pneumonia suspected
- Ribavirin via SPAG machine for infants who are very unwell or at risk of severe disease, e.g. BPD, CHD, CF, immunodeficiency or < 6 weeks old
- ECMO if above management is failing

Complications

- **Bronchiolitis obliterans** – severe persistent airways damage (usually with adenovirus)
- **Macleod syndrome** – persistent overdistension of one lung

INHALATION OF A FOREIGN BODY (FB)

Clinical features

Acute episode	Acute coughing or choking episode followed by
	Stridor (in upper airways), or
	Wheeze (in lungs)
	Positive history of small object inhaled
Chronic symptoms	Respiratory infection not resolving
	Recurrent lobar pneumonias involving the same lobe
	Persistent wheeze

Investigations

CXR	FB radio-opaque only in 10–15% of cases. NB: Peanuts are radiolucent
	Collapse distal to FB
	FB side may be hyperinflated
	Inspiratory (both sides equal) and expiratory film (FB side lung hyperinflated)

Management

Removal of FB using **rigid bronchoscopy** under general anaesthesia.

ASPIRATION (ACUTE AND RECURRENT)

Causes

Acute	Infants with acute viral illness exacerbating existing gastro-oesophageal reflux
	Depressed gag reflex
	Reduced state of consciousness
Recurrent	Neurological swallowing disorder, e.g. cerebral palsy
	Gastro-oesophageal reflux
	Oesophageal incoordination
	Structural anomaly, e.g. tracheo-oesophageal fistula

Clinical features

- Cough, stridor and wheeze
- Pneumonia

Investigations

CXR	Consolidation
	More than one lobe may be involved
	Features of collapse in recurrent aspiration
Other	To elucidate cause, e.g. reflux investigations

Management

Treat acute infection, then identify and treat underlying cause.

ASTHMA

This is an endemic condition affecting up to 1:10. It is a chronic inflammatory disease of the airways characterized by:

- Reversible bronchoconstriction
- Mucosal oedema
- Excessive mucus production

Associations   Atopic conditions (33% have eczema, 50% have allergic rhinitis $\pm$ conjunctivitis)

Chronic clinical features

- Recurrent wheeze ⎫
- Difficulty in breathing ⎬ Both often with exercise
- Nocturnal wheeze with cough
- In long-standing disease there may be chest hyperinflation, pectus carinatum (pigeon chest) and Harrison sulci (a permanent groove in the chest wall at the insertion of the diaphragm)

Clinical features of an exacerbation

- Dyspnoea
- Expiratory wheeze (crackles in younger children)
- Respiratory distress (tachypnoea, recession, tachycardia, cyanosis)

Features of a life-threatening attack

- Unable to speak or feed
- Central cyanosis
- Exhaustion/confusion/decreasing level of consciousness
- Silent chest on auscultation (due to minimal air entry)
- Peak flow $\leqslant$ 30% of predicted
- Hypotension – pulsus paradoxus (fall of inspiratory systolic BP > 10 mmHg from expiratory systolic BP)

Important questions in asthma history
1. What triggers the asthma, e.g. pets, exercise, cold, dust mite, pollen, respiratory infections?
2. How often and severe are the attacks?
3. Does the asthma affect daily living, e.g. school, sport, sleep?
4. Can they measure peak flow properly to monitor asthma?
5. Can they use their device properly (get them to demonstrate)?
6. Do they understand the difference between quick-relief and preventive medications?
7. Do they recognize a deterioration and have a good management plan for this?
8. Do they recognize a severe attack and know to seek medical attention?

Management

Acute attack

- Oxygen
- β-agonist either 10 puffs from an MDI via spacer device or nebulized, as frequently as necessary (initially 15 minutely)

131

- Ipatropium bromide 6 hourly
- Systemic steroids (oral prednisolone 1–2 mg/kg [max. dose 40 mg] or IV hydrocortisone)
- If severe attack, may then need:
- IV infusion or bolus of salbutamol or aminophylline infusion (if on oral theophylline no loading dose)
- Intubation and ventilation if deterioration in general condition, i.e. peak flow, blood gases, drowsiness or tiring, despite above measures

Long-term therapy

This is outlined in the British Guidelines on Asthma Management (summarized below). The lowest step to control the asthma should be used. Management should be reviewed every 3–6 months and a step down in treatment is possible if control is sustained for > 3 months. β-Agonists are used as relievers on all of the steps.

NB: A short course of steroids is usually required to treat an acute exacerbation.

Children under 5 years

Step 1	Step 2	Step 3	Step 4
Mild intermittent	*Regular preventer*	*Add-on therapy*	*Persistent poor contol*
Occasional inhaled β-agonist	Add Inhaled steroid 200–400 µg/day*	2–5 years Consider leucotriene receptor antagonist (LRA)	Refer to respiratory paediatrician
(or LRA if inhaled steroid cannot be used)		< 2 years consider step 4	

School children (5–12 years)

Step 1	Step 2	Step 3	Step 4	Step 5
Mild intermittent asthma	*Regular preventer therapy*	*Add-on therapy*	*Persistent poor control*	*Frequent or continuous use of oral steroids*
Occasional β-agonist inhaled (or other prevention drug if inhaled steroid cannot be used)	Add inhaled steroids (200–400 µg/day*)	Add 1. Long-acting β-agonist (LABA) 2. Assess control: – LABA benefit, but still poor control, ensure 400 µg/day* inhaled steroids – LABA no response, stop LABA, ensure 400 µg/day* inhaled steroids Trial other therapies, e.g. theophylline SR, leukotriene antagonist	Increase inhaled steroids to 800 µg/day*	Use daily steroid tablet in lowest dose to maintain control Ensure high-dose inhaled steroids maintained 800 µg/day* Refer to respiratory paediatrician

*Beclomethasone equivalent.
Ref: British Guideline on the Management of Asthma Thorax May: 63 Suppl 4: iv 1–121.

Asthma medications

Immediate-relief bronchodilators

1. *β-2-agonists, bronchodilator*
Bronchodilators acting directly on the β-2 receptors in the bronchi.

| *Side-effects* | Tachycardia, arrythmias, peripheral vasodilatation, headache, fine |
| *(due to stimulation of β-receptors)* | tremor, excitement, hypokalaemia if used frequently |

Generic name	**Device**
Salbutamol `}` short acting	MDI, tabs, syrup, injection, neb sol, dry powder
Terbutaline	MDI, turbohaler, tabs, syrup, neb sol, injection
Salmeterol `}` long acting	MDI, dry powder
Eformoterol	MDI, turbohaler

2. *Anticholinergics*
Antimuscarinic bronchodilators. Slower onset (30–60 min), last up to 6 h. Rarely used in children < 1 year old. Sometimes used in acute attacks. Examples:

| Ipatropium bromide | MDI, resp sol, dry powder |
| Oxitropium | MDI, resp sol, autohaler |

Long-term preventive medications

1. *Inhaled steroids*
Anti-inflammatory effect on airways. Steroid side-effects minimal unless high dose inhaled or oral steroids given regularly.

Beclomethasone	MDI, dry powder
Budesonide	MDI, dry powder, neb sol
Fluticasone	MDI, dry powder, neb sol

2. *Mast cell stabilizers*

| Sodium cromoglycate | MDI, dry powder, neb sol |
| Necrodomil | MDI |

3. *Methyl xanthines*
Bronchodilators, smooth muscle relaxer. Narrow margin between toxicity (arrhythmias, convulsions) and therapeutic dose.

| Aminophylline | Tabs, injection |
| Theophylline | Tabs, caps, syrup |

4. *Leukotriene receptor antagonists*
Blocks effect of cysteinyl leukotrienes in the airways. Additive effect with corticosteroids.

| Monteleukast | Tabs |

Delivery devices

There are many different devices and routes for the medications suitable for different ages of child, and the most convenient and appropriate is chosen for each child.

- It is most important the parents and child are taught how to use the equipment properly
- The best device to use for *all* children and adults is an **MDI with spacer**
- Some older children prefer for practical reasons to use dry powder devices
- Methods of dispersing medication to the lungs: Metered dose inhaler (MDI) with or without spacer
  Dry powder inhaler, e.g. turbohaler and accuhaler
  Nebulizer
- Two spacer devices exist. By increasing the distance, these slow the aerosol, allowing propellants to evaporate. This reduces the size of the droplets which helps inhalation and traps larger non-respirable particles in the chamber. Also, they reduce the need for coordination between drug release and inhalation. They connect with different medications:
  1. Nebuhaler – terbutaline, budesonide
  2. Volumatic – salbutamol, beclomethasone, fluticasone, ipatropium bromide

VIRAL-INDUCED WHEEZE

- Wheeze only with concurrent URTI
- Usually found in pre-school children
- Individuals are often non-atopic and symptoms resolve by school age
- Management as for acute asthma attack, dependent on severity. Acute bronchodilators when symptoms occur; short course oral steroids may be necessary

PERSISTENT WHEEZE IN INFANCY

- Recurrent episodes of wheeze in infants, sometimes following viral infections
- Usually these children have small airways (boys, child of smoking mother)
- Some resolve in first few years, others go on to become asthmatic

CAUSES OF CHRONIC COUGH

- Asthma
- Recurrent aspiration
- Prolonged infection, e.g. pertussis, mycoplasma, RSV, TB
- Inhaled foreign body
- Habit cough. NB: These will not cough during sleep
- Post-nasal drip
- Lung disease, e.g. cystic fibrosis, bronchiectasis, congenital cysts, primary ciliary dyskinesia
- Immunodeficiency, e.g. HIV, cancer therapy

INFECTION

PNEUMONIA

A common disease of childhood caused by many pathogens.

Clinical features

- Respiratory distress symptoms and signs
- Fever (> 38.5°C) and malaise
- Abdominal pain

Causes

Newborn	Group B β-haemolytic streptococcus, *Escherichia coli, Listeria monocytogenes, Chlamydia trachomatis, Staphylococcus aureus,* CMV
Infants	RSV, adenovirus, influenza viruses, parainfluenza, *Streptococcus pneumoniae, Staphylococcus aureus, Haemophilus influenzae*
Children	*Streptococcus pneumoniae, Mycoplasma pneumonia, Haemophilus influenzae, Staphylococcus aureus,* TB
Immunocompromised	As for children plus *Pneumocystis carinii,* atypical TB

Investigations

This is a clinical diagnosis

CXR	Lobar pneumonia (dense consolidation) or bronchopneumonia (patchy)
Blood tests	Blood cultures, FBC, blood gas if unwell
Oropharyngeal suction specimen	For viral immunofluorescence, M, C & S
Sputum	M, C & S

Management

It is not possible to distinguish between viral and bacterial pneumonia clinically or on CXR, and therefore it is always treated with antibiotics.

1. Humidified oxygen as needed to keep saturation > 92%. Use head box, nasal cannulae, or face mask
2. Therapy with appropriate antibiotic

Complications

- *Pneumococcal pneumonia* – meningitis, pleural effusion
- *Staphylococcal pneumonia* – empyema, lung abscess, pneumothorax

PERTUSSIS (WHOOPING COUGH)

This is an infection caused by the Gram-negative coccobacillus, *Bordatella pertussis*. It is a notifiable disease.

Clinical features

Usually occurs ≤ 5 years of age

Transmission	Droplet
Incubation period	7–14 days
Catarrhal stage	1–2 weeks. Runny nose, conjunctivitis, malaise, highly infectious
Paroxysmal stage	Paroxysms of coughing causing inspiratory whoop and vomiting. The severe coughing can cause conjunctival petechiae and epistaxis. Severe in young babies. Infants may have no whoop, but apnoea following coughing spasms. May last up to 3 months (usually 2 weeks)
Convalescence	1–2 weeks. Resolution of symptoms

Investigations

A clinical diagnosis, confirmed by:

Per nasal swab	PCR and culture
FBC	Lymphocytosis

Management

- Isolate child and give supportive care
- Erythromycin early in disease and for contacts
- Prevention by immunization

Complications

- Lobar pneumonia (causes 90% of deaths)
- Atelectasis, bronchiectasis (late sequela)
- Apnoea, cerebral anoxia with convulsions in young infants
- Rectal prolapse, inguinal hernia, phrenulum tear, periorbital petechiae, subconjunctival haemorrhage (from coughing spasms)

CYSTIC FIBROSIS

- Autosomal recessive disorder. Highest prevalence in Northern Europeans: carrier rate 1:25, 1:2500 affected
- **Chloride** (with passive movement of **sodium** and **water**) is poorly secreted, resulting in viscid secretions
- Due to a defect in CFTR (cystic fibrosis transmembrane regulator) protein, which is a **chloride channel**
- CFTR protein located on chromosome 7. Over 1000 mutations found. Loss of phenylalanine at position 508 (DF508) in 75% of UK cases
- The two main problems are: **Recurrent chest infections** causing chronic lung damage (bronchiectasis)
  Malabsorption (due to reduced pancreatic enzymes) causing faltering growth

Clinical features

General	Faltering growth
Respiratory	Recurrent infections classically in the following order: *Staphyloccocus aureus, Haemophilus influenzae, Pseudomonas aeruginosa*, Cepacia
	Restrictive (and obstructive component in one-third) lung disorder
	Chronic lung damage (bronchiectasis, lobar collapse, pneumothorax)
	Nasal polyps, sinusitis
Cardiovascular	Right heart failure (late feature secondary to severe lung disease)
Pancreas	Decreased pancreatic enzymes in 85% (lipase, amylase, proteases), causing steatorrhoea
	CFRD (CF-related diabetes) – increasing incidence with age (one-third of adults)
Liver	Fatty infiltrate, cholesterol gallstones, cirrhosis, pericholangitis, portal hypertension
Gut	Meconium ileus (15% present with this – soon after birth with delayed passage of meconium and bowel obstruction. Relieved either surgically or with Gastrograffin enema), meconium ileus equivalent
	Rectal prolapse (> 18 months) – resolves rapidly on starting enzyme replacement
	Hepatosplenomegaly, pubertal delay
	Intussusception, constipation
Joints	Cystic fibrosis-related arthropathy
Reproductive	Males infertile (as vas deferens are absent)

Neonatal presentations

- Meconium ileus
- Prolonged neonatal jaundice
- Recurrent chest infections
- Malabsorption with diarrhoea or steatorrhoea
- Faltering growth

Examination findings

General	Poor growth and nutritional state
	Finger clubbing, finger prick marks (from monitoring IDDM)
Respiratory	Hyperinflation, scoliosis, Portacath (NB: Auscultation may be normal if post physiotherapy)
Cardiovascular	Right heart failure
Abdominal	Hepatosplenomegaly, faecal masses, pubertal delay, jaundice, caput medusae, surgical scars, e.g. from meconium ileus, liver transplant, gastrostomy
ENT	Nasal polyps
Joints	Swelling (cystic fibrosis-related arthropathy)
CXR findings	Bronchial wall thickening
	Hyperinflation with flattened diaphragms } All become more marked with increasing disease
	Ring and line shadows, mottling } severity

Diagnosis

This is usually suspected on the basis of failure to thrive and recurrent chest infections.

Sweat test	**Gold standard.** Two tests needed, with ⩾ 100 mg sweat, pilocarpine used
	In CF, **high chloride** (> 60 mmol/L) is diagnostic, **sodium** also high
Immune-reactive trypsin (IRT)	↑. Used < 3 months of age. May be performed on Guthrie test
Gene analysis	PCR technique looking for common mutations. This is possible on the Guthrie test. Also antenatally to screen for maternal mutations for risk of having CF child
Stool	With pancreatic insufficiency elastase is low, chymotrypsin absent and high fat content
Electrolytes	Unwell children have **hypokalaemic alkalosis** secondary to sodium and potassium loss in the sweat. Known as **pseudo-Bartter syndrome**

Causes of a false-positive sweat test	
Dehydration	Addison disease
Hypoproteinaemia (severe)	Hypothyroidism
Eczema	Nephrogenic diabetes insipidus
Ectodermal dysplasia	Congenital adrenal hyperplasia
Flucloxacillin therapy	HIV
Glycogen storage disease type 1	Fuscidiosis
Mucopolysaccharidoses	

Management

Aims of management are to ensure optimal physical and emotional growth, and delay the progress of the pulmonary disease.

Lung disease	Physiotherapy often twice daily (more as necessary)
	Antibiotics (long-term or pulsed as prophylaxis)
	May be nebulized
	Intercurrent infections treated as necessary
	Bronchodilators (useful in 30%)
	Oxygen at night at home if necessary
Gastrointestinal disease	Oral pancreatic enzymes, e.g. Creon®, Pancrease®
	Optimum nutrition: High-calorie, high-protein diet
	Vitamins, bile acids (ursodeoxycholic acid)
	Salt required in hot weather and for babies

Other treatments Mucolytics, e.g. DNase therapy or hypertonic saline
Heart–lung transplantation in end-stage disease
Treatment for complications, e.g. insulin for CFRD
Gene therapy is still in development

Regular review

- General growth and development
- Respiratory pathogens
- Frequency and severity of chest infections and lung function
- Nutrition and gastrointestinal symptoms
- Development of diabetes, liver or joint disease
- Psychosocial problems (school progress, etc.)
- Fertility and genetic counselling

BRONCHIECTASIS

This is a condition of permanent dilatation of the bronchi. It may be localized or diffuse. There are inflamed bronchial walls, decreased mucociliary transport and recurrent bacterial infections.

Causes

- Severe pneumonia
- Post-whooping cough, measles and TB
- Inhaled foreign body
- Cystic fibrosis
- IgA deficiency IgG subclass deficiency
- Primary ciliary dyskinesia

Clinical features

- Chronic productive cough
- Haemoptysis
- Dyspnoea and clubbing after time

Investigations

CXR Hyperinflation and peribronchial thickening of affected area
CT scan thorax Dilated bronchi and thickened walls

Management

- Postural drainage
- Antibiotics (for acute infections or prophylaxis)
- Bronchodilators
- Surgical resection of affected lobe if necessary and possible

IMMOTILE CILIA SYNDROME

A group of inherited conditions caused by an absence of dynein arms (ATPase) on the cilia, which results in defective or absent cilia action. The defective cilia affect the lungs, nose, ears and sperm ducts. First described as **Kartagener syndrome** (situs inversus, chronic sinusitis and immotile cilia).

Clinical features

- Neonatal respiratory distress
- Chronic sinusitis
- Otitis media (conductive hearing loss)
- Chronic productive cough $\pm$ wheeze
- Males infertile (sperm motility poor)

Diagnosis

- Ultrastructural changes of dynein arms on the cilia (**gold standard**)
- Nasal mucosal scrapings – motility decreased
- Mucociliary clearance – time to taste saccharine placed on inferior nasal turbinates (prolonged)
- Liver function tests – obstructive picture
- CXR and CT scan as for bronchiectasis

Management

As for bronchiectasis with ENT involvement.

α_1-ANTITRYPSIN DEFICIENCY

The lung disease in α_1-antitrypsin deficiency generally presents as emphysema at 30–50 years of age, though younger presentation occurs. Hyperinflation is seen on CXR. Management is with aggressive treatment of infections, vaccination for pneumococcus and influenza, bronchodilators if necessary and advice against smoking.

PULMONARY FIBROSIS

This is a rare condition resulting in 'honeycomb' lung seen on CXR. Progression to respiratory failure is inevitable.

Causes

Localized	Widespread
TB	Langerhans cell histiocytosis
Sarcoid (on CXR)	Neurofibromatosis
Systemic sclerosis	Tuberose sclerosis
Post-pneumonia	Rheumatoid lung
	Drugs – busulphan, bleomycin, cyclophosphamide

Management

Supportive, with steroids to alleviate symptoms.

SARCOIDOSIS

A multisystem granulomatous disease, uncommon in children, most usually seen in young adults.

Clinical features

Very variable depending on the organs involved and the severity. Organs involved include:

Lungs   Parenchymal infiltrates, miliary nodules, *restrictive* lung changes
Hilar and paratracheal lymphadenopathy
Eyes   Uveitis, iritis

Joints	Arthritis
Other	Skin rashes, peripheral lymphadenopathy, liver involvement
	Hypercalcaemia may lead to renal damage

Clinical presentation

Young child	Cough, fatigue, weight loss, anaemia, bone and joint pain
Older child	Maculopapular erythematous rash, uveitis, arthritis and minimal lung involvement

Investigations

Biopsy	Of involved area (non-caseating, granulomatous lesions)
Serum	ESR ↑
	Ca ↑
	ACE (angiotensin-converting enzyme) ↑, a measure of disease activity
Urine	Hypercalciuria
Lung function tests	Restrictive defect
CXR/CT scan	Perihilar lymphadenopathy, parenchymal infiltrates

Management

- Regular assessment for lung, renal, eye and other involvement
- Supportive and symptomatic treatment. Steroids may be used
- Prognosis is very variable

FURTHER READING

British Thoracic Society. The British Guidelines on Asthma Management, *Thorax* 1997 Vol 52: Suppl 1, 1–21

Chernick V, Boat TF, Wilmott RW, Bush A *Kendig's Disorders of the Respiratory Tract in Children*, 7th edn. Philadelphia: WB Saunders, 2006

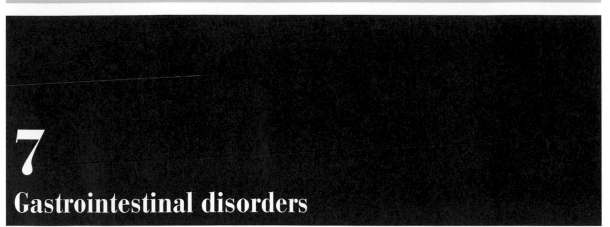

7

Gastrointestinal disorders

- *Physiology*
- *Upper gastrointestinal conditions*
- *Malabsorption*
- *Gastroenteritis*
- *Diarrhoea*
- *Chronic abdominal pain*
- *Peptic ulcer*
- *Inflammatory bowel disease*

- *Constipation*
- *Pancreatitis*
- *Gastrointestinal tract bleeding*
- *Gastrointestinal tract tumours*
- *Faltering growth*
- *Nutritional disorders*
- *Eating disorders*

PHYSIOLOGY

OESOPHAGUS

The oesophagus propels food along with normal peristaltic waves, which are disturbed in motility disorders. It has two sphincters:

Upper oesophageal sphincter (UOS)	Normally closed by the cricopharyngeus muscle
Lower oesophageal sphincter (LOS)	A high resting tone to prevent reflux of gastric contents
	Composed of oesophageal smooth muscle, under vagal and hormonal control
	Intra-abdominal oesophagus also acts as a physiological valve

STOMACH

Function	Food reservoir, mixes food, produces acid, emulsifies fats, intrinsic factor secretion and minimal absorption

Gastrin (hormone)

Released with	Antral distension
	Amino acids in antrum
	Vagal nerve stimulation
	pH > 1.5

Actions   Release of gastric acid, pepsin, IF
                     Gastric emptying
                     Pancreatic bicarbonate release

Stimulation of gastric acid secretion	Inhibition of gastric acid secretion
Vagal stimulation	Low gastric pH
Hormonal stimulation (gastrin)	Higher centres, e.g. fear (sympathetic NS)
Histamine release (H2 receptors on oxyntic cells)	Intestinal peptides – CCK-PZ, GIP, secretin
Pepsin	

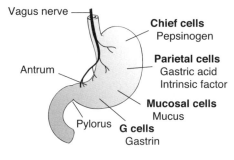

Figure 7.1 The stomach

PANCREAS

Exocrine function (98%)		Endocrine function	
These enzymes are produced in the acinar cells	In islets of Langerhans:		
Enzymes	Maltase, lipases, amylase, nucleases	1. β-cells	Insulin
Proenzymes	Trypsinogen, chymotrysinogens, proaminopeptidase, procarboxypeptidases, co-lipase	2. α-cells	Glucagon
		3. D-cells	Somatostatin
		4. pp-cells	Pancreatic polypeptide

DUODENUM AND JEJUNUM

Function   Digestion, absorption, hormone production and defence organ

Produces 2 L of fluid/day, made from:

• Brunner's glands – bicarbonate juice
• Panneth cells – watery juice
• Enterocytes – digestive enzymes and absorption

Principal gastrointestinal polypeptide hormones

Secretin	Pancreatic bicarbonate release ↑
	Delays gastric emptying, inhibits gastric acid and pepsin secretion
Cholecystokinin-pancreozymin (CCK-PZ)	Pancreatic enzyme and bicarbonate release ↑, gallbladder contraction, inhibits gastric emptying
Gastric inhibitory peptide (GIP)	Insulin secretion ↑, inhibits gastric acid secretion
Motilin	Increases bowel motility
Gastrin	Action as above (p. 141)
Pancreatic polypeptide (PP)	Inhibits pancreatic secretion
	Gallbladder relaxation
Somatostatin	Inhibits secretion and action of many hormones
Vasoactive intestinal peptide (VIP)	Intestinal and pancreatic secretion ↑, inhibits gastric acid and pepsin secretion
Substance P	Increases small bowel motility

Digestive enzymes

Amylase, lactase, sucrase, maltase, isomaltase, lipases and enterokinase.

Absorption

- Passive – water, salts, folic acid, vitamins B and C
- Active – amino acids and monosaccharides
- Released from micelles then passive – fatty acids, cholesterol, monoglycerides, vitamins A, D, E, K

ILEUM

Function is absorption (though this occurs mainly in the jejunum and duodenum), with bile salts and vitamin B_{12} absorbed in the terminal ileum.

Bile acids

Function	Digestion of fats
Bile contains	Bile acids, cholesterol, phospholipids, bile pigments (bilirubin and biliverdin) and protein
Primary bile acids	Cholic acid
	Chenodeoxycholic acid
Secondary bile acids	Deoxycholic acid ⎫
	Lithocholic acid ⎬ From breakdown of primary acids

ENTEROHEPATIC CIRCULATION

This occurs 6–8 times a day. It is increased by parasympathetic stimulation, gastrin and secretin and decreased by sympathetic stimulation and cholestyramine.

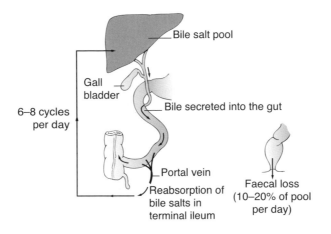

Figure 7.2 The enterohepatic circulation

COLON

Function   Absorption of water, sodium and chloride (passive and active)
          Secretion of potassium, bicarbonate and mucus

Stool is 70% water.

UPPER GASTROINTESTINAL CONDITIONS

GASTRO-OESOPHAGEAL REFLUX

This is the passage of gastric contents involuntarily into the oesophagus. It is the result of an incompetent lower oesophageal sphincter, usually secondary to immaturity.

Associations   Cerebral palsy
          Hiatus hernia
          Thoracic stomach
          Coeliac disease
          Raised intracranial pressure
          UTIs
          Fabricated or induced illness

Clinical features

- Vomiting at end of feeds (± altered blood)
- Crying, food refusal, poor sleeping, irritability
- Usually resolves spontaneously by 12–18 months of age

Complications

- Faltering growth
- Oesophagitis ± oesophageal stricture
- Apnoea, ALTE, SIDS
- Aspiration, wheezing, hoarseness, recurrent chest infections
- Iron-deficiency anaemia
- Seizure-like events, torticollis

Investigations

These are necessary only if there is failure to resolve with simple measures or the reflux is complicated. The investigations complement each other.

Oesophageal pH measurement	% of time pH < 4.0 in 24 h: >10% = abnormal if < 1 year old; > 6% = abnormal if >1 year old
Barium swallow and meal	Looking for malrotation, hiatus hernia, oesophageal stricture
Endoscopy	Looking for oesophagitis, stricture, enteropathy
Other investigations	CXR
	Urine M, C & S
	Hb and iron studies
	Faecal occult bloods
	Remember raised intracranial pressure may cause reflux

Management

Position	Nurse on side, 30° head up
Thicken feeds	Add thickeners, e.g. Carobel, Nestargal, or use prethickened feeds, e.g. Enfamil AR, SMA Staydown
Change feeds	Consider changing feeds to hydrolysate, e.g. Nutramigen, Pregestamil, Peptijunior, or elemental amino acid-based (Neocate)
Drugs	Antacid, e.g. Gaviscon Infant
	Prokinetic, e.g. domperidone
	H_2 blocker, e.g. ranitidine
	Proton pump inhibitor, e.g. omeprazole
Surgery	If medical management fails over a 3-month period, consider an antireflux procedure, e.g. Nissen fundoplication, but only if life-threatening reflux as it normally resolves spontaneously by 12–18 months of age

POSSETTING

This is small-volume vomits that occur during or between feeds. The infant will be thriving and there is no cause for concern. Management is with reassurance.

HIATUS HERNIA

This is herniation of the stomach through the oesophageal hiatus and may be of the sliding type (gastro-oesophageal junction slides into the thorax) or para-oesophageal (a portion of the stomach herniates beside the gastro-oesophageal junction).

Sliding hiatus hernia	Paraoesophageal hiatus hernia
Common type	No reflux occurs
Associated with GOR	Complication of fundoplication (Nissen) Upper abdominal pain common symptom

Management

- Antireflux medication
- Surgery if necessary (rarely so)

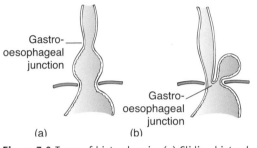

Gastro-oesophageal junction

Gastro-oesophageal junction

(a)   (b)

Figure 7.3 Types of hiatus hernia. (a) Sliding hiatus hernia. (b) Para-oesophageal hiatus hernia

CAUSES OF VOMITING

Gut pathology Medical	Surgical
Possetting (not pathological)	Obstruction:
Overfeeding	• Atresias/stenoses
GOR	• Intussusception
Gastroenteritis	• Malrotation
Food intolerance	• Achalasia
Cyclical vomiting	• Foreign body
Coeliac disease	Acute abdomen from any other cause Other – peptic ulcer
Other pathology	
Acute infection/occult infection e.g. UTI	
Metabolic disorder, e.g. IDDM	
Drugs or deliberate poisoning	
CNS disease, e.g. migraine, ICP	
Psychogenic, e.g. anorexia nervosa, bulimia	
Severe illness	

MALABSORPTION

Malabsorption may be *generalized* or *specific* where individual transport mechanisms or enzymes are defective. Generalized malabsorption presents with **faltering growth** and **steatorrhoea**. Specific malabsorption may present with different features.

CAUSES OF MALABSORPTION

Generalized

Gut	Short gut syndrome, blind loop syndrome, chronic infection (giardiasis, immunodeficiency), coeliac disease, food intolerance, e.g. cow's milk protein
	Diffuse mucosal lesions, e.g. congenital microvillous atrophy
Pancreas	Cystic fibrosis, chronic pancreatitis, Shwachman–Diamond syndrome
Liver	Cholestasis of any cause, e.g. biliary atresia

Specific

Protein	Amino acid transport defects, e.g. Hartnup disease, cysteinuria
Carbohydrate	Disaccharidase deficiencies, e.g. lactase, sucrase-isomaltase
	Glucose-galactose malabsorption
Fat	Abetalipoproteinaemia
Elements	Chloride diarrhoea, acrodermatitis enteropathica (zinc)
Vitamins	Juvenile pernicious anaemia (B_{12})

INVESTIGATIONS

The list is exhaustive and therefore investigations must be symptom led. Some investigations to consider are:

Bloods	FBC, iron studies, bicarbonate, U&Es, creatinine, plasma lipids
	Coeliac screen, CF genotype
Stool	Electrolytes, fats, reducing substances
	Microscopy and culture (cysts, parasites)
	Faecal elastase ($\downarrow$ in pancreatic insufficiency) and α_1-antitrypsin ($\uparrow$ in protein-losing enteropathy)
Sweat test	Cystic fibrosis
Radiology	AXR, CXR, barium studies
Endoscopy	With duodenal/jejunal biopsies and duodenal juice microscopy
Breath tests	Lactose, sucrose and lactulose breath tests (the latter for bacterial overgrowth)

FOOD INTOLERANCES

Dietary protein intolerance (cow's milk protein intolerance)

This is most commonly due to cow's milk protein (CMP) intolerance. Other protein intolerances occur to soya, fish, wheat and eggs.

Associations	Atopy
	IgA deficiency

Clinical features

- Diarrhoea, vomiting, failure to thrive
- Recurrent mouth ulcers, allergic pancolitis

- History of contact allergy or anaphylaxis (rare) to cow's milk, family history of reaction to foods
- Atopic history (eczema, asthma)

Investigations

Diagnosis may be established by:

- Trial of cow's milk protein elimination diet without biopsy, or
- Small intestinal biopsy – patchy partial villous atrophy, eosinophils in lamina propria
- Other investigations: IgE ↑, eosinophilia

Management

Elimination diet using casein-hydrolysate based formula. Breast feeding mothers need to avoid cow's milk and soya protein.

NB: 35–40% of children with CMP sensitivity also have soya sensitivity and need a CMP and soya-free diet, e.g. Nutramigen, Pregestamil, Peptijunior or, increasingly commonly, elemental amino-acid based milk (Neocate). 50% of children recover by 1 year of age and most of the rest by 2 years.

Post-gastroenteritis intolerance

This is a transient condition, occurring after acute gastroenteritis and resulting in persistent diarrhoea (> 14 days). They have usually developed a temporary intolerance to lactose secondary to CMP sensitization and villous damage. Diagnosis is on the history and presence of reducing substances in the stool (positive Clinitest). Test for glucose in the stool (Clinistix) is negative. The condition usually resolves after 2–3 days on a lactose-free diet.

Lactose intolerance

Lactase, the enzyme necessary for digesting lactose (the sugar in milk), appears late in fetal life and falls after age 3. 40% of Orientals have late-onset (classically age 10–14 years old) lactose intolerance.

Causes

- Transient post-gastroenteritis
- Primary lactase deficiency (very rare)
- Late-onset lactase deficiency (common)

Clinical features

After ingestion of lactose: explosive watery diarrhoea, abdominal distension, flatulence, loud audible bowel sounds.

Investigations

- Stool chromatography positive for lactose, i.e. > 1% present
- Lactose hydrogen breath test

Management

- Lactose-free formula feed for infants
- Milk-free diet with calcium supplements for older children

Types of infant formula available	
Milk substitute	Composition
Nutramigen	Casein hydrolysate (hydrolysed protein to peptides of < 15 amino acids)
Pregestamil	Casein hydrolysate (hydrolysed protein to peptides of < 15 amino acids)
Peptijunior	Partial whey hydrolysate (contains some peptides > 15 amino acids)
Neocate	Amino acids

SUCRASE–ISOMALTASE DEFICIENCY

Autosomal recessive, rare. This is a congenital enzyme deficiency of the disaccharidases sucrase and isomaltase and is worth considering as a differential diagnosis in 'toddler's diarrhoea'.

Symptoms are of diarrhoea and bloating. The sugars (sucrose and isomaltase) may be seen in stool chromatography. These are not reducing sugars. Enzyme assays show the specific deficiencies and hydrogen breath test is positive after sucrose ingestion. Management is with dietary sucrose restriction.

GLUCOSE–GALACTOSE MALABSORPTION

Autosomal recessive. This is due to a congenital deficiency of the glucose galactose transport sites. The condition presents with severe diarrhoea, bloating and dehydration. Management is with glucose and a galactose-free diet, using fructose-containing formula.

COELIAC DISEASE

A dietary **gliadin** intolerance resulting in small bowel mucosal damage. Gliadin, a fraction of the protein gluten is in wheat, barley, oats (marginally) and rye.

Associations   HLA-B8 DR3, DR7, DQW2.

Presentation is usually with the introduction of dietary gluten at around 4–6 months of age.

Clinical features

- Faltering growth, anorexia, vomiting, diarrhoea
- Irritable, unhappy
- Abdominal pain, rectal prolapse, smelly stools
- Signs of pallor, abdominal distension, clubbing and malabsorption

NB: Increasingly a more subtle presentation occurs with, for instance, poor height and weight for the familial context, e.g. parents may be on 90th percentiles whilst the child may be on the 25th centiles. Without appreciation of the parental heights, the child's diagnosis of coeliac disease may be missed as they fall within population normal percentiles. Many adults have coeliac disease but are unaware of their diagnosis, e.g. common cause of male infertility.

Associations/other features

- Malabsorption
- **Dermatitis herpetiformis:**   Very itchy vesicles on extensor surfaces. Improves on a gluten-free diet
  IgA Abs in normal and perilesional skin but not active lesions
  Treatment is with dapsone until diet effective
  (All children with dermatitis herpetiformis have coeliac disease)

- Selective IgA deficiency
- IDDM
- Intestinal lymphoma
- Later life: osteopoenia and general increase in bowel carcinoma incidence

Investigations

IgA anti-endomysial and tissue trans-glutaminase Abs	(With total IgA level because in the 1 in 200 or so individuals who have a low IgA there may be false-negative serological results as these antibodies are IgA antibodies, i.e. these antibodies are not seen in IgA-deficient individuals.) Anti-gliadin antibodies are now not considered specific enough for a serologically secure diagnosis
Jejunal biopsy	**Gold standard** Total or subtotal villous atrophy seen on small bowel biopsy by endoscopy
Gluten challenge	Now only necessary in children diagnosed under 2 years of age – transient gluten enteropathy may occur under this age but coeliac disease is diagnosed as a life-long condition after 2 years of age.
Other findings include	Anaemia (dimorphic blood film from iron and folate deficiency) Hypoalbuminaemia

Management

Lifetime gluten-free diet. (This reduces risk of complications such as intestinal lymphoma.)

Causes of villous atrophy on jejunal biopsy

Subtotal/total	Partial
Coeliac disease	Cow's milk protein intolerance
Giardia lamblia	Soya intolerance
Tropical sprue	Post-gastroenteritis enteropathy Immunodeficiency, e.g. SCIDS, chemotherapy

INTESTINAL LYMPHANGECTASIA

This is a group of disorders involving dilatation of the intestinal lymphatic vessels with leakage of lymph into the intestine and peritoneal cavity.

Associations   Noonan and Turner syndromes

Causes

Congenital

Acquired Lymphatic obstruction from abdominal or thoracic surgery, malrotation, right heart failure or constrictive pericarditis, post-Fontan cardiac surgery

Clinical features

- Fat malabsorption with steatorrhoea and features of vitamin E deficiency
- Protein-losing enteropathy (oedema, chylous ascites, hypoalbuminaemia and hypogammaglobulinaemia)

Diagnostic investigations

- Small bowel biopsy – distorted villi with dilated lacteals
- Faecal α_1-antitrypsin $\uparrow$ due to protein-losing enteropathy

Management

High-protein, low long chain (LCT) triglycerides, high medium chain triglyceride (MCT) diet.

ABETALIPOPROTEINAEMIA

Autosomal recessive. Severe fat malabsorption with neuropathy secondary to vitamin E deficiency. Underlying deficiency of microsomal triglyceride transfer protein in the small bowel.

Clinical features

Gastrointestinal	Faltering growth, steatorrhoea, abdominal distension
Neurological	(After age 10 years) Ataxia (spinocerebellar degeneration), loss of proprioception and vibration sense, peripheral neuropathy and retinitis pigmentosa
	Mental retardation and regression

Investigations

- Decreased cholesterol and triglycerides and no vitamin E in serum
- **Acanthocytes** in the blood (spiky red cells)
- Jejunal biopsy (fat accumulation in intestinal cells)

Management

Special diet with increased MCTs and supplements of fat-soluble vitamins (A, D, E and K).

SHWACHMAN–DIAMOND SYNDROME

An inherited autosomal recessive condition, 1:50000 births, female > male, 2:1. Caused by mutation (pseudogene copy) in the SBDS gene on chromosome 7q11.

The syndrome involves:

- Pancreatic exocrine insufficiency (with subsequent malabsorption)
- Haematological dysfunction: Neutropaenia – often cyclic, progression to myeloid arrest can occur
  Neutrophil chemotactic defects
  Thrombocytopaenia (70%), anaemia (50%)
  High HbF
- Skeletal abnormalities: Metaphyseal dysostosis
  Short stature and faltering growth

Management is with pancreatic enzyme replacement therapy and steroids or androgens. Average survival time is 35 years. Stem cell transplant and GCSF have been used.

GASTROENTERITIS

Causes

Viral	Rotavirus (winter epidemics, cause in 60% < 2 years old in winter)
	Norwalk virus, adenovirus (40 and 41), astrovirus

Bacterial	Staphylococcus (exotoxin)	
	Watery diarrhoea	Enterotoxigenic *E. coli* (ETEC, traveller's diarrhoea)
		Vibrio cholerae
	Bloody diarrhoea	Enteroinvasive *E. coli* (EIEC)
		Enterohaemorrhagic *E. coli* (EHEC)
		Shigella, *Campylobacter jejuni,Salmonella enteritidis*, yersinia
Protozoal	Giardia, cryptosporidium, amoebiasis	

Clinical features

- Acute-onset vomiting and diarrhoea
- Abdominal pain and distension
- Mild pyrexia
- Invasive bacterial infection – unwell, high fever, blood and mucoid stool

Differential diagnosis

Acute infection	Septicaemia, meningitis, UTI, respiratory infection
Surgical	Intussusception, appendicitis
Metabolic	Diabetic ketoacidosis
Other	Reye syndrome, coeliac disease

Examination findings

- Assess child for **dehydration**, which is difficult to do accurately (see below). Below 5% dehydration usually there are no obvious clinical findings. Dehydration is usually hyponatraemic or isotonic.
- Other possible findings: Acidosis – hyperpnoea
    Potassium depletion – hypotonia, weakness
    Hypocalcaemia – neuromuscular irritability
    Hypoglycaemia – lethargy, coma, convulsions

Dehydration assessment

	Moderate 5–10%	Severe > 10%
Condition	Restless/lethargic	Drowsy
Eyes	Sunken	Very sunken
Fontanelle	Sunken	Very sunken
Tears	Reduced	Absent
Mucous membranes	Dry	Very dry
Tissue elasticity	Reduced	Absent
Capillary refill time	2–4 s	> 4 s
Pulse	Tachycardia	Thready, very tachycardic
BP	Normal	Normal or low
Urine output	Reduced	Reduced/absent

Hypernatraemic dehydration

- Unusual and potentially serious
- Irritable with doughy skin and relatively good circulation
- Water shifts from intracellular to extracellular and therefore the signs of extracellular fluid loss are reduced
- Rehydration should be slow (over 48 h) to avoid rapid brain rehydration and subsequent raised intracranial pressure

Investigations

These depend on the clinical state of the child.

Stool	Virology, M, C & S, PCR, 'hot stool' for cysts and ova
Bloods	FBC, haematocrit, U&Es, creatinine, glucose, capillary blood gas
	Plasma and urine osmolality as necessary

Management

Mild < 5%	Oral rehydration therapy (ORT) for 24 h or until diarrhoea settles, then milk and light diet
	ORT fluid contains glucose and sodium because they are absorbed across even a damaged mucosa by a joint mechanism and water absorption follows by osmosis NB: Breast feeding can continue with initial ORT
Moderate/severe > 5%	Admit
	If the CRT >3 s or acidotic breathing is apparent, IV rehydration is necessary
	If in shock: IV volume expansion with 20–30 ml/kg 0.9% saline. Then rehydrate over 24 h

---

Rehydration fluids

1. **Deficit** = % dehydration × weight (kg)

2. **Maintenance**

3. **Continuing losses**

Use 5% dextrose/0.45% saline (or 5% dextrose/0.9% saline) depending on the plasma sodium and calculated total body sodium. If severe acidosis (pH < 7.0) treat with bicarbonate (half the deficit).

Maintenance fluid calculation

Weight	Fluid requirements
0–10 kg	100–120 ml/kg/24 h (4 ml/kg/h)
10–20 kg	1000 ml + 50 ml/kg/24 h (2 ml/kg/h) for each kg >10
> 20 kg	1500 ml + 20 ml/kg/24 h (1 ml/kg/h) for each kg >20

Bicarbonate calculation

Half deficit (mmol) = weight (kg) × 5 × 0.3 × (24 − plasma bicarbonate)

Complications

Renal	**Oliguria** (i.e. < 200 ml/m^2/day or < 0.5 ml/kg/h)

<table>
<tr><td></td><td>NB: If prerenal renal failure:</td><td>Urine osmolality > 500</td></tr>
<tr><td></td><td></td><td>Urine Na < 10 mmol/L</td></tr>
<tr><td></td><td></td><td>Urine urea > 250 mmol/L</td></tr>
<tr><td></td><td></td><td>Urine:plasma osmolality ratio > 1.3</td></tr>
</table>

	Management of oliguria: urgent IV volume re-expansion. If no recovery of renal function, then give minimal maintenance fluid plus losses only, with no potassium. Dialysis is necessary if the fluid, electrolyte or acid–base status does not correct. Recovery is seen with the polyuric phase of acute tubular necrosis
	Renal vein thrombosis (haematuria + renal mass, see p. 216)
	Haemolytic uraemic syndrome (see p. 217)
Pulmonary oedema	From fluid overload
Convulsions	Several possible causes: hypernatraemia, hypoglycaemia, febrile convulsions, other electrolyte disturbance and cerebral haemorrhage
	Check blood glucose, U&Es, Mg, Ca and cranial USS and treat accordingly
Prolonged diarrhoea	Diarrhoea > 14 days (see p. 155)

DIARRHOEA

The pathogenesis of most episodes of diarrhoea can be explained by osmotic, secretory or motility disorders or a combination of these. In **osmotic diarrhoea** the underlying mechanism is a high osmotic load of *intra-luminal* content, and in **secretory diarrhoea** the mechanism is active chloride secretion.

Osmotic diarrhoea	Secretory diarrhoea
Common	Rare
Stops when feeding discontinued	Does not stop when feeding discontinued
Reducing substances in stool	Very watery, severe diarrhoea
Stool electrolytes ↓ (Na < 50 mEq/L)	Stool electrolytes ↑ (Na > 90 mEq/L)
Examples	*Examples*
Lactase deficiency	Cholera, toxigenic *E. coli*
Disaccharidase enzyme deficiencies	Congenital chloride diarrhoea
Drugs, e.g. lactulose	Neural crest tumours, e.g. carcinoid, VIP
Maldigestion, e.g. Crohn, CF	Bile salt/fatty acid malabsorption
Transport mechanism disorder, e.g. glucose galactose malabsorption	

Motility disorders

Increased motility	A decreased transit time results in diarrhoea
	Causes include IBS, post-vagotomy and dumping syndrome
Decreased motility	Bacterial overgrowth results in diarrhoea
	Causes include intestinal pseudo-obstruction

Combined mechanisms

This occurs with **mucosal invasion**, resulting in inflammation, decreased colonic reabsorption and increased motility. This is seen in dysentery from bacterial infection, e.g. salmonella, and amoebic infection.

A *decreased* surface area results in both osmotic and motility disorders, as seen in short bowel syndrome.

Causes

Chronic	Acute
Toddler's diarrhoea	Gastroenteritis
Overflow constipation	Systemic infection
Anxiety	Toxic ingestion
Irritable bowel syndrome	
Post-infectious	
Chronic infection, e.g. giardia, cryptosporidium	
Coeliac disease	
Food intolerance	
Pancreatic dysfunction	
Inflammatory bowel disease	
Hirschsprung disease	
Immunodeficiency	
Inborn error of metabolism, e.g. congenital chloride diarrhoea	
Carbohydrate malabsorption, e.g. sucrase isomaltase deficiency	
Congenital lactase deficiency	
Protein-losing enteropathy, e.g. intestinal lymphangiectasia	
Hyperthyroidism	

TODDLER'S DIARRHOEA

A chronic diarrhoea up to 4–5 years of age, with loose stools at a frequency of 3–6 per day, normal growth and nothing abnormal on examination. The cause is not clearly understood and may be due to decreased gut transit time leading to colonic bacterial degradation of partially digested foods and subsequent release of secretagogues.

Management is with reassurance and dietary changes ($\uparrow$ fat, $\downarrow$ fibre, $\downarrow$ juice) to increase gut transit time. The condition usually resolves spontaneously by 3 years.

CHRONIC DIARRHOEA

Prolonged diarrhoea may be due to any of the above causes and the child will quickly become malnourished.

Investigations

Stool	M, C & S, reducing substances, fats and electrolytes
	Faecal elastase (pancreatic insufficiency)
Bloods	FBC (immunodeficiency), electrolytes, ESR, CRP
	Coeliac screen (anti-endomysial IgA, tissue transglutaminase and total IgA)
AXR and CXR	(Obstruction, bronchiectasis)
Sweat test	(Cystic fibrosis)
Trial off oral feeds	(Secretory or osmotic diarrhoea)
Endoscopy	With small biopsy and duodenal juice culture (enteropathy, infection)

Management

Nutritional support while the diagnosis is being arrived at. A hypoallergenic modular feed with supplementation, e.g. Neocate, can be tried first. If enteral feeds fail, then a period of TPN will be necessary.

A trial of metronidazole for 5–7 days may be considered (as giardia is only detected in stool specimens in 20% of cases).

CHRONIC ABDOMINAL PAIN

CAUSES

Psychiatric	Psychogenic recurrent abdominal pain
Abdominal	Constipation, food intolerance (including lactose intolerance), IBD, coeliac disease, Meckel diverticulum, abdominal TB, peptic ulcer, irritable bowel syndrome
Pancreas/liver	Chronic pancreatitis, cystic fibrosis, cholecystitis, chronic hepatitis
Renal	UTI, pyelonephritis, renal calculi
Metabolic	IDDM, porphyria, lead poisoning
CNS	Migraine
Other	Referred testicular pain, ovarian pain, sickle cell crisis

RECURRENT FUNCTIONAL ABDOMINAL PAIN

This is a very common condition. In order to arrive at this diagnosis, a thorough history and examination must be done. It is defined as > 3 episodes of life-altering pain per week for 3 months (Apley's criteria).

Features

- Pain *para-umbilical* and worse on waking
- *No* signs or symptoms of organic abdominal pathology
- Growth normal and good health otherwise
- Girls > boys
- Most commonly age 6–9 years (school-age symptom)
- High achiever personality (doing well at school, anxious)

Features that suggest an organic cause

Pain:	Localized away from the umbilicus
	Waking child at night
	Radiates to back, legs or shoulders
Bowel habit change	
Rectal bleeding or mucus	
Dysuria	
Child unwell (fever, weight loss, faltering growth)	

Management

Thorough history and examination	Pain: site, nature, timing, recurrence rate
	Aggravating factors (? related to school)
	Vomiting, weight loss, bowel habit, urinary problems, headache
	Ask parent(s) and child what they think the cause is
	Take thorough social history (family life, school life)
Any necessary investigations to exclude organic disease	An MSU should be done to exclude a urinary tract infection
	Other investigations only if indicated, e.g. FBC, ESR, CRP, AXR, endoscopy, etc.
Treatment	Explain that although a psychosomatic cause, the pain is *real*
	Reassure parents, child and teachers that no organic cause was found. This can result in the symptoms improving
	Try to avoid medications as these imply there may be something organic
	Rapid recovery is seen in 50%, slow recovery in 25%, and continuation of symptoms in 25%

NB: Other common recurrent pain syndromes are headache and limb pain.

Organic causes of Recurrent Abdominal Pain

Gastrointestinal	Renal
Food intolerances (certain foods trigger attacks, improve on elimination diet)	UTI, pyelonephritis
	Renal or bladder calculi
Inflammatory bowel disease	Hydronephrosis
Coeliac disease	
Peptic ulcer	
Intermittent obstruction	

Liver and pancreas	Other diseases
Cholecystitis	SLE, JCA
Cystic fibrosis	DM
Chronic pancreatitis	Porphyria
Chronic hepatitis	Lead poisoning

PEPTIC ULCER

Duodenal ulcers are seen in children with gastric ulcers being very rare.

Zollinger–Ellison syndrome – multiple ulcers due to a gastrin-secreting tumour (see p. 259).

Association *Helicobacter pylori* infection accounts for 90% of duodenal ulcers in childhood (can be asymptomatic or cause chronic gastritis or peptic ulceration)

Clinical features

- Intermittent abdominal pain, worse at night
- Nausea, vomiting
- Iron-deficiency anaemia, gastrointestinal bleeding

Investigations

- Endoscopy with biopsies
- CLO test on biopsy specimen to detect *H. pylori*; *H. pylori* makes urease, which changes the colour in the agar

Management

- H$_2$ antagonists or proton pump inhibitor, e.g. omeprazole
- *H. pylori* eradication therapy: omeprazole and a combination of two of amoxycillin, clarythromycin and metronidazole for 1–2 weeks – bismuth and tetracyclines are not used under the age of 12 years

INFLAMMATORY BOWEL DISEASE

CROHN'S DISEASE

A disease of chronic inflammation of the bowel, involving any part from the mouth to the anus, classically the terminal ileum, and the rectum is often spared. Incidence increasing, male = female.

Differential diagnosis

- Gastrointestinal TB
- Infectious enteropathies, esp. *Yersinia ileitis*
- Small bowel lymphoma

Clinical features

Gastrointestinal	Abdominal pain, diarrhoea, anorexia, aphthous ulcers
	Abdominal mass, perianal lesions (tags, abscess, fistulae), stricture and fistulae common
Systemic features	Fever, malaise, weight loss, anaemia, nutritional deficiencies, growth retardation, amenorrhoea (primary or secondary)
Extra-abdominal features	See p. 159

Investigations

Bloods	FBC, iron studies, folate, B12, ESR, CRP, LFTs, serum proteins ($\downarrow$)
	Yersinia serology
Stool microscopy and culture	Enterocolitides (salmonella, shigella, campylobacter, *Entamoeba histolytica*)
Plain AXR	Partial small bowel obstruction, **thumb-printing** colon wall
Barium meal and	**Cobblestone appearance** (linear ulcers), deep fissures
follow-through	Strictures and fistulae common, discontinuous disease with normal 'skip' lesions
Upper endoscopy and	
ileocolonoscopy with biopsies	
Histology of lesions	Non-caseating granulomas, transmural inflammation, patchy involvement

Management options

Polymeric elemental diets	Effective as initial therapy instead of steroids. Give exclusive polymeric enteral nutrition, e.g. Modulin IBD, for 8 weeks orally or via NG tube, as tolerated.
Steroids	Oral or IV. High dose for 3–4 weeks, then alternate days and reduce as able
Aminosalicylates	Sulphasalazine, mesalazine or olsalazine for colon disease
	Delayed-release 5-ASA (Asacol) for terminal small bowel disease
Azathioprine	Often now as first line, previously if steroid dependent or not responding
Metronidazole or ciprofloxacin	If fistulae or perianal disease
Tacrolimus/pabecrolimus paste	For perianal disease
TPN	Rarely necessary temporarily
Surgery	Reserved for special indications as recurrence risk high
	Resection of disease unresponsive to medical therapy (wide resection margin with right sub-total hemicolectomy)
	Abscess, perforation, obstruction, bleeding

ULCERATIVE COLITIS

This is a chronic inflammatory disease of the colon with ulceration, classically involving large bowel from the rectum upwards. Small bowel may be involved. Incidence: male = female.

Differential diagnosis

- Crohn colitis
- Amoebic colitis
- Bacillary dysentery

Clinical features

Gastrointestinal	Diarrhoea with blood and mucus
General	Anaemia (iron loss from bleeding), growth retardation (malabsorption rare)
Extra-abdominal features	See below

Investigations

Blood tests	FBC (Hb ↓, leucocytosis), iron studies, B_{12}, LFTs, ESR, CRP, albumin (↓)
AXR	Decreased haustrations
	Dilated colon, NB: **Toxic megacolon** is colon width > 2.5 vertebrae
Double contrast	Continuous pathology, 'collar button ulcers', 'lead pipe' (smooth) colon,
barium (air) enema	backwash ileitis, double contour
Ileo-colonoscopy with biopsies	
Histology of lesions	Mucosal involvement only, gland destruction, crypt abscesses, decreased goblet cells, pseudo-polyps, friability, ulceration

Management options

Aminosalicylates	Oral, e.g. sulphasalazine, mesalazine, olsalazine. For mild colitis and prevention of relapses
Enemas	Aminosalicylate or steroid for proctitis
Steroids	Oral or intravenous at 1–2 mg/kg/day (maximum dose 40 mg) for cases unresponsive to aminosalicylates
Other drugs	Azathioprine, 6-MP, cyclosporin, tacrolimus, metronidazole may be used in steroid-dependent or uncontrolled disease
TPN	In preparation for surgery
Surgery	Colectomy is performed for fulminant disease unresponsive to medical therapy or pancolitis of > 10 years' duration

Complications

- Toxic megacolon
- Fulminating colitis
- Colon cancer (long term), therefore regular colonoscopy after > 10 years' active disease

Extra-abdominal features of Crohn's disease and ulcerative colitis

There are many extra-abdominal features associated with inflammatory bowel disease. Some are more common in Crohn's disease and others in ulcerative colitis.

Crohn's (most commonly)	Ulcerative colitis (most commonly)	Both equally
Erythema nodosum	Pyoderma gangrenosum	Uveitis
Peripheral arthritis	Ankylosing spondylitis	Conjunctivitis
Aphthous ulcers	Sclerosing cholangitis	Fatty liver
Clubbing	Chronic active hepatitis	Cholangiocarcinoma
Episcleritis	Cirrhosis	
Renal stones (oxalate, uric acid)		
Gallstones		

CONSTIPATION

This is a difficulty, delay or pain in defecation. When prolonged, there is overflow diarrhoea due to liquid faeces escaping around a hard lump of faeces in the rectum (rectal faecolith).

NB: Important differential is Hirschsprung disease.

Causes

Non-organic	Coercive potty training in a defiant toddler, lack of privacy
Organic	*Intake* – low-residue diet, dehydration
	Gut – Hirschsprung disease, stricture
	Metabolic – hypothyroidism, cystic fibrosis, hypercalcaemia
	Neuromuscular – cerebral palsy, spinal cord lesions, myotonic dystrophy, absent abdominal wall muscles
	Drugs – narcotics, antidepressants

Complications

Short-term constipation	This quickly resolves with fluids and stool softeners, usually with no sequelae
Long-term constipation	Acquired megacolon (decreased sensation of a full rectum)
	Anal fissures
	Overflow incontinence
	Behavioural problems (fear of defecation, embarrassment of overflow)

Clinical findings

Hard faeces on abdominal examination.

PR	Not always necessary
	Faecal mass, soiled anal region, sacral tuft (spina bifida occulta)
	Sphincter tone ($\downarrow$ in simple constipation, $\uparrow$ in Hirschsprung disease)
AXR	Loaded with faeces
Gut transit study	

Management

1. Positive reinforcement
2. Increase fluids and fibre intake
3. Oral medications: Softener, e.g. lactulose, paraffin oil (also acts as mild stimulant and prevents water reabsorption by coating colonic pits – no fat-soluble vitamin malabsorption has been seen with this therapy)
   Non-absorbed laxative irrigative, e.g. Movicol – non-absorbed polyethylene glycol solution with added electrolytes. NB: Dispensed in adult and paediatric strengths – adult version is twice as strong
   Stimulant, e.g. Senekot, sodium picosulphate
   Bulking agent, e.g. Fybogel
4. Enema if necessary for disimpaction, e.g. phosphate enema
5. Anal fissure treatment with local topical anaesthetic cream and/or GTN ointment

HIRSCHSPRUNG DISEASE

Incidence: 1:5000. Polygenic inheritance, 3–5% recurrence. RET oncogene.

Associations   Down syndrome
Lawrence–Moon–Beidel syndrome
Waardenburg syndrome

This disease is due to the absence of parasympathetic ganglia in Auerbach's and Meissner's plexi. The unopposed sympathetic activity results in hypertonus of the affected segment of bowel. The disease occurs from the rectum upwards.

There are two types:

Short aganglionic segment   Common, male > female

Long aganglionic segment   Rare, male = female, familial

Presentation

Neonatal (> 80%)   Acute obstruction, Hirschprung colitis

Older child   Chronic constipation, history of delayed passage of meconium (> 48 h), faltering growth

Investigations

AXR	Constipation
Barium enema	Narrow aganglionic segment, dilated proximal segment
Rectal biopsy	Rectal suction biopsy (mucosa + submucosa) or full thickness biopsy – surgical transanal
Anorectal manometry	Failure of internal sphincter pressure to drop with rectal distension
Histology of affected bowel	Acetylcholinesterase staining shows *increased* number of hypertrophied nerve bundles that stain positively for acetylcholinesterase

Management

This is surgical, with an immediate definitive repair or a temporary neonatal colostomy with definitive repair at 3–6 months of age. Definitive repair is with direct resection and anastomosis or an endorectal pull-through.

Ultra-short segment disease can be treated with anal dilatation and partial sphincterotomy.

FAECAL SOILING

Faecal soiling is involuntary soiling. Normal bowel control is achieved by around 2 years (girls are quicker than boys).

Soiling by day: Boys > girl (2:1)
                        1–2% 5–12 year olds

Faecal soiling occurs when there is:

- **Faecal retention with overflow incontinence**. This can happen:
  After an episode of diarrhoea, then anal fissure causing painful defecation and constipation
  Due to psychological stress coinciding with toilet training, resulting in refusal to sit on potty
  Due to other disease, e.g. Hirschsprung disease, hypothyroidism
  If the rectum is chronically obstructed with faeces it may enlarge to form a megarectum. Children with megarectum may not sense faecal matter in the rectum, and have diminished urgency to defecate
- **Neurological damage** with failure to establish bowel control, e.g. cerebral palsy, learning difficulties
- **Stress** – normal bowel control but soiling in response to stress only

NB: Important to exclude Hirschsprung disease, which is present from birth. If this is suspected, then full investigation is necessary (see p. 161).

Encopresis is the voluntary passage of faeces in an otherwise healthy child beyond the usual age for toilet training. It is due to non-organic causes.

Management

- Comprehensive history including gastrointestinal and social
- Abdominal (including rectal) and neurological examination
- Plain AXR: faecal retention
- Empty bowel of impacted faeces: microenemas, manual disempaction
- High fibre diet and stool softeners (for soft painless stools)

For encopresis, psychotherapy (child and family therapy) including a behaviour modification programme (positive reinforcement, defined periods of toilet training, remove fear of the toilet, remove control battle between parents and child).

PANCREATITIS

ACUTE PANCREATITIS

This involves inflammation of the pancreas with autodigestion, localized necrosis and haemorrhage. Complications can be severe.

Causes

- Biliary sludging
- Congenital abnormalities
- Blunt abdominal trauma
- Viral infection – mumps, varicella, measles, EBV, coxsackie virus
- Iatrogenic – total parenteral nutrition, steroids, azathioprine
- Diseases associated – HUS, Kawasaki disease, stem cell transplant, brain tumour, metabolic disease such as isovaleric acidaemia

Clinical features

- Abdominal pain (epigastric, radiating straight through to the back), nausea, vomiting, fever
- Tender abdomen, guarding, absent or obstructed bowel sounds, abdominal mass
- **Acute haemorrhagic pancreatitis**: Very unwell, shocked, jaundiced
  Cullen sign (bluish periumbilical region)
  Grey Turner sign (bluish flanks)
  50% mortality with DIC, renal failure, RDS
  Sepsis, gastrointestinal bleeding

Investigations

Serum amylase	> 500 IU/L seen in first 72 h (and/or ↑ serum lipase)
Other bloods	FBC (leucocytosis), glucose (↑), Ca (↓),
	Clotting screen (prolonged clotting), LFTs (↑)
CXR	*Left* pleural effusion, atelectasis
AXR	Ileus, ascites, pseudocyst, pancreatic calcification (in recurrent disease)
USS and/or CT abdomen	Oedematous pancreas, abscess, pseudocyst

Management

1. **Analgesia**
2. Keep NBM with intravenous fluids and nasogastric suctioning until amylase normal. Treat shock if necessary
3. Fluid and electrolyte balance with careful monitoring
4. Surgical drainage if abscess or pseudocyst
5. Possible place for octreotide

CHRONIC PANCREATITIS

Causes

Hereditary	Autosomal dominant. Progressively more severe attacks
Congenital pancreatic or biliary ductal anomalies	Hyperlipidaemia, cystic fibrosis, Wilson disease
Predisposing disorders	Cystinuria, hyperparathyroidism, cystinosis, isovaleric acidaemia, α_1-antitrypsin disease, ascaris

Complications

Pancreatic pseudocysts, calcifications and pancreatic insufficiency.

Investigations

As for acute pancreatitis.
Also check:

- Sweat test and genotype for hereditary pancreatitis
- Stools for ascaris (rare cause), amino and organic acid screen
- ERCP (necessary prior to any surgery), although MRCP may now be preferable as without a therapeutic intention ERCP has a risk-benefit which may not be preferable (5% risk of inducing acute pancreatitis due to the procedure itself, even without any pre-disposing pathology)

Management

Endoscopic treatment with sphincterotomy, pancreatic or biliary endoprostheses and stone extraction is possible as necessary.

GASTROINTESTINAL TRACT BLEEDING

This has many causes, the frequency of which depends on the age of the child.

Causes

Infant	Child	Adolescent
Swallowed maternal blood	Colonic polyps (painless)	Bacterial infections
Haemorrhagic disease of	Anal fissure	IBD
the newborn	Bacterial infections	Anal fissure
NEC	Intussusception	Colonic polyps
Cow's milk protein allergy	Mallory–Weiss tear	Peptic ulcer/gastritis
Anal fissure	HUS	Mallory–Weiss tear
Intussusception	Henoch–Schönlein purpura	Oesophageal varices
Volvulus	Oesophageal varices	Telangiectasia
Meckel diverticulum	Meckel diverticulum	
	Oesophagitis	
	Peptic ulcer/gastritis	
	IBD	
	AV malformation, haemangioma	
	Telangiectasia	
	Sexual abuse	

Clinical presentations

- Haematemesis – fresh blood or 'coffee grounds' (altered by gastric juices)
- Melaena (altered blood per rectum) – tarry smelly stool
- Fresh rectal bleeding
- Massive bleeding with collapse
- Small bleeds with iron-deficiency anaemia

Investigations and management

1. Assess circulation and resuscitate if necessary
2. Bloods – FBC, clotting studies, iron studies
3. Faecal occult bloods
4. Endoscopy – this is the emergency management also. Oesophageal banding for varices. (Sclerotherapy is outdated, and insertion of a Sengstaken–Blakemore tube only in extremis.) Wireless capsule endoscopy is now considered a viable diagnostic alternative in the context of occult or obscure GI bleeding thought to be emanating from the small bowel
5. Laparotomy and/or mesenteric angiography if necessary

Swallowed maternal blood

This is a common event with small babies. Maternal blood is identified with the **APT test**:

Bloody vomit or stool is mixed with water, centrifuged and the supernatant mixed with 1% sodium hydroxide:
If it remains pink = infant blood
If it turns brown = maternal blood

GASTROINTESTINAL TRACT TUMOURS

JUVENILE COLONIC POLYPS

These occur in 3–4% of the population in the colon only. Symptoms usually occur between 2 and 10 years. Uncommon > 15 years. They are usually benign hamartomas (unless they have an adenomatous element).

Presentation

Bright red rectal bleeding, autolysis, prolapse of a polyp, anaemia, abdominal pain (unusual).

Diagnosis

Rectal examination, colonoscopy with polyp removal, barium enema.

FAMILIAL POLYPOSIS SYNDROMES

Familial adenomatous polyposis coli (FAP)

Autosomal dominant, incidence 1:8000, pre-malignant condition. The APC (adenomatous polyposis coli) gene has been identified on the long arm of chromosome 5; many different mutations may occur within this gene, resulting in FAP.

Multiple adenomas on the distal bowel (100–1000), onset < 10 years. Annual colonoscopy needed after age 10 and pan-colectomy after 10 years of disease (usually late teens or early 20s).

Congenital hypertrophy of the retinal pigment epithelium (CHRPE)

Seen in association with APC gene mutations (55–75%). When present, CHRPE lesions are an early clinical marker for familial polyposis coli and may be used in risk assessment.

Turcot syndrome

- APC gene defects
- Primary medulloblastoma
- Multiple colorectal polyposis

Gardner syndrome

- APC gene defect
- Multiple colorectal polyps
- Soft tissue and bone tumours (especially the mandible)
- Extracolonic cancers

Peutz–Jegher syndrome

Autosomal dominant, 50% new mutations.

Syndrome of:

- Mucosal pigmentation (freckles) of lips and gums
- Stomach and small bowel hamartomas
- Malignant tumours (*not* of the GI tract) develop in 50% of patients

ENDOCRINE TUMOURS

APUDomas	These hormone-secreting tumours arise from APUD cells (neural crest cell derivatives of the gastroenteropancreatic endocrine system). They are: • Carcinoid • VIPomas, gastrinoma (see p. 259), somatostatinoma • Mastocytoma (see p. 299) • Medullary carcinoma thyroid
Neurogenic tumours	Ganglioneuroma Phaeochromocytoma (see p. 242)

NB: **APUD** = **a**mine **p**recursor **u**ptake and **d**ecarboxylation

Carcinoid tumours

These tumours of the intestine usually arise in the appendix in children. They are benign or low-grade malignancy and when symptomatic present as appendicitis. Tumours elsewhere in the GI tract are likely to metastasize. They produce the **carcinoid syndrome**, the result of serotonin (5-HT) and other hormone production, when *metastatic*.

Carcinoid syndrome

Clinical features

- All have liver metastases
- Intestinal hypermobility, with watery diarrhoea and abdominal pain
- Bluish-red facial flushing with telangiectasia
- Bronchoconstriction
- Tricuspid incompetence or pulmonary stenosis

Diagnosis

- Urine 5HIAA ↑ (serotonin metabolite)
- Plasma serotonin ↑
- Bradykinin, histamine, tachykinins and/or prostaglandins ↑

Management

- Resection of primary tumour if possible
- Octreotride (somatostatin analogue) inhibits release of gut hormones

FALTERING GROWTH

This is the failure to gain adequate weight or achieve adequate growth during infancy at a normal rate for age. At least two growth measurements needed 3–6 months apart, showing the child falls across two major centiles.

CAUSES

Organic	Non-organic
Inadequate calorie intake	**Undernutrition**
Breast feeding poorly	Parental ignorance
Bottle feeds too dilute	Poverty
Exclusion diets	Poor feeding practice
Cleft palate	
Vomiting/reflux	**Child abuse**
	Psychosocial deprivation
Inadequate calorie absorption	
	Deliberate starvation, laxative administration
Enteropathy, e.g. coeliac, giardia	Parental psychiatric illness
Food intolerance, e.g. cow's milk protein intolerance	
Short gut syndrome	
Pancreatic disease	
Excessive calorie loss	
Vomiting, e.g. gastro-oesophageal reflux, pyloric stenosis	
Protein-losing enteropathy	
Excessive calorie requirements	
Chronic illness, e.g. cardiac, renal, respiratory, GIT	
Thyrotoxicosis	
Malignancy	
Abnormal movement disorder	
Failure of utilization of absorbed calories	
Chromosomal abnormalities, e.g. Down syndrome	
Prenatal growth failure	
Diencephalic syndrome	
Metabolic abnormalities, e.g. hypothyroidism, glycogen storage disease	

MEDICAL MANAGEMENT

History

Include:

- Heights of parents and siblings
- Family history, e.g. atopy
- Pregnancy history, e.g. smoking
- Birth history, e.g. gestation and birthweight
- Dietary assessment
- Social report

Examination

Weight, height ± head circumference, general examination and developmental assessment.

Investigations

The sequence and extent of these is dictated by the clinical history and examination.

NUTRITIONAL DISORDERS

MALNUTRITION

Malnutrition is categorized based on **wasting** (weight for height ratios), indicating short-term effects, and **stunting** (height for age and sex ratios), indicating long-term effects, using standard scores. Traditionally it has been classified into marasmus, kwashiorkor and marasmic kwashiorkor.

Marasmus

This is a mixed deficiency of both protein and calories, resulting in non-oedematous malnutrition. Decreased weight for age and sex ratios (<60% of the mean average).

Features

- Hungry, emaciated child
- Loose, wrinkled skin, 'old man' appearance, decreased skin turgor
- Muscle atrophy and little subcutaneous fat
- Thin sparse hair, hair colour changes unusual
- Hypothermia, bradycardia, hypotension (basal metabolic rate ↓)
- Listlessness

Kwashiorkor

This malnutrition results in oedema which is due to unknown causes, though it has historically been attributed to a disproportionately low protein intake compared with calorie intake. There is a near normal weight for age ratio (weight for age and sex ratio < 80%) and oedema.

Features

- Lethargy, miserable, no appetite
- Oedema – hypoalbuminaemic, overall 'fatness' appearance, moon face
- Hepatomegaly (fatty infiltration)
- Skin lesions (flaking paint rash, ulcers, fissures, pellagra-type rash)
- Thin, red hair and darkened skin
- Cardiomegaly
- Infections, secondary immunodeficiency

Marasmic kwashiorkor (mixed type)

A combined type exists where there are features of both marasmus and kwashiorkor, with a weight for age and sex ratio of < 60% with oedema.

Management of malnutrition

1. Initial rehydration with oral rehydration salts solution (or IV if in shock)
2. Dilute milk for 5 days, increasing volume gradually to 150 ml/kg/day. Look for and treat hypoglycaemia, hypothermia, infection, electrolyte imbalance and micronutrient deficiency
3. High-energy feeds as strength builds up. NB: If feeds are too strong too early, hepatomegaly and a slower recovery result

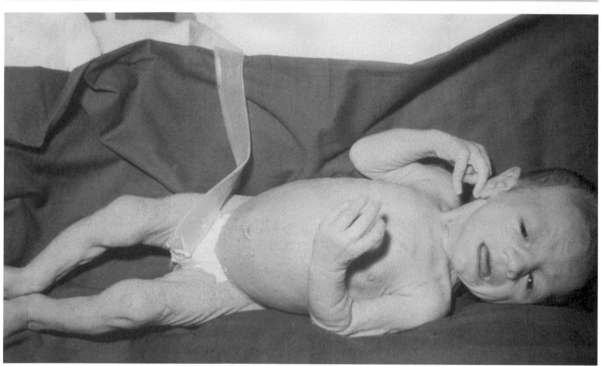

Figure 7.4 Child with severe malnutrition showing a lack of subcutaneous fat stores and muscle wasting

ACRODERMATITIS ENTEROPATHICA (ZINC DEFICIENCY)

This is a disorder of zinc deficiency of various causes.

Causes

Inherited form	Autosomal recessive, rare.
	Due to defective intestinal absorption of zinc
Acquired transient neonatal form	Due to nutritional zinc deficiency from:

- Breast-fed infants in mothers with low zinc levels
- Premature infants with prolonged TPN
- Infants with malabsorption (including cystic fibrosis)

Clinical features

Skin	Persistent *well demarcated* eczematous or psoriaform rash
	Symmetrical distribution
	Perioral, perineum, flexures, eyes, cheeks and nose
	Dystrophic nails, glossitis and stomatitis
Hair	Red with areas of alopecia
Eyes	Photophobia, conjunctivitis, blepharitis, corneal dystrophy
Growth	Faltering growth
Others	Irritability, delayed wound healing, chronic diarrhoea, recurrent bacterial and candida infections

The inherited form develops when weaned from the breast (as breast milk contains a zinc-binding protein and therefore helps zinc absorption) or earlier if bottle fed.

169

Diagnosis

- Low plasma zinc level (< 50 μg/ml)
- Alkaline phosphatase also low (a zinc-dependent enzyme)

Management

Oral zinc supplementation with monitoring of plasma levels.

SCURVY (VITAMIN C [ASCORBIC ACID] DEFICIENCY)

Ascorbic acid is a reducing agent involved in collagen synthesis. It is found in fruit and vegetables, oxidized by heat and leaks into water.

Deficiency features

- Perifollicular haemorrhages, follicular hyperkeratosis and 'corkscrew' hair on back, arms and legs
- Spontaneous bruising and bleeding with subperiosteal haemorrhages of long bones
- Swollen, spongy gums
- Delayed wound healing
- Irritability
- Muscle pain and weakness, pseudoparalysis of the legs
- Anaemia

Diagnosis is made by checking plasma ascorbic acid levels or giving a trial of vitamin C. Management is with oral vitamin C 1 g/day.

PELLAGRA (NIACIN DEFICIENCY)

A lack of niacin (nicotinamide) results in this condition. Niacin forms part of the enzymes NAD (nicotinamide adenine dinucleotidase) and NADP (nicotinamide adenine dinucleotide phosphatase). It is found in fish and meat and in small amount in cereals. Niacin can be made from tryptophan (found in milk and eggs).

Features of deficiency

Dermatitis   Erythema on sun-exposed areas ('Casals' necklace' on the neck), hyperkeratosis, ulcers, progressing to atrophy. Red tongue and angular stomatitis
Dementia   Tremor, depression, encephalopathy, psychosis
Diarrhoea   Also constipation

Management is with oral nicotinamide or vitamin B complex therapy.

Other causes include:

- Isoniazid (causes B_6 deficiency, needed for nicotinamide manufacture)
- Generalized malabsorption, low-protein diets
- Hartnup disease (tryptophan not absorbed)
- Phaeochromocytoma, carcinoid (metabolism of niacin altered)

VITAMIN A DEFICIENCY

Vitamin A (retinol) is found in milk, eggs, liver and green vegetables. Deficiency occurs with dietary deficiency (rare), fat malabsorption, liver disease.

Clinical features

Eyes	Night blindness, xerophthalmia, photophobia, keratomalacia and blindness
Developmental delay	
Growth retardation	
Skin	Follicular hyperkeratosis, dry and scaly

Diagnosis can be confirmed with low vitamin A levels. Management is with oral vitamin A.

BERIBERI (THIAMINE DEFICIENCY)

Thiamine (vitamin B$_1$) is a cofactor for many enzyme reactions. It is found in most foods, especially legumes. Deficiency occurs with dietary deficiency, e.g. polished rice-only diet, alcoholics, and babies breast fed by a deficient mother. Clinical features involve cardiac and neurological problems.

Cardiac features	Dilated heart with cardiac failure and oedema
(wet beriberi)	Tachycardia, tachypnoea, hepatomegaly, QT prolongation
Neurological features	Slow onset
(dry beriberi)	Symmetrical polyneuropathy, commencing with lower limbs (absent lower limb tendon reflexes, paraesthesias, loss of vibration sense)
	CNS involvement (Wernicke–Korsakoff syndrome):

- Occular Nystagmus, papilloedema, lateral rectus palsies
  Conjugate gaze palsies, fixed pupils, ptosis, optic atrophy
- Ataxia Cerebellar signs
- Confusion Irritability, amnesia, apathy and coma

Diagnosis is based on a rapid clinical response to therapy. Management is with IV or IM thiamine if in cardiac failure. Otherwise, oral thiamine is given to the mother and child.

EATING DISORDERS

ANOREXIA NERVOSA

This is predominantly a disorder of Western adolescent girls. Girls > boys, 10:1. Complex family dynamics involved.

Diagnostic criteria

- Fear of becoming obese
- Disturbance of perception of body size, shape and weight
- Refusal to maintain body weight over the age/height minimum (via calorie restriction, obsessive exercise, vomiting, laxatives)
- Amenorrhoea

The typical **psychological profile** includes: overachiever, poor self-esteem, strong-willed, distrustful, uncommunicative, depression, irritability, obsessional (obsessive thoughts of food and body shape in particular) and distorted body image. Family dysfunction with overprotection, conflict avoidance and control battles over food.

Physical features

Bodyweight	Below expected for age/height
Skin	Dry skin, rashes, fine lanugo hair on body and face
Cardiac	Bradycardia, BP ↓ with pronounced postural drop, long QT interval, arrhythmias (may cause sudden death)
Hormones	GH ↑, T3 ↓, rT3 ↑, hypothalamic–pituitary–ovarian disorders (amenorrhoea, LH and FSH ↓) Loss of diurnal variation in cortisol
Electrolyte	Disturbances, e.g. K ↓ and hypochloraemic alkalosis due to vomiting
Other	Hypothermia, constipation, cool peripheries, slowly relaxing reflexes

Management

A combination of expert psychotherapy and nutritional rehabilitation (at home or in hospital) is necessary.

The prognosis is best if treated early, otherwise long-term eating problems are common with a mortality of up to 10% in adulthood.

BULIMIA

This is also predominantly a disorder of adolescent girls, and is more common than anorexia nervosa.

Clinical features

- Episodic high-calorie binge eating
- Followed by self-induced vomiting, laxative abuse and/or episodes of fasting
- Weight is usually normal or mildly overweight
- Teeth enamel erosion, salivary gland enlargement and cheilosis (from recurrent vomiting)
- Electrolyte and cardiac abnormalities as in anorexia nervosa may occur

The diagnosis is made from the history.

Management is with specialist psychotherapy.

OBESITY

Obesity is defined as a body mass index (BMI) > 85th percentile. BMI > 35 = morbid obesity. The International Obesity Task Force (IOTF) has developed specific BMI centile charts.

This is a problem of increasing incidence in the UK.

Causes

Intake and exercise balance	A combination of excessive and poor quality nutrition and inadequate exercise Overfeeding in infants may be secondary to maternal anxiety or postnatal depression Bottle-fed infants more likely to become obese
Other causes	Cushing syndrome Prader–Willi syndrome, Laurence–Moon–Beidel syndrome

Associated problems

- Advanced bone age, increased height (early), early puberty
- Psychological effects (poor self-image, depression)
- Sleep apnoea (severe obesity)
- Obesity throughout life increased
- Long-term effects: hypertension, diabetes, cardiovascular disease

Management of nutritional obesity needs to involve addressing family eating and exercise habits.

FURTHER READING

Walker WA, Hamilton JR, Watkins JB, Durie PR, eds *Pediatric Gastrointestinal Disease*, 3rd edn. Philadelphia: Mosby, 2000

8

Liver disorders

- *Physiology and anatomy*
- *Clinical manifestations in liver disease*
- *Jaundice (icterus)*
- *Metabolic disorders*
- *Congenital hepatic fibrosis*

- *Hepatitis*
- *Portal hypertension*
- *Gallbladder disease*
- *Liver transplantation*

PHYSIOLOGY AND ANATOMY

FUNCTIONS

Protein

Metabolism	Principal site of synthesis of all circulating proteins (except γ globulins), e.g. albumin, coagulation factors (except factor VIII), complement system components, carrier proteins (transferrin, caeruloplasmin), α-fetoprotein, and α_1-antitrypsin. Factors II, VII, IX and X are vitamin K dependent
Degradation	Amino acids are deaminated. Amino acids and ammonia are converted to urea

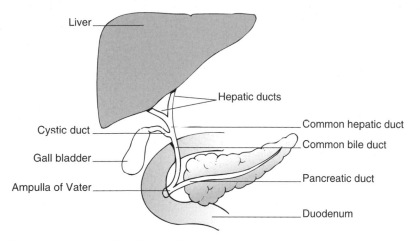

Figure 8.1 Anatomy of the liver and ducts

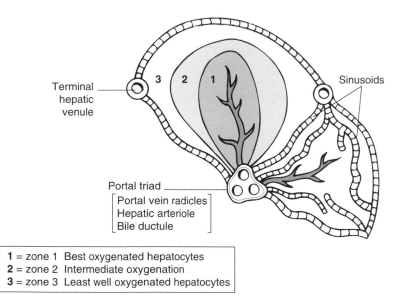

Figure 8.2 A functional liver acinus

Carbohydrate metabolism

Post-prandially, glucose is converted to glycogen and stored, and to fatty acids and transported to adipose tissue. In starvation, glucose is released from glycogen (**glycogenolysis**) and is synthesized from amino acids, lactate and glycerol (**gluconeogenesis**). Preterm infants have inefficient regulation of this.

Lipid metabolism

Synthesis of lipoproteins VLDL and HDL, fatty acid oxidation and cholesterol excretion. Young infants have reduced capacity for hepatic ketogenesis.

Bile

Bile acids	Synthesis from cholesterol
Bilirubin metabolism	See Figure 8.3
Bile secretion	Containing bile acids, water, bilirubin, electrolytes, cholesterol and phospholipids. Neonates have inefficient ileal reabsorption and hepatic clearance of bile acids from portal blood and therefore raised serum levels of bile acids

Hormone and drug metabolism

Many hormones are inactivated in the liver or targeted to the liver. Drugs metabolized by enzymes including the P450 system, e.g. alcohol. Newborns have decreased capacity to metabolize certain drugs.

Immunological function

Involving the reticuloendothelial system of the liver. Kupffer cell (macrophages on endothelium) functions include:

- Phagocytosis
- Secretion of interleukins, TNF, collagenase and lysosomal hydrolases

INVESTIGATIVE LIVER BLOOD TESTS

Laboratory tests examine the **function** of the liver and also markers of **liver cell damage**. As the liver has a very large functional reserve, functional tests alter later in disease.

Albumin	Synthetic function marker
Prothrombin time (PT)	Synthetic function marker. Very sensitive (as short half-life) NB: Must exclude vitamin K deficiency as cause of prolonged PT
Bilirubin	Raised bilirubin level may be: Conjugated = 'direct' reading, or Unconjugated = 'indirect' reading
Aminotransferases (transaminases)	Enzymes in hepatocytes which leak into blood with liver cell damage (also raised in increased red cell degradation) Sensitive markers: 1. Aspartate aminotransferase (AST) – mitochondrial enzyme, also in heart, muscle, kidney, brain 2. Alanine aminotransferase (ALT) – cytosol enzyme, more specific to liver than AST
Alkaline phosphatase (AlkPh)	In canalicular and sinusoidal membranes. Also in bone, intestine and placenta. Isoenzymes used to determine specific origin. Raised in cholestasis, cirrhosis and liver metastases
γ-Glutamyl transpeptidase (γGT)	Microsomal enzyme which increases in cholestasis and is induced by some drugs, e.g. phenytoin, alcohol
Serum proteins	**Albumin** (hypoalbuminaemia as above) **Globulins** (hyperglobulinaemia due to decreased phagocytosis of antigens by Kupffer cells) **Immunoglobulins** (raised in chronic disease)
α-Fetoprotein	Normally produced by the fetal liver. Seen in teratomas, hepatocellular carcinoma, hepatitis, chronic liver disease and in pregnancy with fetal neural tube defects

Immunological tests

- Antimitochondrial antibody (AMA) in primary biliary cirrhosis and autoimmune hepatitis
- Antinuclear (ANA), anti-smooth muscle (ASM) and liver/kidney microsomal (LKMA) antibodies seen in auto-immune hepatitis

Other biochemical alterations – hypoglycaemia, electrolyte imbalance, hyperammonaemia.

CLINICAL MANIFESTATIONS IN LIVER DISEASE

Liver disease may be acute or chronic and may manifest with the following.

ACUTE LIVER DISEASE

- Asymptomatic
- General malaise (fever, anorexia)
- Hypoglycaemia
- Hepatomegaly
- Jaundice
- Pruritis
- Spider naevi and liver palms (rare in acute)
- Encephalopathy, bleeding disorders and renal impairment may occur

CHRONIC LIVER DISEASE

Asymptomatic	
Anorexia	
Liver size	Increased (hepatomegaly), decreased or no change
Jaundice	
Pruritis	Seen in cholestasis, due to conjugated hyperbilirubinaemia
Other skin changes	Palmar erythema, spider naevi (telangiectasia in the distribution of the superior vena cava, < 5 may still be normal), xanthomata, purpura, clubbing
Portal hypertension	An increase in portal venous pressure to > 10–12 mmHg. Caput medusae, varices, splenomegaly
Ascites	Due to hydrostatic pressure from sinusoidal blockade and hypoalbuminaemia
Encephalopathy	Portosystemic encephalopathy (PSE) (a chronic syndrome involving neuropsychiatric disturbance), drowsiness, fetor hepaticus and liver flap. Due to metabolic abnormalities
Endocrine abnormalities	Testicular atrophy, gynaecomastia, parotid enlargement
Renal abnormalities	Secondary impairment of renal function. Hepatorenal syndrome (renal failure of no other demonstrable cause in a patient with cirrhosis)
Gastrointestinal bleeding	Due to coagulation dysfunction and portal hypertension

FULMINANT HEPATIC FAILURE (FHF)

This is an acute clinical syndrome resulting from massive impairment or necrosis of hepatocytes in a patient without pre-existing chronic liver disease. The prognosis is poor with a mortality without transplant of around 70%.

Causes

- Hypoxic liver damage
- Viral hepatitis – combined B and D especially
- Drugs, e.g. paracetamol, sodium valproate
- Metabolic disorders, e.g. Wilson disease, galactosaemia, neonatal haemochromatosis, mitochondrial cytopathy, tyrosinaemia

Clinical manifestations

- Progressive jaundice, fetor hepaticus, fever, vomiting, abdominal pain
- Rapid decrease in liver size with no clinical improvement (ominous sign)
- Defective coagulation
- Hypoglycaemia

- Sepsis
- Fluid overload
- Occult gastrointestinal or intracranial bleeding
- Pancreatitis
- Hepatic encephalopathy with cerebral oedema (lethargy, sleep rhythm disturbance, confusion, progressing to coma)

Poor prognostic features

- Onset of liver failure < 7 days
- $\leq$ 10 years
- Shrinking liver size
- Renal failure
- Paracetamol overdose
- Hypersensitivity reactions of unknown aetiology

Investigations

- PT $\uparrow$
- Transaminases (raised initially, then may decrease with no clinical improvement, indicating little or no functioning liver remaining)
- Ammonia $\uparrow$
- Glucose $\downarrow$
- Hyperbilirubinaemia (conjugated and unconjugated)
- Metabolic acidosis, K $\downarrow$, Na $\downarrow$
- EEG (monitor of cerebral activity, occult seizures may be present)

Management

The aims of management include close monitoring to prevent complications, maintenance of blood glucose > 4 mmol/L, support of the cardiovascular, renal and respiratory systems and close monitoring of CNS function. Liver transplant should be considered early if recovery is considered unlikely.

Specific management includes the following:

- Fluid restriction to 50–75% maintenance (to avoid ICP $\uparrow$)
- Use colloid to maintain intravascular volume
- Sodium and potassium additives depending on electrolytes
- Maintain blood glucose with IV hypertonic glucose as needed
- Monitor with CVP, MAP, urine output, ICP, blood gases, serum electrolyte and glucose status

Cerebral complications	Avoid sedation as this masks encephalopathy
	Monitor for $\uparrow$ ICP and maintain normal ICP with mannitol, hyperventilation, thiopentone and haemofiltration as necessary
	Convulsions may be occult and EEG or cerebral function monitoring should be performed if concern exists. Any convulsions are treated, e.g. phenytoin IV, paraldehyde in oil PR, phenobarbitone IV or thiopentone IV may be required
Renal	Nephrotoxic drugs and arterial hypotension should be avoided. Hepatorenal syndrome may occur
	Established renal failure treated with haemofiltration
Sepsis	Daily culturing for infection and empirical use of broad-spectrum antibiotics with antifungals. Aciclovir if herpetic origin suspected
Bleeding	Vitamin K IV given daily. Avoid invasive procedures if possible
Respiratory	ARDS equivalent may occur

Cardiovascular	Inotropic support as required. Prostacyclin or N-acetyl cysteine may improve microcirculation	
Gastrointestinal	Prophylaxis for stress ulceration with IV ranitidine or omeprazole. GI haemorrhage managed with blood products and emergency endoscopy as necessary	

CIRRHOSIS

This is a histological diagnosis identified by **fibrosis and nodule formation** with **abnormal liver architecture** and results from necrosis of liver cells. It may be macronodular (nodules up to 5 cm), micronodular (nodules < 3 mm) or mixed. Progressive scarring in cirrhosis leads to restricted blood flow with further impairment of liver function and portal hypertension.

Causes

- Acute viral hepatitis
- Metabolic liver disease, e.g. Wilson disease, tyrosinaemia
- Veno-occlusive disease (especially post stem cell transplant)
- Autoimmune CAH, primary biliary cirrhosis
- Idiopathic

The prognosis is variable and the 5-year survival rate is around 50%, depending on the aetiology.

CAUSES OF HEPATOMEGALY

Inflammation	*Hepatitis*	Viral, bacterial, toxic
	Autoimmune	Chronic hepatitis, SLE, sarcoidosis, sclerosing cholangitis
Tumour	*Primary neoplasm*	Hepatoblastoma, hepatocellular carcinoma, haemangioma
	Secondary deposits	Leukaemia, lymphoma, neuroblastoma, histiocytosis
Posthepatic portal hypertension	Hepatic vein obstruction Cardiac failure, pericardial tamponade (constrictive pericarditis, e.g. TB)	
Biliary obstruction	Extrahepatic obstruction	
Haematological	Sickle cell disease, thalassaemia, spherocytosis	
Metabolic disease	*Fatty liver*	Reye syndrome, TPN, CF, IDDM
	Lipid storage disease	Gaucher, Neimann Pick, Wolman syndrome
	Glycogen storage disease	GSD 1, GSD 3, GSD 6
	Other	Wilson disease, haemochromatosis, α_1-antitrypsin disease
Cysts	Polycystic kidney disease, hydatid infection	
Apparent	Chest hyper-expansion due to lung disease, Reidel lobe	

JAUNDICE (ICTERUS)

Serum bilirubin > 35 µmol/L is clinically detectable. Jaundice is traditionally classified as pre-hepatic, hepatocellular and obstructive (cholestatic) but this is inaccurate, as cholestasis occurs in hepatocellular as well as obstructive jaundice. It may help to consider jaundice as:

1. Haemolytic (prehepatic)
2. Congenital hyperbilirubinaemias (hepatocellular)
3. Cholestatic: Intrahepatic (hepatocellular and/or obstructive)
                 Extrahepatic (obstructive)

BILIRUBIN METABOLISM

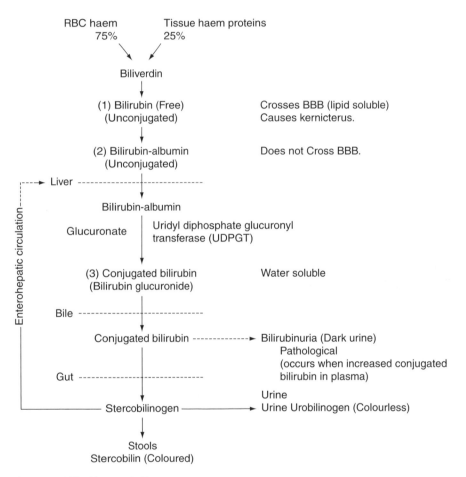

Figure 8.3 Bilirubin metabolism

HAEMOLYTIC JAUNDICE

- Unconjugated bilirubin ↑ (not water soluble, therefore not in urine) = acholuric jaundice, i.e. *no* bilirubinuria. Therefore, urine and stools *normal* colour
- Urine urobilinogen ↑

- Transaminases
- Alkaline phosphatase } Normal
- Albumin

Haemolytic features:

- Plasma haptoglobins ↓
- Lactate dehydrogenase (LDH) ↑
- Reticulocytes ↑
- Bone marrow erythroid hyperplasia
- Spherocytes, red cell fragments, sickle cells may be present

In intravascular haemolysis:

- Haemosiderinuria, haemoglobinuria
- Methaemalbumin
- FDPs ↑, haptoglobins ↓

CHOLESTATIC JAUNDICE

- Conjugated bilirubin ↑ (> 20% total bilirubin)
- Pale stools
- Dark urine (bilirubinuria)

Altered synthetic function and transaminases may sometimes accompany the picture as outlined below.

Intrahepatic may be due to:

- Parenchymal disease (hepatocellular)
- Bile canalicular excretion problem

Additional features

	Intrahepatic	Extrahepatic (large duct obstruction)
AST, ALT	↑↑	(↑)
Alkaline phosphatase	(↑)	↑↑
PT	↑	↑
Albumin	↓	↓
γGT	↑	↑

NEONATAL JAUNDICE

Most neonates develop some jaundice in the first few weeks of life because they have a:

- Relative polycythaemia
- Shortened red cell lifespan (70 days as compared to 120 days in adults)
- Relative immaturity of the liver

Most neonatal jaundice is due to **unconjugated bilirubin** and is **physiological**. Conditions involving haemolysis, e.g. Rhesus disease, excessive neonatal bruising, result in more pronounced jaundice, sometimes severe. Premature infants, sick neonates and those with low albumin levels are at increased risk.

When levels of unconjugated bilirubin are high they exceed the albumin binding capacity of the blood and exist as **free unconjugated bilirubin.** This is harmful to the baby. It is lipid soluble, and therefore can cross the blood–brain barrier where it causes neurotoxicity (known as **kernicterus**):

Immediate effects	Lethargy, irritability, increased tone, opisthotonus
Long-term effects	Sensorineural deafness, learning difficulties and choreoathetoid cerebral palsy

Conjugated hyperbilirubinaemia is *always pathological*, and has many rare causes (see p. 187). Conjugated bilirubin is not toxic to the brain

Causes of unconjugated (UC) neonatal jaundice	
Physiological	
Breast milk jaundice	
Excessive neonatal bruising, e.g. after ventouse delivery	
Haemolytic disease	Blood group incompatibility (Rhesus or ABO) Red cell shape abnormality, e.g. spherocytosis, elliptocytosis Red cell membrane instability, e.g. G6PD deficiency, PK deficiency
Sepsis (UC and C)	
Hypothyroidism (UC and C)	
Congenital hyperbilirubinaemias (UC and C), e.g. Gilbert disease, Crigler Najar types I and II	
Metabolic disease (UC and C), e.g. galactosaemia, fructosaemia	

Causes of neonatal jaundice related to time		
< 24 h of birth	**24 hours–2 weeks**	**> 2 weeks**
Haemolytic disease	Physiological jaundice	Breast milk jaundice
Congenital infection	Prematurity Severe bruising Sepsis Breast milk jaundice Hypothyroidism Haemolytic disease Galactosaemia	Sepsis Haemolysis Neonatal hepatitis Biliary atresia

Management

1 Baseline investigations to assess the severity, type and possible cause of jaundice:
   SBR
   Blood group, Coombs' test and FBC
   Bilirubin conjugated and unconjugated fractions (conjugated is < 20% of total in unconjugated hyperbilirubinaemia, and > 20% in conjugated hyperbilirubinaemia)
   Urine (microscopy, culture and sensitivities)
2. If the serum bilirubin (SBR) exceeds a certain level, treatment is commenced with phototherapy (or exchange transfusion if very rapidly increasing levels). Charts which act as guidelines for the level of bilirubin to commence phototherapy or exchange transfusion have been developed, and vary for different gestations, weights and for ill and sick babies

Phototherapy

Phototherapy does not remove the bilirubin, but works by UV radiation converting the harmful unconjugated bilirubin into water-soluble bilirubin, which can be excreted by the body.

- Whole baby under phototherapy lamp 24 h/day
- Undressed to increase skin exposed to UV
- Eyes are covered to prevent damage (cataracts)
- Extra fluid (30 ml/kg/day) given to prevent dehydration
- Side-effects – loose stools, overheating, dehydration, 'bronze baby syndrome'

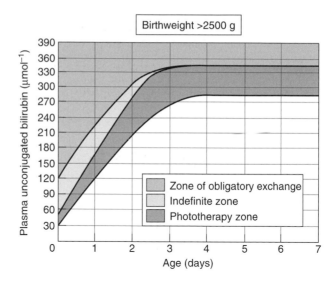

Figure 8.4 Phototherapy treatment chart

Exchange transfusion

Repeated small aliquots of the infant's blood are removed via peripheral arterial line, or umbilical artery or vein, and replaced with O Rh negative blood (or infant's ABO type if mother same group) which will not haemolyse.

Complications   Acidosis, hypoxia, apnoeas and bradycardias, thrombocytopenia and NEC.

Physiological jaundice

- Seen in 65% of term babies and 80% of premature babies
- Commences after 24 h and lasts 5–7 days
- Due to immature fetal liver, postnatal haemolysis and shorter red cell lifespan in infants
- Keep well hydrated
- Phototherapy is needed if the SBR level is high enough ($\geqslant$ 350 µmol/L on day 3)
- Check regular SBRs

Breast milk jaundice

This is a diagnosis of exclusion that is poorly understood. It lasts for several weeks, requires no treatment, and breast feeding should continue. The infant should be investigated to rule out other causes.

Haemolytic jaundice due to Rhesus or ABO incompatibility

- This is due to high levels of haemolysis, resulting in too large a bilirubin load for the immature fetal liver
- Jaundice develops within the first 24 h and rapidly rises
- Mixing of blood, with a few fetal red cells entering the maternal circulation, can result in maternal antibodies developing to the fetal cells if they have a different antigenic component
- This mixing usually occurs at delivery or, if there is a placental bleed, may occur during the pregnancy. The antibodies are therefore usually formed after the first pregnancy, so it is subsequent pregnancies that are affected
- Anti-D injections (as this is the most common form) are therefore given during pregnancy to Rhesus negative women to 'mop up' any fetal red cells in the maternal circulation and prevent antibodies developing

183

It may be caused by:

Rhesus incompatibility Maternal antibodies to Rhesus C, D or E antigen (usually anti-D)
Mother is blood group Rhesus negative, the baby Rhesus positive
Antibodies cross the placenta and cause haemolysis *in utero*
If severe, the infant can become profoundly anaemic and develop hydrops fetalis (see p. 477)

ABO incompatibility Maternal antibodies to red cell A or B antigens develop
Mother is group O, the baby group A, B or AB

Rarer but more severe than Rhesus incompatibility

Management

1. Cord blood is taken for Hb, PCV (to assess severity), fetal blood group, maternal antibodies, Coombs' test and bilirubin level
2. Phototherapy
3. Regular 6-hourly SBR, Hb and PCV levels
4. Exchange transfusion if the bilirubin level becomes high enough
5. Intrauterine exchange transfusions can be done in fetal medicine units in very severe cases

Neonatal conjugated hyperbilirubinaemia

Causes

1. Extrahepatic bile duct obstruction:
   Biliary atresia
   Choledochal cyst

2. Intrahepatic disease:
   Intrahepatic bile duct obstruction Intrahepatic biliary hypoplasia, e.g. Alagille syndrome
   Intrahepatic biliary dilatation (Caroli disease)
   Progressive familial intrahepatic cholestasis (PFIC)

   Hepatocyte injury *Infections*:
   Hepatitis, e.g. HSV, CMV, enteroviruses, hepatitis B and C
   Systemic, e.g. listeria, toxoplasmosis, UTI

   Metabolic disease:
   Galactosaemia, fructosaemia, tyrosinaemia,
   α_1-antitrypsin deficiency
   Glycogen storage disease
   Cystic fibrosis
   Peroxisomal disease
   Inborn error of bile acid biosynthesis

   Other:
   Idiopathic neonatal hepatitis
   Hypothyroidism
   TPN therapy
   Chromosomal
   Hypoxic–ischaemic damage

NB: 'Neonatal hepatitis syndrome' refers to intrahepatic cholestasis of many causes (idiopathic, infectious hepatitis or intrahepatic bile duct paucity).

Examination and investigations

Examination	Liver and spleen size
	Cystic mass below the liver (choledochal cyst)
	Skin lesions, purpura, choroidoretinitis (congenital infection)
	Cataracts (galactosaemia, hypoparathyroidism)
	Cutaneous haemangioma (hepatic haemangioma)
	Situs inversus (extrahepatic biliary atresia)
	Dysmorphic features (trisomy 13, 18 or 21, Alagille syndrome)
	Micropenis, optic nerve hypoplasia (septo-optic dysplasia)
Biochemistry	Fractionated bilirubin (conjugated > 20% of total is pathological)
	LFTs
	Blood glucose, U&E, creatinine
	Galactose-l-phosphate uridyl transferase
	α_1-antitrypsin phenotype
	Metabolic screen (urine and serum amino acids, urine-reducing substances)
	Sweat test if feasible, IRT, CF genotype
	Thyroid function tests
	Cholesterol profile
Haematology	FBC, prothrombin time, blood group
Infection screen	Culture of urine, blood and CSF
	Serology for congenital infection and hepatitis B and C, i.e. HBsAg, VDRL, HIV, other specific viral serology
Urine	Succinylacetone ($\uparrow$ in tyrosinaemia – suspect if parents consanguineous)
Imaging	USS liver and gallbladder (choledochal cyst, biliary tract dilatation)
	TOBIDA scan following 3–5 days of phenobarbitone to help distinguish neonatal hepatitis (usually some excretion) from biliary atresia (no excretion).
	Direct cholangiography at operation
	Other systems, e.g. skeletal X-rays, echocardiography
Liver biopsy	Biliary tract and hepatocellular differentiation (NB: Correct prothrombin time prior to biopsy if abnormal)

Biliary atresia

Incidence 1:15 000–20 000 live births. A condition of *progressive* obliteration of part or all of the extrahepatic biliary ducts (an obliterative cholangiopathy). This leads to chronic liver failure and death. It should be suspected if there is prolonged jaundice beyond 14 days.

Clinical manifestations

- Normal at birth
- Jaundice persisting from day 2
- Pale stools and dark urine
- Hepatosplenomegaly with progressive liver disease

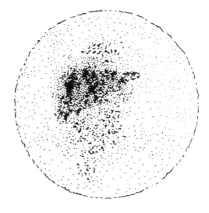

Figure 8.5 TOBIDA scan shows no excretion into the bowel

Investigations

LFTs	Often normal enzymes, with conjugated hyperbilirubinaemia
USS	May be normal, gallbladder may be absent on fasting USS (should be present)
Fasting TOBIDA radioisotope scan	Isotope uptake into liver unimpaired, excretion into the intestine absent
Liver biopsy	Perilobular oedema and fibrosis, proliferation of bile ductules, bile plugs, basic hepatic architecture intact
Laparotomy with operative cholangiography	

NB: It can be difficult to differentiate **biliary atresia** (bile duct proliferation present) from **neonatal hepatitis** (intrahepatic disease with giant cells present).

Management

1. Kasai procedure (hepatoportoenterostomy): Success rate 80%
   Later complications: cholangitis, fat malabsorption, cirrhosis, portal hypertension
   NB: Surgery must be performed < 60 days of life to increase chances of success

2. Liver transplantation usually necessary at a later date

Alagille syndrome (arteriohepatic dysplasia)

Autosomal dominant with variable penetrance, incidence 1:100 000 births. Gene mapping is now possible.

Liver	**Progressive intrahepatic bile duct paucity**, pruritis
Facial dysmorphism	Broad forehead, hypertelorism, deep-set eyes, long nose, small mandible
Eyes	Posterior embryotoxon
CVS	Peripheral pulmonary stenosis, tetralogy of Fallot
Skeletal	'Butterfly vertebrae' (vertebral arch defects)
Renal	Tubulointerstitial nephropathy
Other	Cholesterol ↑, tuberous xanthomas

Zellweger syndrome (cerebrohepatorenal syndrome)

Autosomal recessive. Incidence 1:100 000 births. A peroxisomal disorder.

Liver	Progressive degeneration, hepatomegaly. Absence of **peroxisomes** in hepatocytes
Kidneys	Progressive degeneration, renal cortical cysts
Neurological	Neurological impairment, severe hypotonia, psychomotor retardation
Dysmorphism	Abnormal-shaped head, distinctive facies (similar to Down syndrome)
Skeletal	Stippled calcification of patellae and greater trochanter (chondrodysplasia punctata)
Eyes	Congenital cataracts, hypoplastic, pale optic disc, retinal pigmentary changes

Caroli disease

Autosomal recessive. A congenital cystic dilatation of the intrahepatic bile ducts.

Symptoms are of recurring episodes of acute cholangitis and biliary lithiasis, and there is increased risk of cholangiocarcinoma.

Caroli disease	Isolated ductal dilatations
Caroli syndrome	Ductal dilatations with congenital hepatic fibrosis and autosomal recessive polycystic kidneys

CONGENITAL HYPERBILIRUBINAEMIAS

Unconjugated	Conjugated
Gilbert syndrome	**Dubin–Johnson syndrome**
2–5% population Autosomal dominant Hepatic UDPGT activity (+ other biochemical defects) Asymptomatic LFTs normal Bilirubin levels 50–60 ($\uparrow$ during illness and fasting)	Autosomal recessive Hepatocyte secretion of bilirubin glucuronide $\downarrow$ Bilirubin excretion defective Mild conjugated hyperbilirubinaemia Usually asymptomatic Pigment in the liver $\rightarrow$ black liver
Crigler–Najjar syndrome	**Rotor syndrome**

Type I (autosomal recessive)
 No glucuronyl transferase
 Severe or fatal kernicterus
 Treatment: Neonatal exchange transfusion
           Phototherapy into childhood
           Liver transplant
 	
 Type II (autosomal dominant)
 Decreased glucuronyl transferase
 Neonatal unconjugated hyperbilirubinaemia
 Survive to adults, usually asymptomatic
 Treatment: Phenobarbitone
           Liver transplant
	Autosomal recessive
	 Deficiency in uptake and storage of bilirubin

METABOLIC DISORDERS

WILSON DISEASE (HEPATOLENTICULAR DEGENERATION)

Autosomal recessive. Incidence 1:100 000 births. Gene mapped (ATP7B) to chromosome 13 q14–21.

The underlying problem is a copper transport defect. A defect in the hepatocytes prevents entry of copper into the caeruloplasmin compartment. Copper therefore accumulates in the liver and then escapes to the circulation and other organs such as the brain, kidneys and eyes.

Copper metabolism

Ingested copper is absorbed in the stomach and small intestine and transported bound to albumin to the liver. In the liver it is incorporated into caeruloplasmin for transport to the rest of the body. It is excreted into the biliary system or incorporated into copper storage proteins.

Clinical manifestations

Liver   Manifest > 5 years. Subacute or chronic hepatitis, hepatomegaly ± splenomegaly, fulminant hepatic failure, cirrhosis, portal hypertension, manifestations of chronic liver disease

Brain   Manifest > 10 years. Copper deposition in the basal ganglia. Intention tremor, severe 'wing-beat' tremor later, dysarthria, choreoathetosis, dystonia, behavioural change (bizarre or psychotic), school performance deterioration. Occasionally behavioural changes may be the only manifestation

Kidney   Proximal renal tubular acidosis (Fanconi syndrome), renal failure
Blood   Haemolysis, may be initial presentation, severe
Cornea   Kayser–Fleischer ring is **pathognomonic** (golden brown ring at periphery of cornea due to deposition in Descemet membrane)
Others   Arthritis, endocrinopathies, e.g. hypoparathyroidism

Diagnostic investigations

Urine   24-h copper excretion $\uparrow$
                           24-h copper excretion after penicillamine given $\uparrow\uparrow$
Serum caeruloplasmin $\downarrow$
Liver biopsy   Characteristic histology and periportal copper deposition present
Serum copper   Raised early in disease, may be normal

Management

Symptoms and signs improved with therapy, pre-symptomatic disease treated in relatives.

Copper chelation agents Penicillamine orally. (NB: This is an antimetabolite to vitamin B_6, therefore this is also given)
                           TETA (triethylene tetramine dihydrochloride) if penicillamine not tolerated
Copper intake   Reduce to < 1 mg/kg/day
                           Foods high in copper: liver, nuts, chocolate, shellfish
Liver transplant   If fulminant liver disease

Screening

All family members are screened for pre-symptomatic disease:

- Caeruloplasmin ($\downarrow$)
- Urine copper ($\uparrow$)
- Liver biopsy if diagnosis suspected

Antenatal diagnosis is possible.

HAEMOCHROMATOSIS

Autosomal dominant. 1:300 heterozygotes. Gene (C282Y) on chromosome 6p.

Associations   HLA A3 (72%)
                   HLA B7 (Australia)
                   HLA B14 (France)

A disease of excess iron deposition and absorption. The underlying defect is unknown.

Clinical manifestations

Clinical features rare below age 20 years.

Liver   Fibrosis, cirrhosis, of which 30% will develop primary hepatocellular carcinoma
Skin   Slate-grey discolouration
Pancreas   IDDM, 'bronzed diabetes'
Heart   Cardiomyopathy, arrhythmias
Endocrine glands   Pituitary (failure), growth failure, hypothyroidism, hypoparathyroidism, testicular atrophy
Joints   Chondrocalcinosis (calcium pyrophosphate deposition), asymmetrical, all joints

Investigations

Serum	Ferritin ↑
	Iron ↑
	TIBC (saturated)
Bone marrow	Biopsy (Perls' stain)
Liver biopsy	Fibrosis and iron deposition
	Liver CT/MRI
Desferrioxamine test	Iron excretion increases with chelation

Investigations to assess individual organ damage:

Liver	LFTs, CT/MRI, biopsy
Cardiac	CXR, ECG, echocardiogram
Endocrine	Pituitary function tests, TFTs, GH, parathyroid, adrenal and gonadal function

Management

- Venesection regularly
- Iron chelation therapy with desferrioxamine subcutaneously five nights a week

Neonatal haemochromatosis

An acquired condition secondary to severe prenatal liver disease. Severe liver dysfunction, with liver transplantation usually required. Aggressive chelation and an antioxidant regimen can, rarely, avoid the need for liver transplantation. Diagnosis is most accurate by estimation of extrahepatic iron deposition, e.g. lip biopsy.

Transfusion-induced haemochromatosis

This occurs with multiple chronic transfusions and results in a similar pathology due to the excess iron deposition. Therefore, chelation therapy must be given.

α_1-ANTITRYPSIN DEFICIENCY

Autosomal dominant. Incidence 1:2000–5000 live births. Common in Northern Europeans (1:10 carries a deficiency gene). Gene located on chromosome 14q31–32.3.

This disease is the result of a deficiency of α_1-antitrypsin in varying degrees of severity. α_1-antitrypsin is a protease inhibitor (Pi) made by hepatocytes; it is a glycoprotein and accounts for $\geqslant 80\%$ of the circulating α_1-globulin.

The disease results in:

- Liver disease – childhood onset
- Lung disease – 20–40 year onset

Proteases are inherited as a series of co-dominant alleles (> 20 phenotypes exist). The genetic variants are characterized by their electrophoretic mobilities as medium (M), slow (S) and very slow (Z). Example genotypes are:

PiMM	= normal phenotype
PiSS	= α_1-AT 60% activity
PiZZ	= α_1-AT 15% activity. 1:3400 births. Most clinical disease. 20% have neonatal cholestasis
Pinullnull	= not associated with liver disease. 0% α_1-AT activity

Clinical manifestations

Liver	Very variable. Neonatal cholestasis, transient jaundice in first few months of life, hepatomegaly ± splenomegaly, childhood cirrhosis

189

Respiratory   Emphysema (as for adult)
Skin   Persistent cutaneous vasculitis, cold-contact urticaria, acquired angiooedema

Investigations

- Serum α_1-antitrypsin $\downarrow$
- Liver biopsy (globules of α_1-antitrypsin in the periportal cells)
- Pi phenotype
- Parental genotype

Antenatal diagnosis is possible.

Management

- Liver transplant if severe liver disease.
- Lung disease – give danazol (increases α_1-antitrypsin), enzyme replacement therapy available
- Genetic counselling required for future pregnancies

REYE SYNDROME

A syndrome of acute encephalopathy and fatty degeneration of the liver. The incidence has markedly declined over recent years, due to decreased aspirin use in children and greater recognition of the differential diagnoses. Usual age 4–12 years, mortality 40%.

Associations   Aspirin therapy
                   Viral infections (influenza B, varicella)
                   Mitochondrial cytopathy

Clinical manifestations

- Prodromal URTI or chicken pox
- 4–7 days later: Vomiting +++
                      Encephalopathy
                      Moderate hepatomegaly, no jaundice, not icteric
                      $\pm$ Hypoglycaemia

Clinical staging

Grade	Signs
I	Lethargic, vomiting
II	Confusion, delirium
III	Light coma, decorticate rigidity, seizures
IV	Deeper coma, decerebrate rigidity, seizures
V	Isoelectric (flat) EEG, respiratory arrest

Investigations

Blood   Ammonia $\uparrow$ (> 125 µg/dl)
         AST, ALT, LDH, CK ($\uparrow$)
         Glucose ($\downarrow$, in small children especially)
         Clotting deranged (PT $\uparrow$)

CSF	Normal analysis, raised ICP
Liver biopsy	Fatty infiltration, specific mitochondrial morphology on EM

Management

This is supportive, with correction of hypoglycaemia and coagulation defects, and IPPV intensive care as necessary. It is important to:

- Control raised ICP
- Make sure the diagnosis is correct

Differential diagnoses

- CNS infections
- Drug ingestion
- Haemorrhagic shock with encephalopathy
- Metabolic disease, e.g. fatty acid oxidation defects, organic acidurias, urea cycle defects

CONGENITAL HEPATIC FIBROSIS

Autosomal recessive. This is a congenital disease involving:

Liver disease	Diffuse fibrosis ± abnormal bile ducts
	Hepatosplenomegaly, portal hypertension
Renal disease (75%)	Renal tubule ectasia, ARPKD, nephronophthisis

Clinical features

- Hepatosplenomegaly, bleeding from varices
- Cholangitis (when bile duct abnormal)

Investigations

LFTs	Alkaline phosphatase ↑
	Other LFTs (AST, ALT, bilirubin, albumin and PT) usually normal
Liver biopsy	Needed for the diagnosis

Management

Treatment of varices.

HEPATITIS

VIRAL HEPATITIS

This may be caused by the hepatitis viruses, CMV, EBV, HSV, varicella, HIV, rubella, adenovirus, enteroviruses and arboviruses.

Hepatitis A (HAV)

RNA picornavirus, the commonest cause of viral hepatitis.

Transmission	Faecal–oral (especially water, seafood, poor sanitation)

Clinical features

Incubation (2 weeks)   Infective until just after jaundice appears (while faecal HAV excreted)
Prodrome (2 weeks)   Malaise, nausea, vomiting, diarrhoea, headaches (mild in young children)
Jaundice (2–4 weeks)   Cholestatic jaundice, mild hepatosplenomegaly, symptoms improving
Rare complications   Fulminant hepatic failure, vasculitis, arthritis, myocarditis, renal failure

Investigations

Prodrome	Jaundice
Serum bilirubin (N)	Bilirubin (↑)
Urine bilirubin and urobilinogen (↑)	AST (↑) for up to 6 months
AST (↑↑)	Alkaline phosphatase (↑)
FBC (WCC ↓ with relative lymphocytosis, aplastic anaemia, Coombs +ve haemolytic anaemia) ESR ↑, PT (↑ indicates liver injury) Stool EM positive for HAV	Anti-HAV IgM

Management

Supportive only. No carrier state.

Prevention

- Passive immunization – standard immunoglobulin, three months protection
- Active immunization – vaccine available

Hepatitis B (HBV)

DNA hepadnavirus. Transmission by intravenous, close contact or vertical

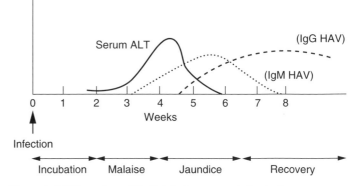

Figure 8.6 HAV serology. (NB: IgG indicates past infection)

Clinical features

These are as for hepatitis A but more prolonged and severe.

Investigations

As for hepatitis A.

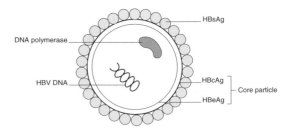

Figure 8.7 HBV particle

Specific markers for hepatitis B:

Antigen	Antibody
HBsAg	Anti-HBsAg
HBcAg	Anti-HBcAg
	IgM anti-HBcAg
HBeAg	Anti-HBeAg

PCR for HBV DNA is also available (indicates continued viral replication)

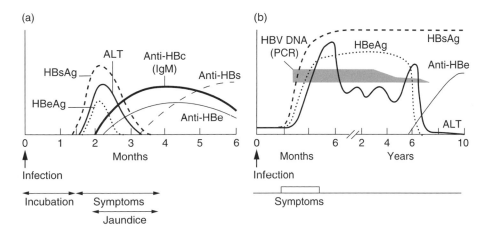

Figure 8.8 HBV serology. (a) Acute infection. (b) Chronic carrier

Clinical course

Most make a full recovery.

Fulminant hepatitis (1%) (Anti-HBcAg diagnostic in this situation)
Chronic infection (10%) HBsAg (normal carrier state)
HBeAg (very infectious)
70–90% asymptomatic carrier → chronic hepatitis, cirrhosis, hepatocellular carcinoma (few)
10–30% chronic hepatitis → cirrhosis → hepatocellular carcinoma
Common among infants infected < 1 year

Carriers may be treated with pegylated interferon-α and lamivudine which may seroconvert them.

Infants of hepatitis B carrier mothers		
These are at risk of contracting hepatitis B.		
If mother is:	HBsAg positive Anti-HBeAb positive	Vaccine within 12 h of birth, 0.5 ml (10 µg) IM thigh Repeat doses of vaccine at 1 and 6 months
If mother is:	HBsAg positive HBeAg positive	Vaccine within 12 h of birth, 0.5 ml IM thigh Hepatitis B immune globulin (HBIG)<1 h, 200 IU, IM, opposite thigh Repeat doses of vaccine at 1 and 6 months

Hepatitis C (HCV)

RNA virus with six subtypes. Types I, II and III common in Europe; Type IV is common in the Far East.

Transmission   Vertical (uncommon); intravenous, close contact

This causes a mild flu-like illness.

Rare complications are aplastic anaemia, arthritis, agranulocytosis, neurological problems. Chronic liver disease occurs in 50% → cirrhosis (25%) → hepatocellular carcinoma (15%).

Diagnosis is with anti-HCV antibody detection (negative until 1–3 months after clinical onset)

Pegylated interferon-α and ribavirin can be given to chronic carriers. No prophylaxis for maternal transmission.

Hepatitis D (HDV)

Hepatitis D virus (delta virus) is an incomplete RNA particle enclosed in the HBsAg. It can only replicate in the presence of hepatitis B infection. Two patterns of infection are seen: **super-infection** in a person already infected with HBV and **co-infection** with HBV. Features are similar but more severe with more fulminant hepatitis occurring than in other viral hepatitis.

Co-infection	Superinfection
Acute hepatitis common	Chronic hepatitis common
Similar to HBV but more severe	Fulminant hepatitis more common
Biphasic AST rise	IgM anti-HDV and IgG anti-HBcAg
IgM anti-HDV and IgM anti-HBcAg	

Transmission   Percutaneous, close contact, vertical

- Diagnosis is by detecting IgM antibody to HDV
- Chronic infection is very serious as 70% get cirrhosis
- α-Interferon therapy causes a remission only

Hepatitis E (HEV)

RNA virus.

Transmission   Enteral route

Clinical illness is similar to hepatitis A though often more severe. NB. Pregnant women have high rate of fulminant hepatic failure (20% vs 2% in others infected) and fatality.

- Diagnosis is by HEV RNA detection in serum or stools
- No effective prophylaxis
- No carrier state exists

CHRONIC HEPATITIS

This is the presence of hepatic inflammation (manifest by elevated transaminases) for > 6 months. There are two subdivisions of chronic hepatitis, distinguished histologically:

Chronic persistent hepatitis   Benign, self-limiting usually
Chronic active hepatitis   Progressive disease with eventual cirrhosis

The clinical manifestations are variable:

- Asymptomatic
- Chronic liver disease
- Hepatic failure

Causes

- Persistent viral infection
- Autoimmune
- Drugs, e.g. isoniazid, nitrofurantoin, sulphonamides, dantrolene
- Metabolic, e.g. cystic fibrosis, Wilson disease, haemochromatosis, α_1-antitrypsin disease

Chronic persistent hepatitis (CPH)

Usual cause	Hepatitis B or C
Histology	Inflammation limited to portal triads, no fibrosis or cirrhosis
Clinical manifestations	Usually asymptomatic, may have non-specific malaise and mild hepatomegaly. Sometimes chronic liver disease occurs
Investigations	Transaminases ↑, bilirubin ↑
	Alkaline phosphatase, albumin, PT all normal
	Autoantibodies negative
	Liver biopsy essential
Management	Interferon-α may help in hepatitis B or C disease

Chronic active hepatitis (CAH)

Usual cause	Hepatitis B or C, autoimmune disease
Histology	Inflammatory infiltrates beyond portal areas, 'piece-meal necrosis' of hepatocytes, fibrosis and necrosis between neighbouring triads, cirrhosis
Clinical manifestations	Very variable, ranging from asymptomatic to cirrhosis or hepatic failure
Associations	Arthritis, rash, nephritis, vasculitis, haemolytic anaemia in autoimmune disease
Investigations	Transaminases ↑, bilirubin ↑, γ-globulins ↑, PT ↑
	Anaemia, thrombocytopoenia, leucopoenia
	ANA ↑, ASM ↑, AMA ↑, LKM (liver–kidney microsomal antibodies) ↑ and IgG ↑ in autoimmune disease
	Liver biopsy essential
Management	Steroids and azathioprine in autoimmune disease
	Course of interferon-α injections in hepatitis B or C
	Liver transplant in end-stage liver disease

PORTAL HYPERTENSION

This occurs when the portal pressure is elevated ≥ 10–12 mmHg (normal = 7 mmHg). Increased portal venous pressure results in collaterals (varices) developing (portosystemic shunting) and a hyperdynamic circulation. These together can cause varices to rupture and result in GI bleeds. Important sites of collaterals (varices):

- Oesophagus
- Anorectal
- Periumbilical (caput medusae. NB: These flow *away* from the umbilicus)
- Retroperitoneal
- Perivertebral/perispinal

Causes

It is caused by obstruction to the portal flow anywhere along the portal system.

Prehepatic	Hepatic	Posthepatic
Small liver, big spleen	*Liver small/large/normal Big spleen*	*Big liver, big spleen*
Portal/splenic vein thrombosis:	**Hepatocellular:**	**Hepatic vein thrombosis**
• Neonatal sepsis	• Cong. hepatic fibrosis	(Budd–Chiari syndrome):
• Dehydration	• Viral hepatitis	• Cong. venous web
• Hypercoagulable state	• Metabolic cirrhosis	• Polycythaemia
Increased portal flow:	• Hepatotoxicity	• Leukaemia
• AV fistula	(TPN)	• Coagulopathy
	(Methotrexate)	• Sickle cell disease
	Biliary tract disease:	• Oral contraceptive pill
	• Sclerosing cholangitis	• GvHD
	• Choledochal cyst	**Veno-occlusive disease**
	• Biliary atresia	(seen in stem cell transplant)
	• Intrahepatic bile duct paucity	**Right heart failure**
		Constrictive pericarditis

Clinical features

- Bleeding oesophageal varices
- Cutaneous collaterals (periumbilical, inferior abdominal wall)
- Splenomegaly (depending on the site of the obstruction)
- Liver size may be normal, enlarged or small, and there may be signs of underlying liver disease
- Haemorrhagic encephalopathy secondary to massive GI bleed

Investigations

USS	Outlining portal vein pathology, direction of flow of the portal system, presence of oesophageal varices
CT/MRI scan	Findings as for USS
Arteriography	Can be done from the coeliac axis, superior mesenteric artery or splenic vein
Endoscopy	Outlining oesophageal and gastric varices

Management

Emergency	Resuscitation (clear fluids and blood)
	Treatment of coagulopathy (FFP, vitamin K, platelets)
	NG tube
	H_2 antagonist or proton pump inhibitor intravenously
	Other drugs if necessary (octreotide, GTN)

Elective
Endoscopy – sclerosis (now virtually never undertaken), elastic band ligation of varices or insertion of, in extremis, Sengstaken–Blakemore tube (gastric balloon only) may be required
Endoscopic obliteration (as above)
Portosystemic shunts, e.g. TIPSS (transjugular intrahepatic porto-systemic shunt), REX shunt (but shunts have complication of encephalopathy)
Liver transplantation (for intrahepatic disease or hepatic vein obstruction)

GALLBLADDER DISEASE

Gallstones are relatively rare in children. They are of the pigment type in 70% of children and cholesterol stones in 20%. Conditions associated with gallstone formation include:

- Chronic haemolysis (sickle cell disease, spherocytosis) (pigment stones)
- Crohn disease
- Ileal resection
- Cystic fibrosis
- TPN
- Obesity
- Sick premature infants

Clinical features

- Intolerance of fatty foods
- Recurrent colicky RUQ abdominal pain
- Acute cholecystitis: RUQ pain, tenderness and guarding, fever, jaundice, nausea, vomiting

Investigations

USS   Liver and gall bladder
Blood LFTs, blood cultures (in acute cholecystitis)

Management

Cholecystectomy (open or laparoscopic, once acute infection subsided)

LIVER TRANSPLANTATION

Orthotopic liver transplant is available for chronic liver disease or acute/subacute liver failure.

Transplant should be considered before irreversible nutritional deficit and growth and developmental delay. Biliary atresia and metabolic liver disease are common indications in children.

Combined small bowel and liver transplantation is now an effective treatment for short-gut or intestinal failure. However, isolated small bowel transplant is recommended unless end-stage liver dysfunction accompanies bowel disease.

Indications and contraindications for urgent liver transplantation

Indications	Contraindications
Deteriorating liver synthetic function INR > 4 ↓ Transaminases reflecting ↓ hepatic mass Blood glucose and albumin ↓ if unsupported Emergent and worsening hepatic encephalopathy Chronic indications also include poor quality of life, severe pruritis, persistent encephalopathy, recurrent hepatic complications, persistent hyperbilirubinaemia ≥ 120 μmol/L.	Irreversible cerebral damage Multisystem disease not correctable by transplant, e.g. peroxisomal disorders

Complications

Early   Renal impairment, hypertension, GI haemorrhage, graft dysfunction, acute rejection
Late   Infection (especially bacterial, CMV and PCP), organ rejection, lymphoproliferative disease

Prognosis

80–90% 5-year survival rate for elective transplantation.

FURTHER READING

Kelly DA *Diseases of the Liver and Biliary System in Children*, 2nd edn. Oxford: Blackwell Publishing, 2003

Shah N, Thomson M The liver in intensive care. In: Henderson J, Fleming P, eds, *Manual of Paediatric Intensive Care*. London: Edward Arnold, 1999

9 Renal disorders

- Physiology
- Urinary tract infection
- Vesicoureteric reflux
- Congenital urinary tract obstruction
- Nocturnal enuresis
- Renal calculi
- Nephrotic syndrome
- Glomerulonephritis

- Haemolytic uraemic syndrome
- Renal venous thrombosis
- Disorders of tubular function
- Congenital structural malformations
- Urate metabolism
- Hypertension
- Renal failure

PHYSIOLOGY

FUNCTIONS OF THE KIDNEY

- Excretion of waste products
- Regulation of body fluid volume and composition (salt and water [and hence BP] and pH balance)
- Endocrine and metabolic (renin, prostaglandins, erythropoietin, vitamin D metabolism)

GLOMERULAR FILTRATION

Glomerular filtration rate (GFR) = the total volume of fluid (plasma) per minute filtered through the glomerulus

$$GFR = \frac{\text{Urine flow} \times [\text{Urine}]}{[\text{Plasma}]}$$ [ ] = concentration of substance

The GFR is very low *in utero* and at birth, and rises to reach adult levels by 18 months–2 years of age.

Normal value = 80–130 ml/min/l.73 m²   (55–75 ml/min/m²)   (Adult)

Approximation = $\dfrac{\text{Height (cm)} \times 40}{\text{Plasma creatinine } (\mu\text{mol/L})}$ (Child)

Renal clearance = volume of plasma from which all of a given substance is removed per minute by the kidneys

Cr clearance = $\dfrac{(\text{Urine Cr} \times \text{Urine (vol/min)})}{\text{Plasma Cr}}$ (Cr = creatinine)

GFR can be estimated using endogenous substances or by injecting a substance and comparing the rate of urinary excretion with the plasma concentration. The ideal substance for this estimation is:

1. Not metabolized
2. Freely filtered, i.e. not protein bound
3. Neither secreted nor reabsorbed
4. The concentration in the plasma remains in a steady state during the collection of urine, i.e. rate of production = rate of clearance

If all these criteria are met then the **renal clearance = GFR**. Substances that may be used for measurement:

Creatinine	Commonly used (endogenous), some tubular secretion
Cystatin	Endogenous substance
Inulin	Gold standard, used for research purposes
Cr EDTA	Used for accurate GFR calculation, but does involve radioactivity
Iothalamate	Non-radioactive assays possible, multipoint using finger prick blood spots increases accuracy

RENAL BLOOD FLOW (RBF)

This is dependent on the BP and the renal vascular resistance. RBF is low at birth and gradually increases to adult levels (25% of the cardiac output). The RBF remains constant throughout a BP range of 80–180 mmHg in adults.

The **countercurrent mechanism** ensures a concentrated environment surrounding the distal collecting duct and thus water is reabsorbed at this point (the amount dependent on ADH status), resulting in more concentrated urine.

RENIN–ANGIOTENSIN–ALDOSTERONE SYSTEM

This system is involved in the control of BP. The juxtaglomerular apparatus (JGA) is made up of specialized arteriolar smooth muscle cells which secrete renin in response to various stimuli. Renin cleaves angiotensin I from angiotensinogen, which is then converted to active angiotensin II. This vasoactive substance results directly in vasoconstriction and also in sodium retention via aldosterone release. These changes mediate an increase in BP and salt and water retention.

ATRIAL NATRIURETIC PEPTIDES (ANP)

These are peptides secreted from the cardiac atria in response to increased stretch, increased pressure and increased osmolality and are involved in cardiovascular and fluid homeostasis. ANP has the following actions:

- GFR ↑
- Na excretion ↑
- H_2O excretion ↑
- BP ↓
- Renin ↓, aldosterone ↓

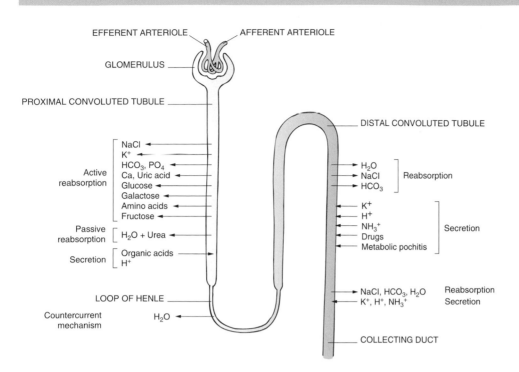

Figure 9.1 Schematic diagram of sites of electrolyte absorption and excretion

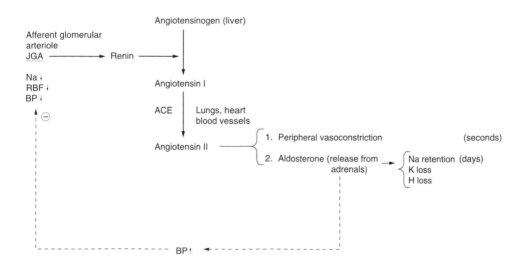

Figure 9.2 Renin–angiotensin–aldosterone system

ACID–BASE HOMEOSTASIS

Normal arterial blood gases:

pH	7.35–7.45	
PO$_2$	10.0–13.3 kPa	(75–100 mmHg)
PCO$_2$	4.8–6.1 kPa	(36–46 mmHg)
HCO$_3$	23–30 mmol/L	
BE	± 2.3 mmol/L	

Anion gap

This is used to evaluate acid–base disturbances. It is the apparent disparity between the total cation (+) and the total anion (–) concentration in the blood. It occurs because some anions are not routinely measured.

Anion gap $= [Na] – [Cl + HCO_3]$

Normal values are 10–12 mmol/L.

The anion gap is useful in metabolic acidosis when the key distinguishing factor is chloride concentration – this will be normal or increased, depending on the cause of the acidosis

Acidosis with normal anion gap (chloride$\uparrow$ compensates for reduced bicarbonate)

Bicarbonate loss $\uparrow$	GIT losses
	Renal losses, e.g. proximal RTA, interstitial nephritis, hypoadrenalism
H$^+$ excretion $\downarrow$	E.g. distal RTA

Acidosis with increased anion gap (chloride normal, other acids must be present to explain the acidosis)

Acid increased	Lactic acidosis
	Ketoacidosis
	Inborn errors of metabolism

Unfortunately, chronic renal failure can cause both a normal or increased anion gap acidosis.

DIURETICS

Drug	Mechanism	Side-effects
Loop diuretics E.g. frusemide	Inhibit Na, K and Cl co-transport in the ascending loop of Henle and increase venous capacitance	Ototoxicity Hypochloraemic alkalosis K $\downarrow$, Mg $\downarrow$, Na $\downarrow$ Impaired glucose tolerance Gout (urates $\uparrow$) Myalgia Allergic nephritis
		Hypercalciuria, with renal stone formation or nephrocalcinosis in neonates

Drug	Mechanism	Side-effects
Thiazide diuretics E.g. bendrofluazide	Inhibit Na and K reabsorption in the early portion of the distal tubule and decrease peripheral resistance	K $\downarrow$, Mg $\downarrow$ Na $\downarrow$ (used in DI) Gout (urates $\uparrow$) Impaired glucose tolerance Serum Ca $\uparrow$
Potassium-sparing diuretics Aldosterone antagonists, e.g. spironolactone	Competitive inhibitors of aldosterone at the distal tubule	Na $\downarrow$ Gynaecomastia Gastrointestinal disturbance Impotence
Other potassium-sparing diuretics, e.g. amiloride	Inhibit Na reabsorption at the collecting duct Inhibit sodium reabsorption at the collecting duct	Na $\downarrow$, K $\uparrow$ Dry mouth Gastrointestinal disturbance
Carbonic anhydrase inhibitors		
E.g. acetazolamide	Interfere with H^+ excretion, resulting in increase in Na excretion in proximal tubule	Metabolic acidosis Cl $\uparrow$, K $\downarrow$
Osmotic diuretics E.g. mannitol, urea glucose	Filtered at the glomerulus but not reabsorbed, creating an osmotic gradient into the tubules, with Na and water excretion	Chills, fever Used in cerebral oedema

RENAL RADIOLOGICAL INVESTIGATIVE TECHNIQUES

Ultrasound scan (USS)

The standard imaging procedure generates information on renal size and growth, structure and dilatation (which may be a marker of obstruction). *No* information obtained on renal function.

Intravenous urography (IVU)

Used to check detailed anatomy, i.e. renal pelvis, calyces, ureters, stones and obstruction. Contrast is given intravenously and is excreted via (and hence outlines) the urinary tract. Rarely needed.

Micturating cystourethrography (MCUG)

Radiolabelled scanning with contrast medium instilled into the bladder via a urethral catheter in place and the urinary tract is visualized while the infant is voiding. A sensitive technique to detect and grade reflux and outline urethral obstruction on voiding with the catheter removed. This is a relatively invasive procedure due to the necessity to place a catheter.

Static nuclear medicine scan (DMSA)

Static renal scanning with technetium-labelled 2,3-dimercaptosuccinic acid (DMSA). DMSA is taken up by proximal tubules and the functional cortical mass is outlined. Normal results range from > 45% one kidney and < 55% the other kidney. The scan is used to detect renal scarring and pyelonephritis (though a single scan cannot differentiate acute from chronic).

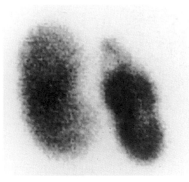

Figure 9.3 A 6-year-old girl presenting with urinary incontinence, both daytime and night-time wetting. Final diagnosis is that of a duplex right kidney with ectopic opening of the upper moiety ureter below the bladder neck and VUR into the lower moiety with damage. This is the right posterior oblique projection of the ^{99m}Tc-DMSA scan showing a defect in the upper pole of the right kidney. In addition, there is a focal defect on the lateral aspect of the lower portion of the right kidney, better seen in the oblique projection

Dynamic nuclear medicine scanning (DTPA and MAG3)

Radioisotope scanning with technetium-labelled diethylenetriaminepenta-acetic acid (DTPA) or mercaptoacetylglycine (MAG3). DTPA and MAG3 are freely filtered through the glomerulus. In a normal scan the isotope is quickly excreted, but with pathology the excretion is delayed. Frusemide is then given to differentiate an obstructed system (where delay continues) from an unobstructed system. Used to detect renal blood flow, function and drainage disorders, and reflux in an older child who can control micturition on demand.

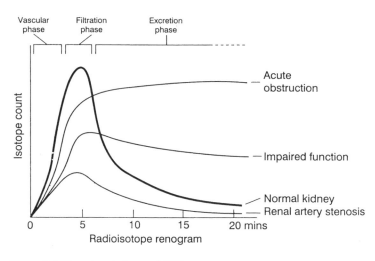

Figure 9.4 Normal and abnormal DTPA scans

URINARY TRACT INFECTION (UTI)

A UTI can present as acute cystitis, acute pyelonephritis, septicaemia or be picked up as asymptomatic bacteriuria. Acute pyelonephritis may lead to renal scarring and changes of chronic pyelonephritis. UTI associated with reflux can cause scarring in a **growing kidney** and this can lead to hypertension and chronic renal failure.

Causes

Predisposing factors	Common bacteria
Female (3% of girls cf. 1% of boys)	*Escherichia coli*
Urinary tract abnormality (50%)	Proteus (boys particularly, triple phosphate stones)
Immunosuppression	*Pseudomonas aeruginosa* (common in structural abnormalities)

Clinical manifestations

Asymptomatic bacteriuria or:

Infant	Sepsis (PUO)
	Faltering growth, gastro-oesophageal reflux
Older child	Dysuria, frequency, nocturia, abdominal pain, incontinence of urine, haematuria, smelly urine
	Systemic infection (PUO)

Diagnosis

1. *Urine sample:* Suprapubic aspiration (SPA) – in infants < 1 year. Standard in sick infants
   Clean-catch urine – infants. Preferred sample. Three samples collected prior to treatment
   Bag urine – infants. Contamination common. Three samples collected prior to treatment
   Catheter sample
   Midstream urine (MSU) – children > 3 years (or younger with patience or if potty-trained)
   Signs of infection (on urinalysis, microscopy and culture):
   - Proteinuria, haematuria (dipstick) ⎫
   - Pyuria (almost always) (microscopy) ⎬ Supportive
   - Organisms on microscopy (microscopy) ⎭
   - Single species growth > 10^5/ml (culture) **Diagnostic**

2. In unexplained fever and sick infants/children – urine sample, U&Es, creatinine, ESR, CRP, blood cultures
3. Urgent USS if there is a known structural abnormality and concern of obstruction or severe localized flank pain (looking for obstructed, infected kidney)

NB: Some infants with posterior uretheral valves, i.e. must be boys, can present with an early UTI – usually with sepsis at 1–2 months of age.

Management

- Antibiotic therapy: If unwell/infant – intravenous (change if necessary when sensitivities known)
  If well child – oral therapy (change if necessary when sensitivities known)
- Optimize hydration
- Commence prophylactic antibiotics until further investigations complete
- Drainage procedures if required

Further investigation in proven UTI

Proven UTI
↓
USS (and abdo X-ray if stones, obstruction, bladder or spinal anomaly suspected)
IVU if concern on USS (rarely needed)
↓
Prophylactic antibiotics until investigations are complete

< 1 year	1–5 years	> 5 years	> 5 years
↓	↓	If abnormal USS/abdo X-ray	Normal USS/
2 months later	2 months later	2 months later	AXR
↓	↓	↓	↓
DMSA (scars?)	DMSA	DMSA	No further
+	↓	↓	investigation
MCUG (reflux/ obstruction?) (especially important in boys)	If abnormal (USS or DMSA) or pyelonephritis or recurrent infection or FH reflux ↓ MCUG (MAG–3 if older or can urinate on demand) (If pyelonephritis, add DTPA)	If abnormal ↓ MAG–3	

Figure 9.5 Further investigation in proven UTI. (This is a baseline protocol; individual units may vary in the detail)

Prevention

- High fluid intake
- Girls to wipe themselves after micturition from front to back
- Empty bladder completely and regularly; may involve double micturition, i.e. empty once and then repeat a few minutes later
- Avoid constipation

VESICOURETERIC REFLUX (VUR)

This is detected on renal investigation, usually following UTI. It is retrograde flow of urine from the bladder into the ureters ± kidney, due to incompetence at the vesicoureteric junction or abnormality of the whole ureter.

- It is very common (1:50–100) and usually resolves spontaneously
- It is familial (multifactorial, several loci found)
- 10–15% improvement in reflux per year

Traditional teaching is that reflux can result in renal scarring (**reflux nephropathy**) because:

1. The renal pelvis is exposed to high pressures (during urination), and
2. The reflux facilitates the passage of bacteria to the renal pelvis

However, many of the kidneys are already abnormal at birth because of combined maldevelopment of the lower urinary tract and kidneys, i.e. urinary tract 'field defect'. 20% of adult ESRF is traditionally said to result from reflux nephropathy, but many of these may have had an underlying developmental defect.

Classification

Grades I–V:

- Grades I and II – spontaneous resolution in 80%
- Grades III and IV – spontaneous resolution in 15%

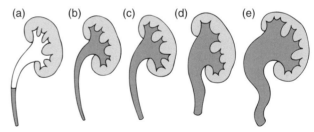

Figure 9.6 Simplest classification is by Scott who divided the types into those with normal calibre or dilated ureters

Management of reflux and renal scarring

1. Long-term prophylactic antibiotic therapy (trimethoprim 2 mg/kg/night). Controversial when to stop (when reflux resolved, no UTIs for a year, or after the age of 35 when new scarring is very rare)
2. MSUs if/when symptomatic
4. Consider circumcision in boys if recurrent UTIs and tight foreskin
5. Cystoscopic injection of reinforcing material around ureteric orifices in the bladder or surgical re-implantation of the ureters (old fashioned) if medical management fails (rarely necessary)
6. If bilateral scarring, perform regular renal growth (ultrasound) and function tests (creatinine, GFR)

Reinvestigate regularly in early childhood looking at:

- Renal growth (USS)
- If condition has resolved (MAG3)
- Any new scars (DMSA).
- BP and urinalysis check 6–12 monthly for life

CONGENITAL URINARY TRACT OBSTRUCTION

NB: Ureteral dilatation does *not* always signify obstruction (congenitally abnormal ureters could be present).

Congenital obstruction may occur at the sites shown in Figure 9.7.

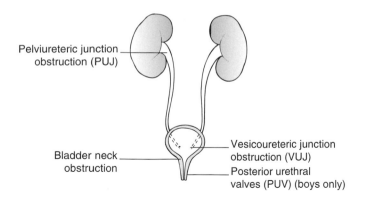

Figure 9.7 Urinary tract obstruction sites

Obstruction results in dilatation of the urinary tract proximal to the obstruction, ± hydronephrosis and hydroureter, ± dysplastic or malformed kidneys, often with peripheral cortical cysts. Intrauterine detection of dilatation on antenatal ultrasound scan is possible.

It is important to assess infants in whom congenital hydronephrosis has been detected in order to check for obstruction and possible renal damage, and then to treat the cause. These infants are commenced on prophylactic antibiotics from birth, which may later be discontinued if all investigations are normal.

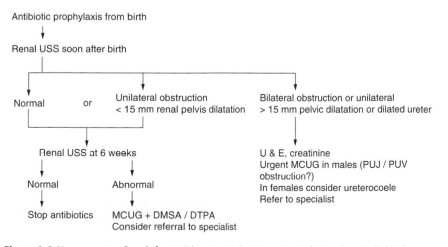

Figure 9.8 Management of an infant with antenatal urinary tract obstruction (individual protocols may vary)

POSTERIOR URETHRAL VALVES (PUV)

This condition is seen in male infants and it is important to recognize it early as prompt surgical treatment can delay/prevent rapid progression to renal failure (though irreversible damage may have already occurred *in utero*).

An outflow obstruction in the posterior urethra causes aberrant bladder development with a thick wall and small capacity. There is bilateral hydronephrosis, there may be associated ureteric and kidney abnormalities and, if severe, oligohydramnios and the Potter sequence can occur. It may present as sepsis during the first few weeks of life.

NOCTURNAL ENURESIS

This is the involuntary passage of urine during sleep.

Incidence   (100% at birth, i.e. normal!)
          5% at 5 years of age
          2–3% at 10 years of age
          < 2% at 15 years of age

It may be primary (always present) or secondary (occurs after continence was achieved). It is due to an inability to wake when the bladder is full, bladder overactivity and/or a high nocturnal urine output.

Causes of pathological nocturnal enuresis

Psychological   > 95%
Organic   UTI
                  Constipation
                  Polyuria, e.g. IDDM, diabetes insipidus, polyuric renal failure
                  Neurological, e.g. spina bifida
                  Renal structural abnormality, e.g. ectopic ureter

Initial investigations and assessment

- History of onset and frequency. Is the child dry during the day? Get parents/child to keep a drinks and toilet diary
- Diet, stress and nocturnal access to the toilet
- Examination of abdomen, genitalia, spine, neurological assessment and growth
- Urine sample: check for glycosuria, proteinuria, infection and early morning urine osmolality
- BP check
- Renal USS if indicated (± AXR)

NB: The history is most important and guides investigations. Organic causes must be ruled out prior to managing it as a psychological problem.

Management options

- Star charts and reward systems (positive reinforcement)
- Alarm pads (negative reinforcement)
- Behavioural programmes, e.g. retention control during the day to increase bladder capacity
- *Drugs (only needed in a very few):*   Anticholinergics, e.g. oxybutinin
                                            Adrenergics, e.g. ephedrine
                                            ADH analogue (desmopressin) for short-term relief

RENAL CALCULI

Unusual in children (overall incidence 1.5:1 000 000).

Clinical features

- None
- UTI
- Haematuria, abdominal pain, renal failure (if bilateral)
- Family history

Classification

Type	Causes
Calcium 80% (oxalate or phosphate) (Male > female) (radio-opaque)	Idiopathic hypercalciuria, primary hyperparathyroidism, vitamin D excess, sarcoidosis, distal RTA, malignancies, immobilization, juvenile chronic arthritis, frusemide
Calcium oxalate (radio-opaque)	Type I and II hyperoxaluria Ileostomies, Crohn disease (intestinal hyperoxaluria)
Uric acid 4% (radiolucent)	Lymphoma, ileostomies, Crohn disease, hyperuricosuria Lesch–Nyan syndrome, G6PD, polycythaemia
Mixed (struvite) 15% (staghorns) (radio-opaque)	Infection with urease-splitting bacteria (e.g. proteus)
Cystine 1%	Cystinuria (weakly radio-opaque)
Xanthine, very rare	XO deficiency (radiolucent)

Investigations

Urine	M, C & S (NB: proteus)
	Urinalysis for pH (distal RTA)
	Amino acid screen (cystinuria)
	Calcium/creatinine ratios or 24-h collection
Blood	Renal function tests (creatinine, HCO_3 especially)
	Calcium, phosphate, alkaline phosphatase
	PTH if concern of hyperparathyroidism
Imaging	AXR, renal USS, IVU
Stone analysis	

Management

- High fluid intake
- Alkalinize the urine to pH 7.5 (cystine and uric acid stones)
- Stone removal via lithotripsy or endoscopically
- Treat cause if possible

NEPHROTIC SYNDROME

Incidence 1:50 000 children. Male > female, 2:1. Typical age 1–6 years.

This condition is characterized by **heavy proteinuria** and the consequences of hypoalbuminaemia.

Diagnostic triad:

1. Proteinuria > 40 (mg/h/m^2)
2. Hypoalbuminaemia < 25 mg/L
3. Oedema

Hyperlipidaemia (LDL ↑, triglycerides ↑) also occurs in most cases.

There are three main types of nephrotic syndrome in childhood:

Minimal change disease (85–90%)	No changes seen under normal microscope, but podocyte foot process fusion on EM
Focal segmental glomerulosclerosis	Focal because not all glomeruli affected (usually deeper ones) and (10–15%) segmental because only segments of each glomeruli affected
Membranous nephropathy (1–5%)	Associated with hepatitis B and malignancy, e.g. lymphomas

Other types of nephrotic syndrome fall into an overlap pattern with nephritis, where there is marked inflammation in the glomerulus (hence there will be additional features such as red and white cells ± casts in the urine, secondary to inflammation). Unlike uncomplicated nephrotic syndrome, it is rare for the plasma albumin to fall below 20 g/dl in these conditions. Causes include:

- Poststreptococcal glomerulonephritis
- HSP
- Anaphylactoid
- Malaria
- SLE
- Drugs, e.g. penicillamine, and heavy metals

Clinical features

Preceding URTI		
General features	Lethargy, anorexia, diarrhoea	
Hypoalbuminaemia	Oedema:	Periorbital in mornings (first sign, often misdiagnosed as allergy)
		Scrotal, sacral, leg and ankle later in the day
	Ascites	
	Pleural effusions with SOB (uncommon)	
Proteinuria	Frothy urine (rare)	
Hypogammaglobulinaemia	Infections (especially encapsulated organisms [pneumococcus])	
	Abdominal pain, e.g. secondary to peritonitis	
Intravascular hypovolaemia	(Abdominal pain, circulatory collapse or venous thrombosis)	

Initial investigations

Urine	Dipstick for proteinuria (+3 or +4)	
	(May have +3 or +4 blood too because sticks are overly sensitive)	
	Albumin:creatinine ratio (> 200 mg/mmol)	
	Na concentration (< 20 mmol/L is an indication of potential hypovolaemia)	
	Microscopy (0 or minimal cells in uncomplicated nephrotic syndrome; red cells, white cells and casts in glomerulonephritis)	
	Selective protein clearance (research only): IgG (large molecule), albumin (small molecule)	
	Low ratio = selective protein leak. Seen in minimal change disease	
Serum	FBC, PCV, ESR (↑ haematocrit or Hb in hypovolaemia, ↑ ESR and WCC in infection)	
	U&E, creatinine, albumin (< 25 g/L), cholesterol and triglyceride (both ↑)	
	Complement factors C3 and C4 (↓) (not in minimal change)	
	ASOT, anti-DNAse B (streptococcal infection)	
	HBsAg (if membranous GN and from Middle/Far East or at-risk group)	
Throat swab	(Streptotoccal infection)	
Renal biopsy	Only if:	1. No response to steroids after 4–6 weeks, or
		2. Atypical features at presentation, i.e. high creatinine, hypertension, or < 1 year of age

Management

1. Oral corticosteroids – 60 mg/m^2/day (2 mg/kg/day) for 4 weeks (irrespective of when they go into remission, i.e. do not shorten the initial course). Then 40 mg/m^2 alternate days for 4 weeks. If no response to steroids consider renal biopsy
2. Oral penicillin prophylaxis
3. Monitor intravascular volume (see below)
4. Daily weight, electrolytes and albumin and fluid input–output chart
5. Diuretics as needed (in hospital only)
6. Monitor proteinuria at home when recovered to assess for a relapse

Features of intravascular hypovolaemia

Orthostatic hypotension, cool peripheries, oliguria, capillary refill time ↑, abdominal pain, tachycardia, significant core–periphery temperature difference, urine sodium < 20 mmol/L, rising haematocrit.

NB: The BP will not fall in these children until there is severe hypovolaemia due to their compensatory mechanisms; therefore, the above features must be regularly assessed.

Give albumin if hypovolaemic (4.5% albumin if in shock, 20% albumin 0.5–1 g/kg with diuretics over at least 4 h if not in shock).

Complications

- Hypovolaemia (see above)
- Infection: classically pneumococcal peritonitis, although Gram-negative sepsis is becoming commoner due to penicillin prophylaxis. (Due to low immunoglobulins)
- Intravascular thrombosis – renal vein thrombosis and DVT (due to hypovolaemia, hypercoagulable state with a low antithrombin III)
- Hypercholesterolaemia
- Acute tubular necrosis – if severe hypovolaemia

Prognosis

Steroid-sensitive disease: $^1/_3$ resolve with no relapses
$^1/_3$ have occasional relapses
$^1/_3$ have regular relapses

Steroid-resistant disease   Alternative immunosuppressive therapy needed, which may include cyslophosphamide and/or cyclosporin
Up to 50% progress to chronic renal failure

If well, follow-up yearly, checking particularly BP and growth.

CONGENITAL NEPHROTIC SYNDROME

This is the development of nephrotic syndrome presenting antenatally or within the first month after birth.

Causes

Genetic   Various mutations found
Finnish type (nephrin gene defect, autosomal recessive). Gene testing available
Denys–Drash syndrome (WT1 gene mutation)
Post-infective   Congenital syphilis, congenital toxoplasmosis

Clinical features

- Large oedematous placenta
- Proteinuria
- Clinical deterioration with oedema in the first weeks of life due to the increase in GFR (and therefore protein excretion)

Management options

1. Supportive therapy until large enough for renal transplantation (> 10 kg)
2. Reduce the GFR with NSAIDs and ACE inhibitors, then unilateral nephrectomy, or bilateral nephrectomy with dialysis as necessary. Transplant when big enough (> 7–10 kg).

Death may occur from the complications (CRF, peritonitis, respiratory infections and strokes).

GLOMERULONEPHRITIS

This is a term covering several diseases involving **inflammation of the glomerulus**. It is often immune-mediated. There are two major mechanisms of immunological injury:

1. Deposition of circulating antigen–antibody immune complexes (95% of GN)
2. Deposition of antiglomerular basement membrane antibody (anti-GBM, 5% of GN, e.g. Goodpasture syndrome)

HISTOLOGICAL CLASSIFICATION OF GLOMERULAR PATHOLOGY

This may be asked about in exams.

	Histology	Common presentation	Common causes
Predominantly presenting as glomerulonephritis *Proliferative GN*			
Diffuse	Endothelial and mesangial cell proliferation Glomerulus packed with cells. Deposits of C3 and Ig	Acute nephritis	Poststreptococcal
Focal segmental	Some glomeruli normal, some have proliferative changes	Haematuria Proteinuria	Berger, SLE, HSP, shunt nephritis, SABE, PAN
With crescents (rapidly progressive GN)	Crescents (macrophages and epithelial cells) in most glomeruli	Renal failure	Goodpasture, PAN, Wegener
Membranoproliferative (mesangiocapillary, MCGN)	Type I: Mesangial cell proliferation Subendothelial immune complex deposits, BM splitting, C3 ↓, C4 N Type II: Mesangial cell proliferation Intramembranous immune complex deposits C3 stain only	Haematuria, proteinuria Nephritic, nephrotic, CRF	Idiopathic, Shunt nephritis

	Histology	Common presentation	Common causes
Predominantly presenting as nephrotic syndrome			
Membranous GN	Thickening of GBM due to immune deposits	Nephrotic in adults	Idiopathic Penicillamine Hepatitis B SLE, malaria
Minimal change nephropathy NB: Not a true GN	Fusion of podocytes of epithelial cells on EM (normal glomerulus on LM)	Nephrotic in children	Idiopathic
Focal segmental glomerulosclerosis	Glomerulosclerosis	Proteinuria Nephrotic	Idiopathic Diabetes CRF in 50%

ACUTE NEPHRITIC SYNDROME

This has four major characteristics:

- Haematuria
- Proteinuria
- Oliguria
- Volume overload leading to hypertension ($\uparrow$ circulating volume) and oedema ($\uparrow$ extravascular fluid)

Other features are red cell casts and white cells in the urine.

General investigations

Urine	Urinalysis (protein, blood, casts)
	M, C & S (haematuria, proteinuria, casts, features of infection)
Serum	FBC, ESR
	U&E, creatinine, LFTs
	Complement levels (C3 and C4)
	Viral titres and ASOT
	HBsAg, ANA
Throat swab	M, C & S (features of infection)

Management

This is supportive.

1. Fluid restriction – insensible loss (300–400 ml/m^2/day) + urine output
2. Sodium restriction – difficult in children, hence often use 'no added salt' diet
3. Hypertension management, e.g. frusemide to correct volume overload
4. Penicillin if positive throat swab or nephrotic picture, i.e. low albumin
5. Dialysis if necessary, e.g. marked hyperkalaemia

CAUSES OF PROTEINURIA

Proteinuria may be mild or heavy. Microalbuminuria is defined as 20–200 mg/day and is not detectable on dipsticks. Proteinuria may also be detected by measuring the albumin:creatinine ratio on a spot urine (normal = < 0.1).

Physiological	Pathological
Orthostatic, i.e. proteinuria only when standing upright) Exercise induced (transient) Febrile (transient)	Tubular disease: • Hereditary tubular dysfunction • Acquired tubular dysfunction Glomerular disease: • Glomerulonephritis • Nephrotic syndrome Other: • Urinary tract infection • Drugs • Tumours, e.g. lymphoma • Stones

POST-STREPTOCOCCAL GLOMERULONEPHRITIS

Typically this presents as the nephritic syndrome 6–10 days after a Group A β-haemolytic streptococcal URTI or 14–21 days after streptococcal skin infection.

Investigations

General investigations for glomerulonephritis and specifically: anti-streptolysin O titre (ASOT) (positive), anti-DNase B antibodies($\uparrow$), C3($\downarrow$), C4 (N), throat swab (M,C & S). Renal biopsy only if atypical, i.e. severe BP $\uparrow$, rising creatinine.

Management

- 10-day course of penicillin if positive throat swab
- Supportive therapy as for nephritic syndrome (NB: steroids unhelpful)

Prognosis

Spontaneous resolution in > 95%. NB. Haematuria can continue for up to a year, but *not* significant proteinuria.

HENOCH–SCHÖNLEIN PURPURA (HSP)

This is a vasculitic syndrome affecting small vessels. Male > female, 2:1, age 3–10 years. Mostly in late winter and early summer. Often there is a preceding URTI.

Clinical features

The four classical features are **rash**, **joint** involvement, **abdominal pain** and **haematuria**.

Rash	Often the first sign. Vasculitic (macular, becoming purpuric). Typically on buttocks, extensor surfaces of lower limbs and pressure points, e.g. sock line. Recurs over weeks
Joints	Non-destructive arthritis of weight-bearing joints (hips, knees, ankles)
Abdominal pain	Bloody stool due to intussusception. Pancreatitis, ileus, protein-losing enteropathy, GI bleeding from vasculitic Lesions
Haematuria	Secondary to GN
Renal	Glomerulonephritis (focal segmental) in 80%
Oedema	Forehead, genitalia, hands and feet, periarticular
Other organs	CNS, testis, pancreas, parotids, muscles, lungs (haemoptysis)

Renal disease

- Microscopic haematuria in 80%
- Nephritic syndrome
- Nephrotic syndrome

Investigations

- General investigations for nephritic and/or nephrotic syndrome
- ESR ($\uparrow$)
- IgA ($\uparrow$ in > 50%)
- Clotting and platelet screen (may be deranged)

Management

- Treat any suspected infection (particularly streptococcal disease)
- Supportive therapy for arthralgia, rash, fever and malaise
- Renal disease: Standard treatment of nephritis or nephrotic syndrome
  Renal biopsy if severe hypertension or increasing creatinine
  If crescentic disease, plasma exchange is used
- Abdominal disease – early use of steroids has been used for abdominal pain but is controversial and may mask signs of intussusception

Prognosis

Generally good, although 5–10% progress to chronic renal disease. Low albumin is a sign of a poor prognosis.

IGA NEPHROPATHY (BERGER NEPHROPATHY)

This condition is *not* inherited. Male > female, 2:1. A focal segmental glomerulonephritis with IgA deposits in the mesangium.

Clinical features

- Microscopic haematuria
- Macroscopic haematuria *during* infections (NB: not after)

Specific investigations

- Complement (normal C3)
- Serum IgA ($\uparrow$ in 20%)
- Renal biopsy

Management

- No specific therapy
- Follow-up for life essential

Prognosis

- End-stage renal failure develops in 25%
- Poor prognosis is associated with BP $\uparrow$ and proteinuria

SYSTEMIC LUPUS ERYTHEMATOSUS NEPHRITIS

This is a systemic vasculitis with protean manifestations (see p. 000). Renal disease may involve various types of nephritis, classified by the WHO into five classes. They include focal and diffuse disease, and proliferate and membranous disease.

Characteristically both C3 and C4 levels are depressed in active disease, ESR is high and CRP normal. Renal biopsy should be considered if haematuria and proteinuria develop in SLE.

Immunosuppressive therapy (steroids, cyclophosphamide and plasma exchange if necessary) is used in the management.

The renal disease may burn out.

GOODPASTURE DISEASE

Rare before teenage years. This disease may follow a URTI and involves:

- Severe progressive glomerulonephritis
- Pulmonary haemorrhage in smokers (intermittent haemoptysis, anaemia, massive bleeding)
- Antibodies to lung and glomerular basement membrane (GBM)

NB: Goodpasture syndrome is the clinical picture of pulmonary haemorrhage and glomerulonephritis seen in a systemic disorder, e.g. SLE, PAN.

Diagnosis is confirmed by renal biopsy.

Therapies include immunosuppression, pulsed methylprednisolone and plasmapharesis. Patients may die in the acute stage of pulmonary haemorrhage or commonly progress to chronic renal failure.

ALPORT SYNDROME

A hereditary disease of collagen IV (part of the glomerulus basement membrane). X-linked dominant, autosomal dominant or spontaneous mutation (20%). Worse in males.

Clinical features

Hereditary nephritis	Microscopic haematuria (macroscopic with infections), proteinuria, ESRF (by 20–30 years)
Sensorineural deafness	High frequency, progressing to the whole speech range
Ocular defects (15%)	Cataracts, anterior lenticonus, macular lesions

The disease generally presents as haematuria and a young patient may show none of the above features. Parents and siblings of an affected individual should be screened for disease by urine dipstick at least.

Typical '**basket weave**' appearance (splitting of the BM) on electron microscopy of renal biopsy. Anti-GBM nephritis can occur in a transplanted kidney in these patients because of immune reaction to 'normal' collagen IV in the transplant.

CAUSES OF HAEMATURIA

Urinary tract infection	
Glomerulonephritis	Alport syndrome
	IgA nephropathy (Berger)
Congenital malformations	
Trauma	
Haematological	Coagulopathy

	Thrombocytopenia
	Sickle cell disease
	Renal venous thrombosis
Exercise induced	
Drugs	E.g. anticoagulants, aspirin
Renal stones	
Tumours	Renal or urinary tract (both rare)

HAEMOLYTIC URAEMIC SYNDROME (HUS)

The commonest cause of acute renal failure in children in the UK. A potentially life-threatening disease involving:

- Acute renal failure
- Microangiopathic haemolytic anaemia
- Thrombocytopaenia

Causes

Diarrhoea-positive HUS	
E. coli	Verotoxin-producing *Escherichia coli* 0157 (10% of these infections develop into HUS)
Other bacteria	E.g. shigella (shigatoxin), salmonella, campylobacter
Diarrhoea-negative HUS	
Familial	Poor prognosis if presents < 1 year, recurrent episodes. Complement factor H deficiency
Bacteria/viruses	Pneumococcus, coxsackie, echovirus, varicella
Drugs	Cyclosporin (post transplant), oral contraceptive pill
Other	SLE, postpartum

The most common causes are diarrhoea-positive disease and familial, the prognosis of the former being much better. Features and management of diarrhoea-positive disease are outlined.

Clinical features in diarrhoea-positive disease

- Usually < 5 years
- Bloody diarrhoea, may resolve, with 5–10 days later oliguria, pallor, lethargy and petechiae
- NB: Hypertension and hyperkalaemia are major causes of mortality
- Other organ damage – CNS (fits, coma), colitis, pancreatitis
- A high presenting WCC is associated with a poor prognosis

Investigations

Serum	FBC and film (microangiopathic haemolytic anaemia, platelets $\downarrow$)
	Coagulation screen (normal)
	U&E, creatinine, calcium, phosphate (changes of acute renal failure)
Urine	Urinalysis (mild haematuria and mild proteinuria)
Stool	M, C & S

Management

Therapy is supportive, as needed.

Fluid status	Careful assessment – twice daily weights
	Diuretics may be needed
Hyperkalaemia	Salbutamol nebulizers or IV, insulin and dextrose, etc.
Dialysis	

| Transfusions | Blood and rarely platelets |
| Cerebral involvement | Consider plasma exchange |

NB: Long-term follow-up is essential, looking for **hypertension** and **chronic renal failure**.

RENAL VENOUS THROMBOSIS

Causes

Neonate/infant	Asphyxia, dehydration, sepsis, maternal IDDM
	Hypercoagulable state, e.g. protein S or C deficiency, prothrombotic mutations (factor V Leyden)
Older child	Nephrotic syndrome, cyanotic CHD, contrast angiography
	Hypercoagulable state

Clinical features

| Neonate | Gross haematuria and unilateral or bilateral flank masses |
| Older child | Micro/macroscopic haematuria and flank pain |

Bilateral thrombosis will also result in acute renal failure.

Investigations

USS	IVC (to check extension) and renal (renal enlargement)
Radionucleotide imaging	Reduced renal function
Doppler flow studies	
Prothrombotic screen	(Up to half have inherited procoagulant defect)

Differential diagnoses

| Causes of haematuria | IgA nephropathy, Alport syndrome, glomerulonephritis |
| Causes of renal enlargement | Cystic kidneys, Wilms tumour, abscess, haematoma, hydronephrosis |

Management

| Unilateral | Supportive therapy with fluids, electrolyte management and treatment of infection |
| Bilateral | Fibrinolytic agents, e.g. heparin, urokinase, TPA |

Prognosis

The kidney becomes atrophic and should be removed if:

- Hypertension develops
- Repeated UTIs occur

DISORDERS OF TUBULAR FUNCTION

RENAL TUBULAR ACIDOSIS (RTA)

This is a condition of **systemic acidosis** caused by renal tubular dysfunction. Three types of RTA exist: types I, II and IV (type III was reclassified as a variant of type I).

- Types I and II result in a **hypokalaemic** hyperchloraemic metabolic acidosis
- Type IV results in a **hyperkalaemic** hyperchloraemic metabolic acidosis

The urine pH should be measured with a glass electrode within 20 min of collection; dipsticks are not accurate enough.

Ammonium chloride loading can help distinguish between types I and II in mild acidosis by increasing the serum acidification and accentuating the defect (type II *can* then acidify the urine).

Type I – distal RTA

This is due to a **failure of H⁺ excretion** by the distal tubule (and urine pH *cannot* be < 5.5). There is a normal anion gap because chloride is increased to compensate for the acidosis.

Causes

Isolated	Autosomal dominant, autosomal recessive, sporadic	
Secondary	Interstitial nephritis:	Obstructive nephropathy
		Pyelonephritis
		Medullary sponge kidney
		Transplant rejection
		SLE nephritis, Ehlers–Danlos and Marfan syndrome
		Cirrhosis
		Nephrocalcinosis
		Sickle cell nephropathy
	Toxins:	Lithium
		Amphotericin B

Biochemical findings

Serum	$HCO_3 \downarrow$, $K \downarrow$, $Ca \downarrow$, $Cl \uparrow$
Metabolic acidosis	(Normal anion gap)
Urine	pH *cannot* be <5.5
	Hypercalciuria (stones)

Clinical findings

- Growth failure
- Nephrocalcinosis
- Renal stones
- Osteomalacia (no clinical rickets)
- Underlying disease

Management

- Bicarbonate supplements as sodium citrate solution or bicarbonate tablets
- Potassium supplements

Type II – proximal RTA

This is due to a **failure of proximal tubular bicarbonate reabsorption**. The serum bicarbonate falls until the bicarbonate threshold is reached (15–18 mmol/L) where no more HCO_3 loss occurs (because less HCO_3 is filtered and this level can all be reabsorbed distally). Because the distal tubular acidification mechanisms are intact, the urine *can* be acidified (pH 5.5) when there is acidosis or when given ammonium chloride.

Causes

Isolated	Autosomal dominant, sporadic
Secondary	Fanconi syndrome:
	Primary
	Secondary

Biochemical findings

Serum	$HCO_3 \downarrow$, K $\downarrow\downarrow$, Cl $\uparrow$
Metabolic acidosis	*(Anion gap normal)*
Urine	pH may be 5.5
	$HCO_3 \uparrow$

Renal loss of other substances in Fanconi syndrome

Clinical findings

- Growth failure
- Rickets, polyuria, polydipsia (in Fanconi)
- Underlying disease
- No renal calcification

Management

Often more difficult to treat and severe than distal RTA.

- Bicarbonate supplements +++
- Potassium supplements

Type IV

In type IV there is hyperkalaemia plus acidosis secondary to failure of bicarbonate reabsorption ± aldosterone deficiency.

Causes

- Adrenal disorders (A $\downarrow$, R $\uparrow$, renal function N) – Addison, CAH
- Hyporeninaemic hypoaldosteronism (A $\downarrow$, R $\downarrow$, renal function $\downarrow$):   Interstitial nephritis (commonest cause)
  Obstruction
  Pyelonephritis
  Diabetes mellitus

- Pseudohypoaldosteronism (A $\uparrow$, R $\uparrow$) – distal tubule unresponsive

Key: A = aldosterone, R = renin.

Biochemical findings

Serum	K $\uparrow$ Cl $\uparrow$
	Renin $\downarrow$ or $\uparrow$, aldosterone $\downarrow$ or $\uparrow$
Metabolic acidosis (Anion gap normal)	
Urine	Ammonium $\downarrow$
	pH may be <5.5

Clinical findings

Features of:

- Primary renal disease
- Adrenal disease

Management

- Bicarbonate supplements
- Potassium reduction, e.g. diuretics

FANCONI SYNDROME

This is a generalized defect in proximal tubular function. A hyperchloraemic hypokalaemic metabolic acidosis results (a type II proximal RTA).

Causes

Congenital	Acquired
Idiopathic (primary)	Heavy metals
Cystinosis	Drugs
Lowe syndrome	Chemotherapy, e.g. ifosfamide
Galactosaemia	Hyperparathyroidism
Tyrosinaemia type I	Vitamin D deficiency
Hereditary fructose intolerance	Interstitial nephritis
Wilson disease	Glue sniffing
Cytochrome C oxidase deficiency	

Clinical features

- Underlying disease
- Failure to thrive
- Rickets
- Polyuria, polydipsia, dehydration

Investigations

Urine   There is excessive urine loss of: water, i.e. low specific gravity, glucose, amino acids, PO_4, HCO_3, Na, Ca, K, urate

Plasma   Cl ↑, K ↓, PO_4 ↓, hypouricaemia
Metabolic acidosis with normal anion gap

Management

Diagnose and treat underlying disease:

- Rickets – large doses of vitamin D, phosphate supplements
- Acidosis – bicarbonate supplements
- Dehydration – extra salt and water, especially in hot weather

CYSTINOSIS

Autosomal recessive condition due to cystine accumulation in lysosomes of the kidneys, bone marrow, liver, spleen, lymph nodes, leucocytes, cornea and fibroblasts.

Clinical features

Infantile form   Fanconi syndrome from 3 months of age
CRF by 10 years
Blonde hair, fair skin
Photophobia (eye crystals) and decreased acuity
Hypothyroidism, diabetes

Growth retardation
Dementia (later)
Adolescent form   Milder and later-onset renal disease
Adult type   No renal disease

Diagnosis

- Fibroblast or leucocyte cystine concentration ($\uparrow \times 100$)
- Cystine crystals in bone marrow, rectal mucosa, lymph nodes
- Slit-lamp examination of the eyes (corneal cystine crystals)
- Genetic studies – gene analysis if family mutation known

Management

1. Phosphocysteamine (lowers intracellular cystine)
2. Phosphocysteamine eye drops
3. Fanconi treatment
4. Renal transplantation (when in ESRF)

Long-term complications

These include CNS problems, myopathy, swallowing difficulty and pancreatic dysfunction (endo- and exo-crine).

Antenatal diagnosis

- Cystine $\uparrow$ in amniotic fluid cells
- DNA analysis (the gene is now known)

CYSTINURIA

Incidence 1:650. This is an inborn error of reabsorption at the proximal tubule of the dibasic amino acids, resulting in increased renal excretion of them: **c**ystine, **o**rnithine, **a**rginine, **l**ysine (COAL).

NB: There is no systemic amino acid deficiency because they are synthesized in the body.

Clinical features

- None
- Renal stones (< 3% people affected), leading to haematuria, obstruction, CRF

Diagnosis

Urine and stone analysis.

Management

- Alkalinize the urine
- High water intake
- D-penicillamine may help if the above methods are failing

BARTTER SYNDROME

Autosomal recessive. This is a condition of renal potassium wasting with hypokalaemia, alkalosis, aldosterone $\uparrow$, but normal BP. The pathophysiology is defective chloride transport channels (NaK_2Cl – frusemide-sensitive channels) in the ascending limb of the loop of Henle. There are elevated renin and aldosterone levels with juxtaglomerular apparatus (JGA) hyperplasia.

Clinical features

- Growth failure
- Weakness
- Vomiting, constipation
- Polyuria, polydipsia, salt craving
- Dehydration
- Normal BP

Investigations

Serum	K $\downarrow$, Cl $\downarrow$, Mg $\downarrow$, (Na $\downarrow$ in severe cases)
	Ca $\uparrow$
	Metabolic alkalosis
	Aldosterone $\uparrow$, renin $\uparrow$, prostaglandin E$_2$ $\uparrow$ (occasionally)
Urine	Excess K and Cl loss (sometimes Na and Ca loss also)
Renal biopsy	Hyperplasia of JGA

Management

- Oral K supplements
- NaCl supplements
- Indomethacin (reducing the GFR reduces the sodium delivery)

GITELMAN SYNDROME

A similar condition often confused with Bartter syndrome, involving hypomagnesaemia, hypokalaemia and hypo-calciuria, with normal growth. Caused by a defect in thiazide-sensitive NaCl channels in the distal tubule. Treatment includes magnesium supplements.

CONGENITAL STRUCTURAL MALFORMATIONS

DEVELOPMENT OF THE URINARY TRACT AND STRUCTURAL MALFORMATIONS

Normal development of the urogenital tract (nephrogenesis)

Understanding the normal development of the urogenital tract helps in understanding the mechanisms involved in congenital urinary tract abnormalities. Three pairs of 'kidneys' arise sequentially from mesoderm lateral to the spinal cord in early embryogenesis: the pronephros, mesonephros and metanephros. The first two degenerate (although mesonephric structures become incorporated into the male reproductive tract) whilst the metanephros goes on to form the definitive kidney.

Aberrant early development

These are caused by defects in interaction between ureteric bud and metanephric mesenchyme:

- Dysplastic kidneys: mostly sporadic, 10% may have family history. When they have multiple large cysts, these are called multicystic dysplastic kidneys – *not* the same as polycystic (see p. 225)
- Kidney abnormalities as part of sporadic or genetic malformation syndromes, e.g. VATER (Vertebral, Anal, Tracheo-oEsophageal, Renal or Radial anomalies) syndrome or Kallmann syndrome, respectively

Defects in terminal maturation

Early nephron and collecting duct development is normal, but there is later dedifferentiation, i.e. reversal of differentiated state, with cyst formation and loss of normal adjacent structures – polycystic kidney disease (AR or AD) (see p. 225).

DYSPLASTIC KIDNEYS AND RENAL AGENESIS

Renal dysplasia is a histological term: the kidney contains undifferentiated cells and metaplastic structures such as smooth muscle and cartilage.

This is usually due to an early developmental problem leading to aberrant interaction between epithelial cells in the ureteric bud and the surrounding mesenchyme cells. Later, lower urinary tract obstruction can also cause dysplasia (but this is usually less severe since the initial development is normal).

Dysplastic kidneys

- May be large and multicystic, normal size or small
- Initially large kidneys may become small and then disappear *in utero* (= false appearance of **renal agenesis**)
- May be unilateral or bilateral
- Associated with other renal abnormalities, often with obstruction, i.e. atretic ureters or lower urinary tract abnormalities
- Associated with extrarenal abnormalities

If urine flow is reduced bilaterally or completely blocked, it causes the **Potter sequence** of severe oligohydramnios (from any cause), resulting in:

- Pulmonary hypoplasia
- Abnormal facies – wide-spaced eyes, epicanthic folds, broad flat nose, low-set ears, small chin
- Limb abnormalities

Diagnosis

- USS (antenatal or postnatal): Bright hyperechogenic kidneys (large and multicystic kidney disease [MCKD], normal size or small)
  Oligo- or an-hydramnios
- Abdominal mass in newborn
- Later finding (incidental scanning, family scanning, hypertension or renal failure)

	Unilateral dysplasia	Bilateral dysplasia
Incidence	1:3000–5000 births	1:10 000 births
Diagnosis	May be incidental finding prenatal detection variable (depends on severity)	Normally diagnosed *in utero* because decreased liquor volume
Other kidney	Abnormal 30–50% (structural or VUR)	
Other renal anomalies		May be present
Extrarenal anomalies	Less common	More common < 35%
Chromosomal defects	Rare	About 10%
Prognosis	Good *if normal other kidney*:	*Poor* if ↓ liquor, small kidneys

Unilateral dysplasia	Bilateral dysplasia
Slight risk of: • CRF • Tumour in dysplastic kidney • Hypertension Generally involute without problems *If abnormal other kidney*: Increased risk of BP↑, CRF, UTI	(Often die in neonatal period from pulmonary hypoplasia and renal failure) *In less severe disease*: • Chronic failure in long term • Recurrent UTIs • Hypertension

NB: Screen siblings and parents:

• Renal USS (autosomal dominant inheritance of many conditions)
• Diabetes (maternal diabetes associated with renal agenesis, and renal cysts and diabetes syndrome)

POLYCYSTIC KIDNEYS

Polycystic kidney disease is caused by defects in terminal maturation of the renal system, with an initially normal nephron and collecting duct, and later cystic dilatation of these and loss of adjacent normal structures.

Polycystic kidney disease may be recessive (ARPKD) or dominant (ADPKD).

Autosomal recessive polycystic kidney disease (ARPKD)

Gene: fibrocystin on 6p. Incidence 1:40 000 births.

Presentation

In utero   Large hyperechogenic kidneys on USS ± oligohydramnios
At birth   Massive kidneys (abdominal mass)

Clinical features

Renal   Bilateral symmetrical renal enlargement with numerous microscopic corticomedullary cysts
          Gradually develop BP↑ and slow decline in renal function
Liver   Bile duct proliferation, portal fibrosis and portal hypertension
Lungs   Pulmonary hypoplasia ± Potter phenotype

Prognosis

Death in neonatal period (5%) or if survive, reasonable prognosis with slow decline (50% in ESRF by end of childhood).

Autosomal dominant polycystic kidney disease (ADPKD)

Two genes found:

85% PKD1 (polycystin-1), Ch 16p
15% PKD2 (polycystin-2), Ch 4q (milder disease, later onset)

Incidence 1:600, i.e. very common indeed.

Presentation

Late childhood or adulthood with ESRF or hypertension or loin pain, haematuria and renal masses. (Some forms present earlier in childhood or antenatally).

Clinical features

Renal   Bilateral large kidneys with large corticomedullary cysts
                   Hypertension
                   Renal stones, renal neoplasms
                   Chronic renal failure
Other organs Cysts may occur in the liver, pancreas, spleen, ovary
                   Cardiac valve defects
                   Intracerebral arteries (Berry aneurysm)

NB: Prenatal diagnosis of both ARPKD and ADPKD possible with chorionic villous sampling if index case details/mutation known.

DUPLEX KIDNEY

Incidence 1:100 (very common).

Two ureteric buds develop on one side.

ECTOPIC KIDNEY

- The kidney fails to ascend from the pelvis, e.g. pelvic kidney
- Usually normal function as long as the other kidney is normal
- Increased risk of UTI

HORSESHOE KIDNEY

- Aberrant fusion of the two kidneys at the lower poles
- Incidence 1:500
- May also be dysplastic
- Increased incidence of UTI, stones and PUJ obstruction

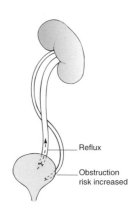

Figure 9.9 Ureteric duplication

HYDRONEPHROSIS

Hydronephrosis is dilatation of the renal pelvis. Relatively common.

May be associated with:

- Reflux (see p. 206)
- Obstruction (see p. 207)
- Renal dysplasia/hypoplasia (see page 224)

NB: Bilateral significant hydronephrosis (> 15 mm) detected antenatally must be investigated urgently since it may indicate lower urinary tact obstruction, such as posterior urethral valves in boys which often needs rapid corrective surgery. There is argument over the size of dilatation that needs full investigation, but > 15 mm definitely does.

BLADDER EXSTROPHY

Incidence 1:40 000 births. Male > female. This condition is very variable in its features and severity. Due to failure of growth of the lower abdominal wall, and a breakdown of the urogenital membrane.

Classical features

- Bladder protrudes from the abdominal wall and its mucosa is exposed
- Pubic rami and recti muscles separated
- Umbilicus displaced downwards
- Epispadias (with undescended testes in boys and clitoral duplication in girls)
- Anteriorly displaced anus, rectal prolapse

The condition results in urinary incontinence, broad-based gait, increased incidence of bladder cancer and sexual dysfunction. Management involves complex surgery.

PRUNE BELLY SYNDROME (EAGLE–BARRETT SYNDROME)

Incidence 1:40 000 births.

An association of:

- Deficient abdominal wall muscles
- Undescended testes
- Urinary tract abnormalities (typically dilated ureters, large bladder, patent urachus)

The condition is thought to be due to severe urethral obstruction early in intrauterine life. Other organ abnormalities may be present.

The infants may have severe oligohydramnios and pulmonary hypoplasia and be stillborn. Of those who survive, 50% develop renal failure from reflux and dysplastic kidneys.

URATE METABOLISM

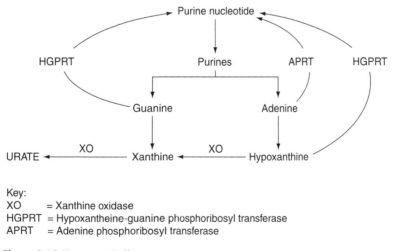

Key:
XO   = Xanthine oxidase
HGPRT = Hypoxantheine-guanine phosphoribosyl transferase
APRT   = Adenine phosphoribosyl transferase

Figure 9.10 Urate metabolism

HYPERURICAEMIA

Urates are poorly soluble and precipitate in the tissues. Joint crystallization causes classic painful gouty arthritis, subcutaneous tissue precipitation results in gouty tophi (ears, bursae, tendons). Plasma urate is usually normal during acute gout attacks. Kidney precipitation causes renal stones and disease.

Causes

Synthesis ↑	Primary gout
Turnover ↑	Tumour lysis syndrome
	Psoriasis
	Starvation
	Polycythaemia
Excretion ↓	Renal dysfunction
	Thiazide diuretics
	Acidosis
	Low-dose salicylates
	Glycogen storage disease type 1
	G6PD deficiency

Management

Acute	High fluid intake, then colchicine and NSAIDs if necessary
Chronic	XO inhibitors, e.g. allopurinol
	Uricosuric drugs, e.g. probenicid, high-dose salicylates

LESCH–NYHAN SYNDROME

X-linked recessive. This is a condition where purines cannot be recycled due to a deficiency of HGPRT, with consequent raised uric acid levels. It results in mental deficiency, self-mutilation, gouty tophi and arthritis, athetosis and spasticity.

XANTHINURIA

Autosomal recessive, uncommon. This condition of XO deficiency results in decreased plasma urates and xanthine renal stones because xanthine is insoluble in acid urine.

HYPERTENSION

This is persistent elevation of BP (systolic or diastolic) > 95th centile and is present in 1–3% of children.

Causes

Essential	(Rare in children, v. common in adults)
Secondary	Renal – parenchymal disease or renal vascular disease
	Cardiovascular – coarctation, renal artery stenosis
	Hormonal – Cushing syndrome, phaeochromocytoma, CAH
	Drugs, e.g. steroids

Clinical features

- Usually asymptomatic
- May have headaches and blurred vision if severe
- Examine for renal masses and bruits, coarctation and eye changes (papilloedema, retinal haemorrhages)

Investigations

Renal	Urinalysis, M, C & S
	U&E, creatinine, Ca, PO_4, FBC
	Renal USS with Doppler studies, renal function tests, e.g. DMSA

Cardiovascular	Echocardiogram, ECG, fasting lipids
Hormonal	Urine HVA and HMA, oxysteroids, 24-h cortisol
	Plasma renin, aldosterone, cortisol, 21-β-hydroxylase
Ophthalmological examination	

Management options

Emergency	Nifedipine:	Oral (not sublingual, which can cause precipitant fall)
	Sodium nitroprusside:	Infusion with care to avoid precipitious BP fall
	Labetalol:	Infusion with care
Long-term	Treat underlying cause	
	Drug therapy, e.g. vasodilators, diuretics, β-blockers, ACE inhibitors	

RENAL FAILURE

This is a failure to maintain adequate fluid and pH balance due to renal insufficiency. Other features include impaired erythropoietin production, impaired vitamin D hydroxylation and hypertension.

ACUTE RENAL FAILURE

Causes

These may be **prerenal** due to local or general circulatory failure, **renal** due to renal parenchymal damage or **postrenal** due to outflow obstruction. Prerenal will convert to intrinsic renal failure if not promptly treated.

Prerenal	Renal	Postrenal
Circulatory failure:	HUS	Bilateral obstruction, e.g. congenital such as PUV, stones
Hypovolaemic (burns, haemorrhage, dehydration)	GN, e.g. HSP, post-streptococcal	
	Interstitial nephritis	Neurogenic bladder
	Drugs, e.g. anticancer	Trauma
Septic	Pyelonephritis	
Cardiac	Vasculitis	
Renal artery or vein occlusion	Myoglobinuria	
	Tumour lysis syndrome	
	Untreated prerenal failure progressing to ATN	

Clinical features

Acute renal failure (ARF) presents as oliguria (< 1 ml/kg/h or 300 ml/m^2/day) with oedema, hypertension, vomiting, lethargy, electrolyte disturbance and metabolic acidosis. (NB. Oliguria is 0.5 ml/kg/h in neonates.)

Acute tubular necrosis (ATN)

This is the most common pathophysiological finding in established ARF. It is the result of ischaemic tubular damage secondary to hypoperfusion.

Oliguria   Initially
Polyuria   During the recovery phase

The prognosis for full renal recovery is good, though it depends on the severity of the underlying cause.

Acute cortical necrosis (ACN)

Cortical necrosis is irreversible loss of renal function with glomerular damage that heals with scarring (glomerulo-sclerosis). Any cause of ATN, if severe, can lead to ACN.

Criteria to distinguish prerenal from renal causes

	Prerenal	Renal
Urine osmolality (mosmol/L)	> 500	< 350
Urine Na (mmol/L)	< 20	> 40
Urine specific gravity	> 1.020	< 1.010
Urine:plasma urea ratio	> 4.1	< 4.1
Urine:plasma osmo ratio	> 1.2	< 1.2
Fractional excretion filtered Na	< 1%	> 1%

(The normal response in normal kidneys is to retain sodium and water if the BP or renal perfusion falls.)

Management

Fluids	In oliguric phase, restrict to insensible loss (300 ml/m^2/day) + ongoing losses
	In polyuric phase, maintain input and electrolytes (as above)
	Twice daily weights, regular electrolytes
Hyperkalaemia	An emergency if ECG changes are present (see below)
Hyperphosphataemia	Give a phosphate binder, e.g. calcium carbonate
Hypocalcaemia	Give calcium and 1-α calcidol
Metabolic acidosis	Give bicarbonate. Give dialysis if no response and pH < 7.25
Hypertension	Correct for fluid overload, antihypertensives
Nutrition	Restrict protein, K, Na and PO$_4$
Anaemia	Transfuse as necessary (but watch K carefully)
Dialysis	Indicated if severe hyperkalaemia, hyponatraemia, metabolic acidosis, fluid overload, symptomatic uraemia or medical management not tolerated

Management of hyperkalaemia

Drug	Onset	Mechanism
10% calcium gluconate	Immediate	Stabilizes cardiac membrane
Salbutamol (nebulized or IV)	Few min	Shifts potassium into cells
8.4% NaHCO$_3$ (IV)	Few min	Shifts potassium into cells
Fluid bolus with frusemide (IV)	Minutes	Renal excretion of potassium
Glucose (I ± insulin)	30 min	Shifts potassium into cells
Calcium resonium (oral or rectal)	30 min (rectal) 2 h (oral)	Potassium excretion through gut
Dialysis	Rapid (haemodialysis) Slower (peritoneal)	Removes potassium

CHRONIC RENAL FAILURE

This occurs with decline in renal function over months or years.

Causes

- Congenital malformations
- Glomerulonephritis
- Inherited nephropathy
- Systemic illness

Clinical features

- Malaise
- Growth failure
- Polyuria, nocturia, oliguria (if late or acute on chronic), proteinuria
- Uraemia, itching, anorexia, nausea, vomiting, skin colour change, polyneuropathy (paraesthesia), restless legs syndrome, myoclonic twitching, mental slowing, coma. Rare in children
- Symptoms of anaemia
- Oedema (peripheral and pulmonary)
- Renal bone disease (osteodystrophy – renal rickets)

Investigations

Urine	Urinalysis, M, C & S, osmolality
	24-h electrolytes and protein
Plasma	U&E, creatinine ($\uparrow$), phosphate ($\uparrow$), ionized calcium ($\downarrow$), bicarbonate ($\downarrow$), PTH ($\uparrow$)
	FBC and film (anaemia)
Radiology	Left wrist X-ray (bone age and osteodystrophy), renal USS, renal function tests
GFR	Estimate from creatinine or measure formally ($\downarrow$)

Management

Diet	High energy, low protein (<1.5 g/kg/day) (controversial as children need to grow)
	NG or gastrostomy feeds may be needed (nausea)
Osteodystrophy	Manifest as PO_4 $\uparrow$, Ca $\downarrow$ and secondary hyperparathyroidism
	Aim is for the PTH to be in the normal range
	Use dietary phosphate restriction
	Calcium carbonate (lowers PO_4)
	Vitamin D supplements (1-α-OH-cholecalciferol)
Sodium and acidosis	Sodium supplements (unless low urine output)
	Bicarbonate supplements (2 mmol/kg/day)
Anaemia	Erythropoietin therapy (subcutaneous)
Hormones	GH if growth fails to improve with optimal nutrition
Dialysis	
BP $\uparrow$	Diuretics, nifedipine, β-blockers, etc

DIALYSIS

This is necessary in **end-stage renal failure (ESRF)**. There are two methods.

Peritoneal dialysis

Peritoneal membrane used as a semi-permeable membrane. The **dialysate** is run through a tube into the peritoneal cavity and the fluid changed regularly to repeat the process.

- CAPD (continuous ambulatory peritoneal dialysis); 2–4 cycles/day done manually
- CCPD (continuous cycling peritoneal dialysis); dialysis occurs only at night with 8–12 cycles done by machine

Major complication is peritonitis.

Haemodialysis

This is technically more difficult. Access is obtained using an indwelling main venous catheter (most common in children) or by creating an A-V fistula. Blood is directed through the dialysis machine where the semi-permeable membrane is located. Performed on average three times per week for 3–4 h per session. Complications: line infections and sepsis.

RENAL TRANSPLANTATION

This is a preferred option to dialysis as lifestyle is markedly improved.

Transplant	Cadaveric or live related donor kidney (HLA-matched)
	In the iliac fossa (attached to the common iliac vessels)
	Intra-abdominally in a small child
Immunosuppression	See below
Complications	Rejection (acute or chronic)
	Infection (CMV, varicella)
	Hypertension
	Drug side-effects (see below)
	Post-transplant tumours, e.g. post-transplant lymphoproliferative disease (PTLD) which is EBV driven

Common side-effects of immunosuppressant drugs in renal transplantation

Cyclosporin	Tacrolimus	Azathioprine	Mycophenolate mofetil
Gum hyperplasia	GI upset	Myelosuppression	Nausea and vomiting
Hypertrichosis		Hepatotoxicity	
Nephrotoxicity			

FURTHER READING

Avner ED, Harmon W, Niaudet P *Pediatric Nephrology*, 5th edn. Baltimore: Williams & Wilkins, 2003

Webb NJA, Posthlethwaite RJ *Clinical Paediatric Nephrology*, 3rd edn. Oxford: Oxford University Press, 2003

10

Endocrinology, growth and puberty

- *Hypothalamus and pituitary*
- *Adrenal glands*
- *Thyroid gland*
- *Parathyroid glands*
- *Polycystic ovary syndrome*
- *Glucose metabolism*
- *Pancreatic tumours*

- *Endocrine syndromes*
- *Growth*
- *Puberty*
- *Sexual differentiation syndromes – ambiguous genitalia*
- *Endocrine tests*

HYPOTHALAMUS AND PITUITARY

PHYSIOLOGY

The anterior lobe of the pituitary develops from Rathke's pouch from an invagination of the oral endoderm. The posterior pituitary is part of a single functional unit called the neurohypophysis which comprises the neurons of the hypothalamus, the neuronal axons (the pituitary stalk) and the neuronal terminals in the posterior lobe of the pituitary.

PITUITARY TUMOURS

Pituitary tumours constitute an important cause of pituitary disease, and they include the following conditions:

- Craniopharyngioma
- Cushing syndrome (see p. 239)
- Non-functioning tumour
- Prolactinoma
- Pituitary gigantism
- Nelson syndrome

Clinical features

They present with symptoms of one or both of:

1. Space-occupying lesion:
   - Raised intracranial pressure symptoms and signs such as headache, papilloedema, vomiting

233

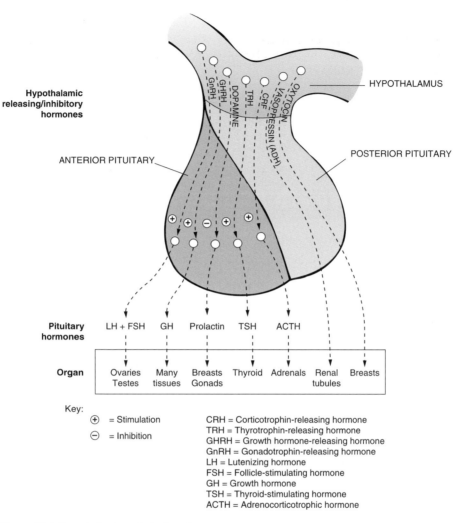

Figure 10.1 Hypothalamic and pituitary hormones

- Visual field defects (bitemporal hemianopia)
- Hydrocephalus (if CSF flow is interrupted)
- Pressure on hypothalamic centres (appetite, thirst, somnolence/wakefulness, precocious puberty)
- Cavernous sinus thrombosis (III, IV, VI cranial nerve lesions)
- Diencephalic syndrome
2. Hormonal excess or deficiency

Examination and investigations

The following should be performed:

- Visual field testing
- Cranial nerve testing
- MRI or CT scan
- Hormonal investigations (showing a deficiency or an excess)

Treatment is with drugs, radiotherapy and/or surgery.

CRANIOPHARYNGIOMA

This is one of the most common supratentorial tumours in children. It arises from a remnant of the connection between Rathke's pouch and the oral cavity. It is often large and cystic and 50% occur under the age of 20 years. Calcification is seen in most cases on skull X-ray.

Presentation

- Headaches, visual field defects and hydrocephalus (compression of the third ventricle)
- Hormonal effects of hypopituitarism: Growth failure, pubertal delay
  Diabetes insipidus
  Hypothyroidism (due to TH deficiency)
  Adrenocortical deficiency (due to ACTH deficiency)

Essential examination and investigations are as above for pituitary tumours.

Treatment

This is with surgical removal (transfrontal or transsphenoidal). Postoperative radiotherapy is used if resection is incomplete or recurrence occurs. Postoperative hormonal deficiency is common and is treated with supplementation as necessary.

PITUITARY GIGANTISM

This is a very rare condition and usually caused by an acidophil adenoma of the pituitary producing excess growth hormone (very rarely due to excessive GHRH). The tumours are mostly microadenomas and most skull X-rays are normal. If the epiphyses are open, pituitary gigantism results, and if they are closed, acromegaly results.

Presentation

- Space-occupying effects
- Hormonal effects: Rapid growth, delayed epiphyseal fusion and eventual tall stature
  Hypogonadism and delayed sexual maturation
  Hypopituitarism (partial or complete of the anterior pituitary), hyperprolactinaemia
  Diabetes mellitus

Essential examination and investigations

As for pituitary tumours. Specific hormonal tests are:

- GH levels ($\uparrow$)
- Glucose tolerance test (fail to suppress GH, 25% have a diabetic result)
- Insulin-like growth factor (IGF-1) levels $\uparrow$
- Prolactin levels (may be raised)
- Pituitary function tests (anterior pituitary)

Treatment

- Surgery
- Radiotherapy
- Octreotride (a somatostatin analogue)
- Bromocriptine

PROLACTINOMA

This is the most common pituitary tumour that occurs in adolescence. They are mostly large tumours (macroadenoma) but may be small (microadenoma, < 10 mm) producing excess prolactin. They are mostly post-pubertal and are twice as common in girls.

Presentation

- Space-occupying effects (headache, visual field defects, nausea, vomiting)
- Hormonal effects: Galactorrhoea, amenorrhoea
Hypogonadism, impotence, delayed puberty
Hypopituitarism

Investigations are those of pituitary tumours in general, plus serum prolactin level. Prolactin levels are usually grossly elevated (> 2000 ng/ml).

Treatment

- Medical (bromocriptine or carbagoline)
- Surgical removal of tumour

Other causes of hyperprolactinaemia

- Stress
- Primary hypothyroidism
- Hypothalamic disease (acromegaly, craniopharyngioma)
- Polycystic ovaries
- Drugs (cimetidine, metoclopramide, oestrogens, opiates)
- Pregnancy, suckling
- Liver failure, cardiac failure, renal failure

HYPOPITUITARISM

This can be a deficiency of either hypothalamic or pituitary hormones. It may also be selective or multiple, with growth hormone being the most common hormone affected. Panhypopituitarism is the deficiency of all anterior pituitary hormones. Vasopressin (ADH) and oxytocin will only be affected significantly if the hypothalamus is involved or there is a very large pituitary lesion.

Causes

Congenital	Septo-optic dysplasia (absence of septum pellucidum and optic nerve hypoplasia)
	Kallman syndrome
	Genetic deficiency of GHRH or GH (several types)
	Empty sella syndrome
	Holoprosencephaly, anencephaly
Destructive	Neoplastic (pituitary/hypothalamic, e.g. craniopharyngioma, meningioma, glioma, secondary deposits)
	Infective (meningitis, encephalitis, TB, toxoplasmosis)
	Traumatic (post surgery or radiotherapy, NAI, traumatic delivery)
	Infiltration (Langerhans' cell histiocytosis, haemochromatosis, sarcoidosis)
Functional	Emotional deprivation, anorexia nervosa, starvation

Clinical features

These are dependent on the extent of the disease. Growth hormone deficiency is the most common, resulting in growth failure. Secondary hypothyroidism and adrenal insufficiency (secondary to TSH and ACTH deficiency, respectively) may be present. Hyperprolactinaemia, diabetes insipidus and deficiency of gonadotrophins may also be present.

If congenital, it may present as an emergency with apnoea, hypoglycaemia and cyanosis, and male infants may have a microphallus. The child has a distinctive facies. When long-standing, there is 'alabaster skin' which is pale and hairless. Sexual maturation is delayed or absent and symptomatic hypoglycaemia with fasting occurs in 10–15%.

Investigations

Pituitary function tests need to be done.

Treatment

This involves treating any underlying disease and replacing hormones as necessary.

DIABETES INSIPIDUS

This is characterized by polyuria and polydipsia and is due to a *deficiency* of vasopressin (ADH) (**cranial diabetes insipidus**) or a *renal insensitivity* to it (**nephrogenic diabetes insipidus**).

Clinical features

- Polydipsia, polyuria, nocturia
- Anorexia, dehydration, lack of perspiration and production of large quantities of pale urine
- Rapid weight loss, constant wet nappies and collapse in infants

Investigations

These show a *mismatch* between urine and plasma osmolalities.

1. **Osmolalities:**
2. Plasma osmolality normal or high, and plasma Na high
   Urine osmolality low: EMU osmolality < 280 (normal > 700)
   Specific gravity 1.001–1.005
2. **Formal water deprivation test:**
   Deprive patient of water until either a mismatch between urine and plasma osmolality is demonstrated or >5% weight loss or urine osmolality > 700 mmol/kg
   Observe failure to concentrate urine; then give DDAVP and observe a rise in urine osmolality
3. A failure of response to exogenous ADH (DDAVP) indicates nephrogenic diabetes insipidus
4. Plasma ADH measurement is possible, and if inappropriately low for plasma osmolality indicates cranial DI
5. Cranial MRI scan

Causes

Cranial		Nephrogenic	
Congenital	Autosomal dominant	*Congenital*	X-linked recessive
	DIDMOAD	*Renal tubule*	Renal tubular acidosis
Newborn	Asphyxia, IVH	*Other*	Nephrocalcinosis
	Listeria, meningitis	*Metabolic*	Hypokalaemia

Cranial		Nephrogenic	
Infection	TB meningitis	*Drugs*	Demeclocycline, glibenclamide, lithium
Tumour	Craniopharyngioma		
Infiltration	Langerhans cell histiocytosis Sarcoidosis		
Ablation	Surgery, cranial DXT		
DIDMOAD = diabetes insipidus, diabetes mellitus, optic atrophy and deafness. Also known as Wolfram syndrome			

Treatment

Cranial diabetes insipidus   DDAVP (desmopressin = ADH analogue) intranasal, oral or IM
Nephrogenic diabetes insipidus Sensitize the renal tubules with thiazides, carbamazepine or chloramphenicol

NB: If initial MRI is normal, it should be repeated at 5-yearly intervals, as anatomical detection of a tumour may be delayed by many years.

Differential diagnosis

- Psychogenic polydipsia (compulsive water drinking). Here the urine will concentrate on water deprivation testing; however, there may be a decreased ability to concentrate urine if the condition is prolonged
- Water intoxication (fictitious or induced illness)

SYNDROME OF INAPPROPRIATE ADH SECRETION (SIADH)

In this condition plasma levels of ADH are *inappropriately high* for the osmolality of the blood.

Clinical features

- Often vague features
- Appetite loss (early), nausea, vomiting, confusion, irritability, fits and coma
- No evidence of dehydration, no oedema, normal blood pressure

Investigations

Plasma   Electrolytes: Na $\downarrow$ (115–120 mmol/L), Cl $\downarrow$
                           Bicarbonate (N)
           Osmolality low (< 280 mmol/L)
           Hypouricaemia
Urine   Osmolality normal
           Na > 30 mmol/L, i.e. sodium excretion continues

Causes

CNS   Meningitis, encephalitis, brain abscess, head injury, birth asphyxia, hypoxic–ischaemic encephalopathy, IVH, subdural haematoma, SLE vasculitis, brain tumour, Guillain–Barré syndrome
Tumours   Lymphoma, cancer of the thymus, Ewing sarcoma
Lungs   Pneumonia, cystic fibrosis, IPPV, lung abscess
Metabolic Acute intermittent porphyria
Drugs   Carbamazepine, vincristine, cyclophosphamide, chlorpropramide, morphine
Infections Rotavirus, TB

Treatment

1. Fluid restrict
2. Daily weight, sodium and osmolality measurements
3. Demeclocycline (dimethylchlortetracycline) therapy to desensitize the kidney
4. If severe: hypertonic saline with furosemide is given under close observation

ADRENAL GLANDS

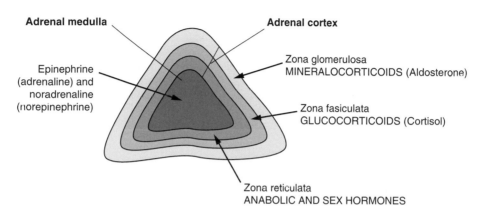

Figure 10.2 Adrenal gland

Glucocorticoid axis

Relative strength of glucocorticoids	
Cortisol (hydrocortisone)	1
Prednisolone	4
Dexamethasone	25

CUSHING SYNDROME

This results from a state of increased circulating glucocorticoids.

Causes

ACTH dependent   Pituitary tumour (basophilic adenoma (20%) or microadenoma (80%)). NB. This is **Cushing disease**

Ectopic ACTH production (extremely rare)

ACTH independent   Adrenal adenoma or carcinoma (most often < age 5 years)

Exogenous steroids – the *commonest* cause

Clinical features

- Appearance: Round face, large red cheeks – 'moon face'

        Truncal obesity – 'buffalo hump', 'lemon on sticks'

Striae and bruises due to protein breakdown

Masculinization signs due to androgen production (acne, hirsuitism and clitoral hypertrophy)

- Growth impairment
- Pubertal delay
- Weakness, headache, mental disturbance
- Impaired glucose tolerance, diabetes (glycosuria)
- Hypertension
- Osteoporosis
- Hyperpigmentation – seen with high ACTH only

Investigations

These are divided into those investigations to establish the *diagnosis* and those to establish the *cause* of Cushing syndrome. NB: Random cortisol is of *no* benefit.

Diagnosis	Underlying cause
1. Serum – Na ↑, K ↓, alkalosis	1. ACTH level:
2. Cortisol circadian rhythm: – 08:00 and 24:00 cortisol – Normal = low at midnight and high in the morning – Cushing = high midnight levels	< 10 ng/L = ACTH independent 20–80 ng/L = normal/high in ACTH dependent > 100 ng/L = high in ectopic ACTH
3. Urine 24 h free cortisol (↑)	2. Low and high-dose dexamethasone suppression tests
4. Overnight dexamethasone suppression test	3. CRF test (exaggerated ACTH response = pituitary-dependent **Cushing disease**)
	4. Adrenal CT scan
	5. Pituitary MRI scan

Treatment

The options available include surgical removal of a pituitary lesion, radiotherapy to the pituitary, resection of adrenal adenoma and reduction of exogenous steroids where possible. Medical therapy with inhibitors of adrenal steroid biosynthesis, e.g. ketoconazole.

NB: **Nelson syndrome** is the occurrence of a pituitary tumour many years after bilateral adrenalectomy, causing high ACTH levels and hyperpigmentation. It is very rare.

PRIMARY HYPERALDOSTERONISM

This is due to an adenoma of the zona glomerulosa in 60% of cases (known as **Conn syndrome**) and an adrenal cortical carcinoma in a minority. Approximately 30% are due to bilateral adrenal hyperplasia (secondary aldosteronism).

Secondary aldosteronism has several causes:

- Ascites – nephrotic syndrome, liver cirrhosis, CCF
- Hypovolaemia secondary to diuretic abuse
- Renal artery stenosis
- Wilms tumour

Clinical features

- Proximal muscle weakness, polyuria, polydipsia, nocturnal enuresis (all due to hypokalaemia)
- Hypertension with no oedema (due to hypernatraemia)

Investigations

- Plasma electrolytes – K $\downarrow$ Na $\uparrow$, metabolic alkalosis (20% have normal K at presentation)
- Plasma renin $\downarrow$ (NB: Secondary aldosteronism–renin $\uparrow$)
- Urine aldosterone metabolites
- Urine Na:K ratio $\downarrow$ (normal = 2:1 mmol/kg/24 h)

Treatment options

- Prednisolone (suppresses the hyperaldosteronism)
- Spironolactone (aldosterone antagonist)
- Surgical resection

ADRENOCORTICAL INSUFFICIENCY

This is deficiency of all the adrenal cortical hormones, but cortisol causes the main effects.

Causes

Acute	Sudden steroid withdrawal
	Birth asphyxia
	Severe hypotension (causing adrenal infarction)
	Sepsis (e.g. **Waterhouse–Freidrichson syndrome** of adrenal haemorrhage secondary to meningococcaemia)
	Trauma
Chronic	Primary (ACTH $\uparrow$):
	• Congenital adrenal hyperplasia
	• Destruction of adrenal cortex (**Addison disease**), due to autoimmune disease or TB
	• Leukaemia, HIV infection
	• Drugs, e.g. ketoconazole
	• Adrenoleukodystrophy (adrenocortical insufficiency, with demyelination in CNS)
	Secondary (ACTH $\downarrow$):
	• Pituitary or hypothalamic disease
	• Long-term steroid therapy

Clinical features

Acute disease	Presents as an **adrenal crisis:** drowsiness and coma, peripheral shutdown, cyanosis, tachycardia, tachypnoea, hypotension. Fatal if not rapidly treated
Chronic disease	
Baby	Apathy, drowsiness, vomiting, faltering growth, hypoglycaemia and dehydration leading to eventual circulatory collapse and coma
Older child	Weakness, fatigue, anorexia, nausea, vomiting, abdominal pain, diarrhoea and faltering growth (except in congenital adrenal hyperplasia where height velocity is increased due to excessive androgen production)
	Postural hypotension and salt craving.
	Hyperpigmentation of buccal mucosa, skin creases and scars occur (with primary disease secondary to ACTH $\uparrow$)

Investigations

Serum electrolytes	Na ↓, K ↑, glucose ↓
Serum hormones	Cortisol ↓
	ACTH ↑ (primary disease)
Synacthen test	Short and long if necessary

Treatment

Adrenal crisis	IV fluids and salt replacement
	Hydrocortisone IV
	Antibiotics if necessary
Long-term therapy	Daily hydrocortisone and fludrocortisone

PHAEOCHROMOCYTOMA

This is a sympathetic nervous system tumour arising from chromaffin cells, secreting catecholamines. Mostly noradrenaline is released but some adrenaline is also released. Males > females 2:1. Very rare.

- 90% adrenal medulla tumour
- 10% along the sympathetic chain
- 25% multiple
- 10% malignant
- 10% recur

Associations	MEN II
	Neurofibromatosis

Differential diagnosis

- Autoimmune disease
- Renal artery stenosis

Clinical features

The symptoms are frequently intermittent.

General	Palpitations, sweating, tremor, headaches, panic attacks, nausea and vomiting, weight loss
Cardiovascular instability	Tachycardia, bradycardia, hypertension, orthostatic hypotension

Investigations

1. 24-h urine catecholamines increased (vanillymandelic acid [VMA] and metanephrins). NB: Dietary vanilla interferes with this test
2. MIBG scan (metaiodobenzylguanidine – a specific chromaffin tissue isotope scan)
3. Abdominal CT scan
4. Serum catecholamines

Management

Surgical resection of the tumour under α (phenoxybenzamine) and β (propranolol) blockade.

THYROID GLAND

PHYSIOLOGY

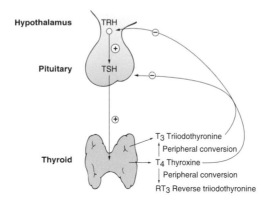

Figure 10.3 Thyroid axis

In plasma 99% of T4 and T3 is bound to thyroid binding globulin (TBG), and thyroid binding pre-albumin (TBPA) and albumin. Only the free form is active; 0.05% is in the free active form.

In acute or chronic illness, thyroid function is affected, with RT3 ↑, TBG ↓, TSH ↓. This results in low total and free T4 and T3 with a normal or low TSH, known as **sick euthyroid syndrome**.

Thyroxine (T4) and antithyroid drugs cross the placenta.

GUTHRIE TEST FOR HYPOTHYROIDISM

This is a measurement of TSH, taken as a capillary blood sample on day 6. An elevated level (> 5–10 mU/L) is abnormal and indicative of hypothyroidism. False-negative results occur with:

- Prematurity or sick euthyroid syndrome
- TBG deficiency (congenital or acquired)
- Secondary or tertiary hypothyroidism

Grossly elevated levels of TSH are most likely due to severe congenital hypothyroidism. Mildly elevated TSH levels (5–20 mU/L) in the presence of normal free T4 levels require close monitoring as they may represent transient hyper-thyrotropinaemia.

If the result is repeatedly equivocal (TSH 20–30 mU/L), thyroxine should be commenced and at a later date the thyroid function reassessed with a repeat TSH measurement and thyroid imaging.

HYPOTHYROIDISM

Causes

Primary   (Thyroid gland dysfunction – TSH ↑, thyroxine ↓)
Congenital
Atrophic autoimmune thyroiditis (thyroid microsomal antibodies)
Hashimoto thyroiditis (goitre and microsomal antibodies, associated with Turner syndrome)
Iodine deficiency (goitre, occurs in mountainous areas)

Treatment of hyperthyroidism or radiotherapy for lymphoma or leukaemia

Drugs – amiodarone, iodine-containing medications

Secondary or   (TSH ↓, thyroxine ↓)
tertiary   Pituitary disease (secondary)

Hypothalamic disease (tertiary)

Congenital hypothyroidism

Incidence 1:4000.

Causes

Thyroid dysgenesis (90%)	Aplasia ($^1/_3$)
	Ectopic ($^2/_3$) – lingual, sublingual or subhyoid thyroid
Dyshormonogenesis (8%)	(Inborn error of thyroid hormone production), e.g. Pendred syndrome (goitre, sensorineural deafness and hypothyroidism)
Transient disease	Due to placental transfer of antithyroid antibodies (maternal autoimmune thyroid disease) or antithyroid drugs

Diagnosis usually on Guthrie test with elevated TSH, confirmed with low serum T4.

Clinical features

Physical features	Macroglossia, wide-spaced eyes, flat nasal bridge, swollen eyelids, large fontanelles, dry skin, umbilical hernia, short broad fingers
Other	Hypotonia, somnolence, feeding difficulties, hoarse cry, noisy breathing, apnoeas, constipation, distended abdomen, dry skin, cutis marmorata, ± goitre (20%)
	Bradycardia, cardiomegaly, cardiac murmurs, low-voltage ECG with prolonged PR interval
	Prolonged neonatal jaundice (unconjugated)
	Mental retardation

Clinical features of acquired hypothyroidism

NB: Thyroid dysgenesis and ectopic thyroid can present later, as acquired.

- Deceleration of growth
- Delayed ossification
- Skin and hair – dry skin, lateral third eyebrow missing, hair dry and thin
- Cold intolerance
- Low energy levels
- Constipation
- Proximal myopathy, ataxia, slow reflexes
- Mental slowness at school often occurs late
- Headaches, precocious puberty and galactorrhoea (seen in secondary and tertiary disease)

Investigations

Thyroid function tests are performed and enable differentiation of primary from secondary and tertiary disease. Other abnormalities seen on blood testing are hypercalcaemia, hypercholesterolaemia and hyperprolactinaemia.

Treatment

This is with thyroxine replacement, giving oral thyroxine 10–15 µg/kg/day.

HYPERTHYROIDISM

Causes

Graves disease	Most common childhood cause
	TSH receptor antibodies (TRSAb – thyrotrophin receptor stimulating antibodies) cause thyroid hormone production
	Diffuse toxic goitre
	Thyroid eye signs (see below) and pretibial myxoedema (occur only in Graves disease)
	Female > male 5:1. HLA-B8, DW3 association
	Autoimmune association (vitiligo, IDDM, RhA, ITP, Addison)
Transient neonatal	Secondary to transplacental antibody transfer in maternal Graves disease, lasts 6–12 weeks
Solitary nodule/adenoma	Plummer disease, toxic uninodular goitre
de Quervain thyroiditis	Acute disease with tender goitre
	Viral origin (mumps, coxsackie, adenovirus)
Reidel thyroiditis	Dense thyroid fibrosis including neck vessels and trachea
Thyrotoxicosis facticia	Ingestion of thyroxine
Tumours	Ovarian teratoma, choriocarcinoma, hydatidiform mole

Clinical features

Usually of gradual onset.

Neurological	Hyperactivity, emotional lability, short attention span
Gastrointestinal	Increased appetite with no weight gain
Skin	Smooth skin, increased sweating, tremor
General	Goitre (usually), heat intolerance
Cardiovascular	Tachycardia, palpitations, dyspnoea, hypertension, cardiomegaly, atrial fibrillation (rare)
Eye signs	Exophthalmos, lid retraction, lid lag, impaired convergence, ophthalmoplegia

Thyroid crisis

This is acute-onset hyperthyroidism and presents as tachycardia, hypertension and restlessness, progressing to delirium, coma and death if not rapidly treated.

Neonatal hyperthyroidism

These babies are classically premature, have IUGR, goitres, exophthalmos, microcephaly. They are irritable, hyperalert and may have tachycardia, tachypnoea, hyperthermia, jaundice, hypertension and progress to cardiac decompensation.

Investigations

1. Free T4 and T3 elevated
2. TSH decreased
3. TRS Abs found in Graves disease

Treatment options

Medical	Antithyroid drugs (propylthiouracyl or carbimazole) or radioactive iodine
	Symptomatic control with β-blockers (propranolol)
Surgery	Subtotal thyroidectomy
	Complications – hypoparathyroidism (transient or permanent), vocal cord paralysis

GOITRE

Goitre is an enlargement of the thyroid gland.

Child may be euthyroid, hypothyroid or hyperthyroid.

Causes

Congenital	Dyshormonogenesis
	Congenital hyperthyroidism
	Maternal antithyroid drugs (hypothyroid usually)
	Maternal iodine-containing drugs, e.g. amiodarone (hypothyroid usually)
	Iodine deficiency (rare)
	Thyroid teratoma
Older child	Colloid goitre (euthyroid, unknown cause, prepubertal girls)
	Autoimmune, e.g. Hashimoto thyroiditis
	Graves disease
	Infective thyroiditis
	Iodine deficiency or iodine-containing drugs
	Antithyroid drugs
	Multinodular goitre (seen in McCune-Albright disease)
	Thyroid tumour (rare)

Investigations

1. Assess the goitre for size, consistency, diffuse/nodular, tenderness. NB: Infants may have respiratory difficulties due to the large gland
2. Check thyroid status
3. Additional investigations may include USS thyroid, thyroid scan and fine needle aspiration

THYROID TUMOURS

These are rare in children and are associated with previous thyroid irradiation as an infant. They present as solitary thyroid nodules ± cervical lymph node metastases. Female > male, 2:1.

Types			
Papillary	70%	Young people, slow growing, local	Good prognosis
Follicular	20%	Early metastases (lungs, bone)	Good prognosis
Medullary	5%	Often familial, e.g. Marfan, MEN II, calcitonin ↑	Poor prognosis
Anaplastic	< 5%	Aggressive	Very poor prognosis

The investigations necessary are lymph node biopsy, thyroid ^{131}I scan (carcinoma usually appears as 'cold' nodules, i.e. decreased concentration of isotope) and thyroid function tests. Treatment is with subtotal or near-total thyroidectomy with or without radiotherapy.

PARATHYROID GLANDS

CALCIUM PHYSIOLOGY

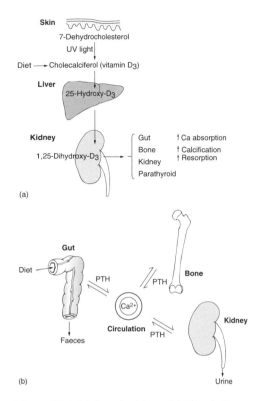

Figure 10.4 Calcium physiology. (a) Vitamin D metabolism and actions. (b) Calcium exchange

Parathyroid hormone (PTH)

This results in ↑ plasma calcium (increasing gut absorption and renal tubular reabsorption of calcium and increasing 1, 25(OH)$_2$D$_3$ synthesis,) and ↓ plasma phosphate (renal PO$_4$ excretion and bone absorption).

Calcium

50% albumin bound:50% free ionized calcium (available). Correct plasma calcium for albumin (if albumin > 40 g/L – corrected level is *lower)*.

Calcitonin

32 amino acid polypeptide, secreted by the C-cells of the thyroid gland.

- Decreases serum calcium (inhibits osteoclasts, ↑ renal calcium excretion)
- Decreases serum phosphate (↑ renal phosphate excretion)

Vitamin D analogues

Vitamin D   = calciferol (D3)
α-Calcidol = 1-α hydroxycholecalciferol
Calcitriol = 1, 25-dihydroxycholecalciferol $(1,25(OH)_2D_3)$

HYPOCALCAEMIA

Causes

PTH↓ (Ca ↓, PO$_4$ ↑)   Primary parathyroid aplasia or hypoplasia
(**Hypoparathyroidism**)   DiGeorge syndrome (parathyroid and thymus hypo- or a-plasia, cardiac
                               abnormalities, auricle hypoplasia, T cell immune defect, abnormal facies – see p. 30)
                               Autoimmune (vitiligo and candidiasis associated)
                               Surgical (post-thyroidectomy)
                               Pseudohypoparathyroidism. NB: PTH ↓ (see below)
PTH ↑ (Ca ↓, PO$_4$ ↓)   Rickets due to:
                               • Intake vitamin D ↓
                               • Metabolism vitamin D ↓
                               • (Renal, liver) excretion calcium ↑

Clinical features

- Seizures
- Cataracts, soft teeth, horizontal lines on toe and finger nails
- Muscle cramps, paraesthesia, stiffness
- Laryngeal and carpopedal spasm, tetany
- Chovstek's sign (facial muscle twitching on tapping facial nerve)
- Trousseau's sign (tetanic spasm of hands and wrist with BP cuff > above diastolic pressure for 3 min)
- Long QT interval, papilloedema

Investigations

Serum   Calcium (↓)
        Phosphate (↓ or ↑)
        Alkaline phosphatase (↓ or ↑)
        Magnesium level (should be normal but necessary to exclude hypomagnesaemia as cause of hypocalcaemia)
        PTH (↓, N or ↑)

Treatment

Emergency therapy   10% calcium gluconate IV stat dose, then 0.5–1 ml/min
                     NB: Calcium gluconate = 8.9 mg/ml
                         Calcium chloride = 27 mg/ml
Long-term   Oral calcium supplements and vitamin D supplements (calcitriol or α-calcidol)

PSEUDOHYPOPARATHYROIDISM (PHP)

A condition of hypocalcaemia, hypophosphataemia and elevated PTH levels, usually associated with the physical features listed below. It is due to end-organ resistance to PTH, secondary to a variety of biochemical defects subdivided into four groups. Group 1a has decreased stimulatory G (Gs) protein activity.

Clinical features

- Short stature, stocky with a round face
- Short 4th and 5th metacarpals
- Brachydactyly, bow legs, dimples overlying MCP joints
- Subcutaneous calcium deposits
- Mental retardation, calcification basal ganglia
- Cataracts, optic atrophy, dental anomalies
- Tetany, stridor, convulsions

Investigations

Serum   Ca $\downarrow$, PO_4 $\uparrow$, alkaline phosphatase $\uparrow$, PTH $\uparrow$

Diagnosis on decreased response in urine cAMP and phosphate after PTH infusion.

Pseudopseudohypoparathyroidism (PPHP)

This is the *clinical phenotype* of PHP with as yet *no* demonstrable biochemical defect, possibly due to incomplete expression of PHP.

PHP	Ca $\downarrow$, PO_4 $\uparrow$, alk. phos. $\uparrow$, PTH $\uparrow$	+ phenotype
PPHP	Normal biochemistry	+ phenotype

RICKETS

This is a failure in mineralization of growing bone. It is most commonly secondary to nutritional causes. In fully developed bone this is called osteomalacia (**osteopenia** is the condition of the actual bones).

Daily vitamin D requirement is 400 IU.

Causes

Vitamin D intake inadequate	Nutritional:
	- Prematurity (p. 464)
	- Breast-fed infants more at risk
	- Poorly fed infants (malnutrition)
	Malabsorption – coeliac disease, steatorrhoea, cystic fibrosis
	Inadequate sunlight exposure (especially dark-skinned)
Metabolism of vitamin D	Renal disease. NB: PO_4 $\uparrow$
	Liver disease
	Anticonvulsants, e.g. phenytoin (metabolizes vitamin D)
Phosphate excretion increased	Familial hypophosphataemic rickets
	Vitamin D-dependent rickets – type I, type II (receptor defect)
	Fanconi syndrome

Clinical features

- *Head* – large fontanelles with delayed closure (> 2 years). **Craniotabes** (ping-pong ball skull), frontal bossing
- *Chest* – **rachitic rosary** (enlargement of costochondral junctions). Harrison groove or sulcus, pigeon chest
- Broad wrists and ankles
- Short stature, kyphosis, small pelvis, coxa vara, bow legs, knock knees, late dentition with enamel defects, greenstick fractures
- Muscular weakness, pot belly

Investigations

1. Biochemical investigations. NB. Classic nutritional rickets: check alkaline phosphatase, calcium, phosphate and PO_4–Ca product (low).

	Ca	PO$_4$	PTH	Alk. phos.	25(OH)D$_3$	1,25(OH)$_2$D$_3$
Nutritional	N, ↓	↑ or ↓	↑, N	↑	↓	↓
Hypophosphataemic	N, ↓	↓	N	↑	N	↓
Vit. D-dependent type I	↓	↓	↑	↑	N	↓
Vit. D-dependent type II	↓	↓	↑	↑	N	↑

2. X-ray of left wrist (or left knee if < 2 years).
   X-ray findings are: Widened epiphyseal plate
   Cupping and fraying of the metaphysis
   Increased joint space
   Line of calcification seen when healing
   Also: cysts, subperiosteal erosions, fractures, Looser's zones, osteopenia if severe

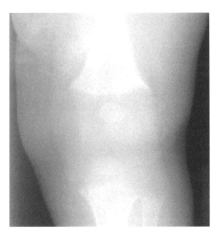

Figure 10.5 X-ray changes of rickets in the knee. Note prominent cupping and fraying

Treatment

This is with vitamin D in the necessary form.

Nutritional rickets   Calciferol (D$_3$)
Renal disease   α-Calcidol (1α-OHD$_3$) or calcitriol (1,25(OH)$_2$D$_3$)

Familial hypophosphataemic rickets (vitamin D-resistant rickets)

X-linked dominant.

Underlying problem

- Defective proximal tubular reabsorption of phosphate
- Reduced $1,25(OH)_2D_3$ synthesis

Treatment is with $1,25(OH)_2D_3$ and oral phosphate supplements.

Vitamin D-dependent rickets

Autosomal recessive. Characterized by a calcium deficiency with secondary hyperparathyroidism and a renal tubular acidosis. There are two types:

Type I   Low $1,25(OH)_2D_3$ levels
Type II   High $1,25(OH)_2D_3$ (receptor defect)

Treatment is with $1,25(OH)_2D_3$. (Type 1 has good response.)

HYPERCALCAEMIA

Causes

PTH $\uparrow$ (Ca $\uparrow$, PO_4 $\downarrow$)   Primary hyperparathyroidism (hyperplasia or adenoma. NB: MEN I and II)
     Tertiary hyperparathyroidism (PTH $\uparrow$ after long-standing secondary hyperparathyroidism now treated)
     Ectopic PTH (other tumours)
PTH $\downarrow$ (Ca $\uparrow$, $PO_4\uparrow$)   Vitamin D $\uparrow$ (TB, lymphoma, sarcoidosis, berylliosis, excess intake)
     Malignancy (leukaemia, lymphoma, neuroblastoma)
     Hypothyroidism (vitamin D metabolism decreased)
     Hyperthyroidism
     Williams syndrome (7q-, hypercalcaemia, supravalvular aortic stenosis, AVSD, peripheral pulmonary stenosis, stellate iris, cocktail party manner, typical facies – see p. 12)
     Familial hypocalciuric hypercalcaemia (PTH inappropriately normal, autosomal dominant, usually asymptomatic)

Clinical features

- **Stones** (renal), **bones** (pain), **abdominal moans** (ulcers), **psychiatric groans**
- Anorexia, vomiting, constipation, peptic ulcers, pancreatitis
- Corneal calcification, conjunctival injection
- Polyuria (nephrogenic DI from nephrocalcinosis)
- Chondrocalcinosis (30%), subperiosteal bone erosions
- Hypertension, hypokalaemia, arrhythmia
- Convulsions and cardiac arrest with high calcium levels (> 3.75)

Investigations

Serum   Calcium, phosphate, alkaline phosphatase and renal function PTH levels
Hand X-ray

Management

Severe	IV bisphosphonates (etidronate, pamidronate)
	Hydration and furosemide
Mild	Oral phosphates (diarrhoea) and/or calcitonin
	Steroids (sarcoidosis)

Hypoparathyroidectomy if necessary (primary hyperparathyroidism).

POLYCYSTIC OVARY SYNDROME (PCOS)

This is a common condition of adolescent girls, the essential features of which are:

- Large polycystic ovaries (in arrested follicular development)
- Increased circulating androgens and high LH:FSH ratio

It is also known as the Stein–Levanthal syndrome. The onset is usually around puberty and the cause is not well understood.

Clinical features

- Secondary amenorrhoea, irregular menstruation
- Obesity
- Hirsutism
- Mild virilization with acne
- Anovulatory infertility
- Insulin resistance

It often presents purely with menstrual irregularities or acne, with none of the classical 'fat, hairy' girl features present.

Investigations

Pelvic USS	Enlarged ovaries with multiple 3–5 mm cysts arranged circumferentially and increased stroma
Hormones	Raised LH:FSH ratio (2:1)
	Free circulating androgens ↑
	Testosterone ↑ or normal
	(Plasma LH ↑, FSH normal or ↓)
	Mild hyperprolactinaemia

NB: Must rule out differential diagnosis of adrenal disorders.

Treatment options

Treatment is symptomatic.

Irregular menses/virilization	Ovarian suppression with the oral contraceptive pill or cyproterone (an antiandrogen), or
	Pituitary ACTH suppression with prednisolone
Infertility	Ovarian wedge resection and clomiphene

GLUCOSE METABOLISM

Blood glucose is generally maintained in the non-fasted state between 3.5 and 8.0 mmol/L. Glucose may be manufactured from glycogen, fat or protein by a process called **gluconeogenesis.**

- Glucose is consumed by the brain as a primary source of energy
- Muscle may utilize glucose for energy or store it as glycogen
- Adipose tissue is also a store for glucose and uses glucose for triglyceride synthesis
- The liver is the principal site for glucose storage, where it is kept as glycogen

The maintenance of a constant blood glucose level is under the control of the hormone insulin.

- High insulin levels → blood glucose level ↓, by increasing glucose utilization and decreasing glucose production
- Low insulin levels have the converse effect
- Other hormones are involved and have the opposite effect to insulin – glucagon, adrenaline, cortisol and growth hormone

Insulin is produced by the pancreatic β-cells as proinsulin. Proinsulin is broken down into C peptide (biologically inert) and insulin during the secretory process. The insulin then travels in the portal circulation to the liver where it exerts its main action.

DIABETES MELLITUS

Diabetes mellitus is a chronic state of hyperglycaemia due to a deficiency of insulin or of its action. It is the most common endocrine disorder in childhood and adolescence.

Subtypes of diabetes mellitus:

Type I diabetes mellitus	Insulin deficiency due to insufficient endogenous insulin. Exogenous insulin necessary for maintenance of life
	Most common form in childhood
Type 2 diabetes mellitus	Mainly due to failure of insulin action (insulin resistance)
	Strongly associated with obesity
	Uncommon in childhood, though incidence rising, particularly in adolescents
	100% concordance in identical twins
	Insulin may be required to correct hyperglycaemia
	Ketosis is uncommon but occurs
Other types	Maturity onset of diabetes in the young (MODY)
	Syndrome-associated, e.g. DIDMOAD (see Renal chapter)
	Mitochondrial disease, e.g. Kearns Sayer syndrome
	Pancreatic disease, e.g. cystic fibrosis
	Post pancreatic surgery for persistent hyperinsulinaemia of infancy (PHHI)
	Neonatal diabetes mellitus (very rare)

Type 1 diabetes mellitus

This develops as a result of destruction of the pancreatic β-cells with consequent insufficient insulin production. It is thought that an environmental insult, e.g. viral illness, results in an antigen cross-reacting in genetically susceptible individuals. There is evidence of both genetic, autoimmune and environmental, e.g. viral, factors contributing:

Genetic	Father has type 1 DM – 1:20 risk for child
	Mother has type 1 DM – 1:40 risk for child
	Sibling has type 1 DM – 1:20 risk
	50% identical twin concordance
Autoimmune	80% have islet cell antibodies (ICA) on presentation
	Association with other autoimmune diseases and certain HLA types
Environmental	Seasonal variation

Prevalence 1:300 in the UK and rising. Presentation most common in spring and autumn.

Clinical presentations

- Short history (2–4 weeks) of: Polyuria (osmotic diuresis
                                   Polydipsia (dehydration)
                                   Weight loss (fluid depletion and muscle and fat breakdown)
- Ketoacidosis
- Asymptomatic glycosuria

Diagnosis

Symptomatic   Random venous plasma glucose ≥ 11.1 mmol/L or
                  Fasting plasma glucose ≥ 7.0 mmol/L or
                  2 h plasma glucose ≥ 11.1 mmol/L 12 h post glucose load (NB: in children need to adjust the
                  dose of glucose in relation to body weight) (An oral glucose tolerance test)
Asymptomatic   Venous plasma sample in diabetic range and confirmation with repeat glucose test in diabetic
                  range on another day (fasting, random or 2 h post glucose load)

NB:

- Whole blood glucose differs from plasma glucose. The whole blood glucose measures 10% lower than plasma glucose
- Glycosuria occurs in 1% of the population (secondary to low renal threshold)
- **Impaired glucose tolerance** = during a formal (75 g) oral glucose tolerance test (OGGT), fasting plasma glucose <7.0 mmol/L and 2 h venous plasma glucose > 7.8 mmol/L but < 11.1 mmol/L

Management

Multidisciplinary approach necessary. Great deal of support necessary for child and family.

Diet   This should be high in unrefined carbohydrates – slow absorption profile (low glycaemic index [GI]), there-
            fore fewer glucose swings
            Calories ideally obtained as 55% CHD, 35% fat and 15% protein
            Refined CBH (high GI) cause rapid swings in blood glucose levels
Insulin   Subcutaneous insulin injections given in the thigh, arm, abdomen or buttocks
            Rotated to prevent lipoatrophy or lipohypertrophy
            Different regimens available to suit different lifestyles
            Twice-daily regimen (used in younger children):
            am before breakfast, give ⅔ daily dose as:
                Short-acting ⅓
                Medium-acting ⅔
            pm before tea, give ⅓ daily dose as:
                Short-acting ⅓
                Medium-acting ⅔
            Multiple-dose pen injection regimen (used in older children). A basal background insulin is given, usually
            in the evening, and a short-acting insulin is given pre-meals. This is less rigid, allowing more flexibility

Insulin types			
	Onset	**Peak**	**Duration**
Ultra-short-acting insulin analogues, e.g. Humulog, Novorapid	10 min	60 min	3–4 h
Short-acting (crystalline, soluble), e.g. Actrapid, Humulin S	30 min	2 h	5–6 h
Medium- or long-acting (mixed with zinc or protamine), e.g. Monotard, Humulin I	2 h	6–8 h	10–16 h
Long-acting insulin analogues, e.g. Glargine, Detemir	2 h	None	22–24 h
	(plateau reached after 3–4 days of once-daily administration)		

Blood glucose monitoring

- Regular capillary blood glucose monitoring done at home to assess control
- Urine glucose unreliable due to variable renal threshold and inability to detect hypoglycaemia
- Glycosylated Hb (HbA1c) or fructosamine give an indication of blood glucose levels over the previous 12 and 6 weeks, respectively

Dawn phenomenon   Increase in glucose (and insulin requirement) around 4 am due to GH surge

Somogyi phenomenon   Rebound hyperglycaemia after hypoglycaemia at night due to *too much* insulin given to counteract 4 am GH surge

Exercise and illness

Exercise   This increases the demand for glucose and, as insulin levels are fixed, a sugar snack prior to exercise helps provide the energy boost

Illness   Insulin utilization rises during illness, though as food intake generally falls, the requirements may not rise

Recent developments

- Increased usage of continuous subcutaneous insulin infusion (pump therapy)
- Continuous glucose monitoring
- Inhaled insulin (not licensed < 18 years age)
- Artificial pancreas
- Stem cell technology

Problems

- Hypoglycaemia – symptoms usually occur with plasma glucose levels <3 mmol/L. 'Hypos' – sweaty, dizzy and irritable. Treat with oral glucose (drink or gel) or glucagon injection
- Weight increase
- Behavioural problems – non-compliance common in adolescence. Labelled 'brittle diabetes'
- Insulin resistance – usually due to obesity
- Skin – lipoatrophy/lipohypertrophy occur at injection sites
- Necrobiosis lipoidica diabeticorum (annular areas of waxy, atrophic skin usually on shins)

Long-term complications

These are all due to micro- and macro-vascular disease.

Diabetic eye disease	Retinopathy (simple and proliferative), cataracts
Renal disease	Initially microalbuminuria, then proteinuria, then gradual decline in renal function to ESRF
Neuropathy	Peripheral neuropathy (sensory loss in extremities), mononeuropathy of a cranial or peripheral nerve, autonomic neuropathy (orthostatic hypotension)
Feet	Ulcers due to neuropathy and microvascular disease
Cardiovascular	BP ↑, stroke, myocardial infarction, limb amputation

Diabetes clinic checks

General health		
Growth	Height and weight. Pubertal onset (may be delayed)	
Monitoring	Blood sugar booklet review. Look for hypos, high levels, and 'too perfect'	
	HbA1c level	
Blood pressure		
Psychiatric health	Compliance issues particularly	
Eye check	Visual symptoms and acuity	Annually after > 5 years of disease if diagnosed prepubertally or > 2 years if diagnosed post-pubertally
	Ophthalmologist review	
Urine	Laboratory check for microalbuminuria	

Diabetic ketoacidosis

This is a state of **uncontrolled catabolism** associated with insulin deficiency, resulting in:

- **Hyperglycaemia**
- **Osmotic diuresis and dehydration**
- **Lipolysis** resulting in free fatty acids broken down to ketone bodies which cause a metabolic acidosis

Causes

- New presentation of diabetes
- Intercurrent illness
- Interruption of insulin therapy

Clinical features

- Hyperventilation (Kussmaul respiration to correct metabolic acidosis)
- Dehydration
- Nausea and vomiting, abdominal pain
- Eventual drowsiness and coma

Management

1. General resuscitation if necessary
2. Bedside glucose (BM stix) and urinalysis for ketonuria
3. Blood for blood glucose, urea, electrolytes, FBC, CRP and PCV and arterial/venous blood gas
4. Blood and urine cultures, a CXR, and if clinically indicated a lumbar puncture
5. Keep child nil by mouth (due to gastric stasis and vomiting), place NG tube if impaired consciousness, and record fluid input–output chart
6. Admit to HDU if necessary
7. Give fluid and insulin therapy under close observation of clinical state and blood parameters

Fluid   Circulating volume expansion with a bolus of 10–20 ml/kg 0.9% saline
Then rehydrate calculated volume deficit + maintenance fluids over 48 h with 0.45% saline, adding K when electrolyte results back (with careful monitoring – risk of hypokalaemia as K pushed back into the cells)
Change fluid to 0.18% saline 4% dextrose when blood glucose < 12 mmol/L
Bicarbonate infusion in severe acidosis or if evidence of decreased myocardial contractility

Insulin   Insulin infusion of soluble insulin 0.01–0.1 units/kg/h to reduce blood glucose at a rate of <5 mmol/L/h
Check blood glucose hourly, and U&Es 2 hourly
When able to eat, transfer to subcutaneous insulin regimen of 0.5–0.7 units/kg/day

NB: Although serum K initially high, this is usually due to K leaking out of the cells and total body K is greatly *depleted*. There is a risk of **hypokalaemia** and **hypophosphataemia** as K and PO_4 are pushed back into the cells with insulin treatment.

HYPOGLYCAEMIA

Hypoglycaemia is defined as a blood glucose level of < 2.6 mmol/L. As glucose levels fall, the insulin concentration falls and lipolysis and ketogenesis are activated. With a blood glucose level of < 2.2 mmol/L, the plasma insulin should be undetectable.

Clinical features

Neonate   Apnoea, cyanosis
Hypotonia, lethargy, poor feeding and seizures
Older child   Pallor, anxiety, nausea, tremor, sweatiness, headache
Tachycardia
Diplopia, decreased acuity
Dizziness, poor concentration, behavioural change
Seizures, reduced consciousness, coma

Causes

Transient neonatal hypoglycaemia (common)	
Substrate deficiency	Prematurity and IUGR (low levels of liver glycogen, muscle protein and body fat, and poorly developed enzyme system for gluconeogenesis)
Hyperinsulinaemia	Infant of diabetic mother
Persistent hypoglycaemia (rare)	
Hyperinsulinism	Persistent hyperinsulinaemic hypoglycaemia of infancy (PHHI, nesidioblastosis) Insulinoma Beckwith–Wiedemann syndrome Diabetic child given relatively too much insulin Deliberate exogenous administration (fictitious or induced illness)
Hormone deficiency states	Growth hormone, ACTH and adrenaline deficiency Addison disease, hypopituitarism
Substrate deficiency	Ketotic hypoglycaemia

Metabolic	Carbohydrate metabolism disorder, e.g. galactosaemia, hereditary fructose intolerance, fructosaemia Glycogen storage disease (types I, III, VI, IX) Fatty acid oxidation defect, e.g. carnitine deficiency (primary or secondary), LCAD Organic acidaemia, e.g. MSUD (maple syrup urine disease)
Other	Poisoning (aspirin, alcohol) Liver failure, Reye syndrome

Persistent hyperinsulinaemic hypoglycaemia of infancy (PHHI, nesidioblastosis)

This is a developmental disorder where there are hyperplastic, abnormally dispersed β-cells, resulting in inappropriately high levels of plasma insulin. (See below for management.)

Ketotic hypoglycaemia

These children are unable to tolerate a prolonged fast. It may represent the low end of the spectrum of a child's ability to tolerate a fast.

- Presents between 18 months and 5 years and resolves spontaneously by 8–9 years
- Occurs when a child misses an evening meal or is unwell, causing a relatively prolonged fast, and they are difficult to arouse in the morning or may have a seizure. Hypoglycaemia, ketonaemia, ketonuria and plasma insulin levels are appropriately low
- These children have low alanine levels (a substrate released from muscle during fasting), so may have a defect in this mechanism. They also have a low muscle bulk and therefore have a low supply of substrate

Investigations

Essential investigations in the event of a hypoglycaemic episode (which may be induced by fasting):

- BMStix – blood glucose, U&E
- Plasma insulin, cortisol, growth hormone, proinsulin (and C-peptide if exogenous administration is suspected)
- β-OH-butyrate, acetoacetate, FFAs, alanine
- Ammonia, LFTs
- First urine sample for ketones, organic and amino acids, non-glucose-reducing substances

Management

Neonates

If able to feed	Oral glucose (breast milk or formula)
If unable to feed or reduced consciousness	3–5 ml/kg 10% glucose bolus IV, and then infusion of 10% glucose 5 ml/kg/h until blood sugars stable

Older child

Conscious	Sugary drink
Reduced consciousness	3–5 ml/kg 10% glucose bolus IV, and then infusion of 10% glucose 5 ml/kg/h until blood sugars stable

PHHI is treated with diazoxide and a thiazide diuretic. Second-line treatment is with octeotride and/or glucagon. Subtotal pancreatectomy is indicated if medical management fails.

NB: Normal infants produce 5–8 mg glucose/kg body weight/min of glucose in the fasting state. This falls to 1–2 mg/kg/min in older children. A neonate with hyperinsulinism may require up to 10–20 mg/kg/min.

PANCREATIC TUMOURS

These arise from APUD cells (amine precursor uptake and decarboxylation) in the pancreas. They are extremely rare in children.

INSULINOMA

This is an islet cell adenoma that secretes insulin. It presents insidiously with recurrent fasting hypoglycaemia.

Diagnosis

- Failure to suppress insulin with fasting hypoglycaemia
- MRI scan, coeliac angiography (v. difficult in infants) to locate tumour

Treatment

Surgical excision.

GLUCAGONOMA

This is a pancreatic tumour of the α-cells producing glucagon. The result is diabetes mellitus. A necrotic migratory erythematous rash is characteristic.

Diagnosis

Serum glucagon $\uparrow$.

NB: Enteroglucagonoma is a glucagon-secreting tumour of the right kidney and jejunal villi hypertrophy.

VIPOMA

This is a pancreatic tumour, secreting VIP (vasointestinal polypeptide).

VIP $\rightarrow$ Intestinal secretion $\rightarrow$ Diarrhoea

Diagnosis

- Serum VIP $\uparrow$
- PHI (peptide histidine isoleucine) also raised

Treatment

- Octreotide
- Surgical resection (if possible)

GASTRINOMA (ZOLLINGER–ELLISON SYNDROME)

Always malignant and slow growing. It is a tumour of the G-cells of the pancreas, which produce gastrin.

Gastrin $\rightarrow$ Gastric acid $\rightarrow$ Peptic ulcers (stomach, duodenum, jejunum)

The symptoms are those of peptic ulcers plus diarrhoea secondary to abnormally low intestinal pH.

Diagnosis

- Serum gastrin $\uparrow$
- Acid studies (high output)
- Ocreotide-labelled isotope scan

Treatment

- Omeprazole (proton pump inhibitor)
- Octreotide
- Surgery if possible

ENDOCRINE SYNDROMES

AUTOIMMUNE POLYGLANDULAR SYNDROME TYPE 1

An autosomal recessive disorder caused by mutations in the autoimmune regulator (AIRE) gene on chromosome 21 involving:

- Hypoparathyroidism
- Addison disease
- Mucocutaneous candidiasis

Additional features occurring with variable frequency include:

- Hypothyroidism
- IDDM
- Pernicious anaemia
- Ovarian failure
- Alopecia areata
- Chronic active hepatitis
- Ectodermal dystrophy

POLYGLANDULAR AUTOIMMUNE SYNDROME TYPE 2 (SCHMIDT SYNDROME)

This classically involves the association of:

- Addison disease
- Hypothryoidism
- IDDM
- Ovarian failure

The sequence of glandular involvement is variable.

MULTIPLE ENDOCRINE NEOPLASIA

Autosomal dominant. The association of a number of endocrine tumours.

MEN I	MEN IIa
Parathyroid	Adrenal (phaeochromocytoma, Cushing)
Pituitary (prolactin or GH or ACTH)	Thyroid (medullary carcinoma)
Pancreas	Parathyroid hyperplasia
(Thyroid)	
(Adrenal)	
Fasting calcium level ($\uparrow$?)	Calcitonin level $\uparrow$ (medullary ca. thyroid)
	Look for phaeochromocytoma
	MEN IIb is the same as MEN IIa, with Marfanoid features and multiple neuromas

Prophylactic total thyroidectomy is performed if the child is known to carry the gene for MEN II.

GROWTH

Growth phases

Infantile phase	Birth–2 years	Rapid, and rapidly decelerating growth rate
		Nutrition dependent
Childhood phase	2 years–puberty	Constant growth rate (5–6 cm/year)
		Hormone dependent
Pubertal phase	Puberty	Accelerated rate to a peak, then slowing to stop
		GH and sex hormone dependent
		Linear growth complete when epiphyses fused

Assessing growth

Essential growth measurements:

- Single **height, weight** (and **head circumference** < 2 years) are measured and plotted to assess:
  Growth is within **normal range** for parents and age-appropriate general population
  Any **discrepancies** between height, weight and head circumference
- Growth pattern plotted over 6–12 month period assessing:
  Rate of growth
  Deviations across centiles

Other measurements may be taken for specific reasons, e.g. sitting height, skinfold thickness.

Growth charts

Charts for height, weight and head circumference from extreme prematurity (23 weeks) to 20 years. There are nine equidistant centile lines $2/3$ of a standard deviation apart (0.4th centile to 99.6th centile – equivalent to $\pm$ 2.67 standard deviations from the mean).

Children falling outside the expected range for their parents (target centile range) or below the 0.4th centile or above the 99.6th centile should be formally assessed (4 in 1000 normal children though will be below the 0.4th centile).

Predicted eventual adult height

Predicted eventual adult height is an estimate made on the basis of the child's height and bone maturation (bone age).

The **mid-parental height centile** (median expected height for any child) and the **target centile range** (range of normal height for a particular child) are calculated from parental heights. They give a rough guide to the expected adult height of the child.

Boy	Expected height (mid parental height centile) = $\dfrac{(\text{mother's height} + 12.5\ \text{cm}) + \text{father's height}}{2}$
Girl	Expected height (mid parental height centile) = $\dfrac{(\text{father's height} - 12.5\ \text{cm}) + \text{mother's height}}{2}$

Bone age (skeletal maturity)

This shows how far the skeleton has matured and can give an idea of potential height, and clues as to the cause of short stature.

Delayed bone age in absence of pathology = slow maturation = more potential growth.

Bone age is assessed by rating a number of epiphyseal centres (and hence the rate of ossification) in a wrist X-ray (left wrist or left knee if < 2 years). This is then compared to chronological age.

Causes of delayed bone age	Causes of advanced bone age
Familial delayed maturation	Growth advance
Delayed puberty	Precocious puberty
Severe illness	Excessive androgen production
Hypothyroidism	Hyperthyroidism
GH deficiency	

Catch-up growth

This is rapid growth in babies who had IUGR and after an illness.

Chronological age = age since birth
Post-conceptional age = age since conceived

NB: Most low birthweight and premature babies should have their growth charts adjusted for their post-conceptional age until the age 2 years, as they will have 'caught up' by then.

Growth velocity

- This is a sensitive indicator of growth problems, and is the 'gold standard' for assessing whether growth is progressing normally. It is age-dependent
- Two measurements are needed 4 months apart (though measurements over 12 months are desirable before clinical decisions are made). The difference between the two height measurements is divided by the time interval between them to give the growth velocity in cm/year and is plotted on a growth velocity chart at the mid-point in time
- Growth velocity should remain between the 25th–75th velocity centiles for height to remain normal

SHORT STATURE

Short stature is height < 2nd centile (approximately 2 standard deviations below the mean). Height velocity < 25th centile is abnormal.

Causes

Familial	Most common cause
	Expected height calculated from parental heights
Constitutional delay	'Slow grower'. Delayed bone age, usually delayed puberty and family history of this pattern. Final height falls within predicted centile range
Psychosocial deprivation	Small child (may also be underweight)
	May have biochemical picture of GH deficiency
Chronic illness	Any chronic illness, also inadequate nutrition

Endocrine (rare)	Growth hormone deficiency:	Isolated GH synthesis or release defects
		Pituitary deficiency/hypopituitarism/hypothalamic defect
		Post-cranial irradiation or chemotherapy
		Laron dwarfism (GH insensitivity)
	Hypothyroidism	
	PHP and PPHP (see p. 249)	
	Cushing syndrome (usually iatrogenic)	
Chromosomal/gene abnormality	Turner syndrome, Down syndrome, Prader–Willi syndrome, Noonan syndrome, Bloom syndrome	
IUGR	Russell–Silver dwarfism	
Skeletal dysplasias	Achondroplasia and hypochondroplasia	

Investigations

These are determined by the history and clinical findings.

General	Bone age
	TFTs
	FBC, ESR, bone profile
	Urinalysis
Specific	Karyotype
	Coeliac screen
	Insulin-like growth factor 1 (IGF-1) and IGF-binding protein 3 (IGFBP3)*
	USS uterus and ovaries
	CT or MRI brain
	Skeletal survey
	Pituitary provocation tests

*IGF-1 levels correlate well with GH status and this together with IGFBP3 are the initial screening tests for suspected growth hormone deficiency. Random GH levels are unhelpful because GH is secreted in a pulsatile manner and is likely to be low in normal children during the daytime.

Treatment

Dependent on underlying cause. Children with GH deficiency, Turner syndrome, Prader–Willi syndrome and those who have suffered from IUGR can be treated with daily recombinant GH injections.

TALL STATURE

Tall stature is height > 98th centile. It is much less common as a clinical problem than short stature, mainly because of perceived social acceptability.

Causes

Familial	Most common cause. Tall expected height (from parental height)
Hormonal	Precocious puberty ⎫ In these two conditions the final height is *short* although child taller than
	CAH ⎭ their peers while growing because the growth spurts are reached earlier
	Pituitary gigantism (GH secreting tumour – rare)
	Hyperthyroidism
Syndrome	Klinefelter syndrome (XXY)
	Marfan syndrome
	Homocystinuria
	Soto's syndrome ('cerebral gigantism' – learning difficulties, clumsiness, big hands and feet, large ears, prominent forehead)
	Beckwith–Wiedemann syndrome (see p. 17)

Investigations

These are determined by the history and clinical findings.

General	Bone age
	Karyotype
	TFTs
Specific	IGF-1 and IGFBP3[*]
	USS uterus and ovaries
	MRI brain scan
	Homocystine
	17-OH-progesterone and urine steroid profile

Treatment

Depends on the underlying cause. It is possible to treat/limit final height in those with familial tall stature by inducing puberty early (using oestrogen therapy in girls and testosterone therapy in boys), which limits the childhood growth phase and causes premature fusion of the epiphyses.

PUBERTY

Pubertal staging

Pubertal stage is assessed using the sexual maturity rating devised by Tanner in 1962.

Boys	G (1–5), P (1–5), A (1–3), testicular volume (2–25 ml)
Girls	B (1–5), P (1–5), A (1–3), menarche

G Genitals (boys)

Stage 1	Preadolescent
Stage 2	Scrotum pink and texture change, slight enlargement of penis
Stage 3	Longer penis, larger testes
Stage 4	Penis increases in breadth, dark scrotum
Stage 5	Adult size

B Breasts

Stage 1	Preadolescent
Stage 2	Breast bud
Stage 3	Larger but no nipple contour separation
Stage 4	Areola and papilla form secondary mound
Stage 5	Mature (papilla projects, areola follows breast contour)

P Pubic hair

		A Axillary hair	
Stage 1	Prepubertal	Stage 1	No hair
Stage 2	Few fine hairs	Stage 2	Scanty hair
Stage 3	Darkens, coarsens, starts to curl	Stage 3	Adult hair pattern
Stage 4	Adult type, smaller area		
Stage 5	Adult distribution		

Puberty onset (timing variable)

Girls	(8–13 years)	Breast stage 2	(First sign – breast development)
Boys	(9–14 years)	Testes 4 ml	(First sign – testicular enlargement)

Pubertal growth spurts

Girls	At breast stage 3
Boys	At testicular volume 10–12 ml

Definitions

Menarche	Commencement of menstruation. Occurs at breast stage 4. Average = 12.2 years
Thelarche	Breast development
Adrenarche	Pubic and axillary hair development

PRECOCIOUS PUBERTY

Gonadotrophin-dependent precocious puberty	Development of secondary sexual characteristics at a young age in a normal progression accompanied by a growth spurt, leading to full sexual maturity from activation of the **central axis**
Gonadotrophin-independent precocious puberty	Gonadotrophin-independent development, and there may be an unusual progression of sexual maturity. Isolated premature thelarche, adrenarche and menarche can occur as separate clinical entities

Girls	Development of secondary sexual characteristics < 8 years is abnormal
	Menarche < 10 years warrants investigation
	Mostly *familial* cases
Boys	Development of secondary sexual characteristics < 9 years is abnormal
	Mostly *pathological* causes, e.g. CAH, intracranial tumours, dysgerminomas

Causes

True **(Gonadotrophin dependent, hypothalamic-pituitary-gonadal axis activated) LH ↑, FSH ↑**
Familial
Central:
- Congenital, e.g. neurofibromatosis, hydrocephalus
- Acquired, e.g. post-sepsis, surgery, DXT
- Brain tumours
Hypothyroidism

False **(Gonadotrophin-independent, excess sex steroids not driven centrally) LH↓, FSH↓**
Adrenal:
- Congenital adrenal hyperplasia
- Adrenal tumour
Gonadal:
- Ovarian tumour
- Testicular tumour (Leydig cell)
McCune–Albright syndrome (see below)
Hypothyroidism
Exogenous sex steroids

Examination and investigations

Always check:

- Clinical pubertal staging
- Bone age
- Pelvic USS (girls) or orchidometer (boys)
- Features of intracranial mass – visual fields and optic discs

NB: In boys, have a low threshold for cranial imaging (? tumour) and α-FP and hCG measurement (? testicular tumour) due to high incidence of pathological causes.

Treatment

This depends on the underlying condition. True precocious puberty can be treated with GnRH analogues, and false precocious puberty with androgen inhibitors (boys) or oestrogen inhibitors (girls).

McCune–Albright syndrome (polyostotic fibrous dysplasia)

This is a syndrome of endocrine dysfunction with hyperpigmentation and skeletal fibrous dysplasia. It is due to a defect in the G-protein controlling cAMP in cells, which results in activation of receptors with a cAMP mechanism and autonomous glandular hyperfunction. The syndrome involves:

Endocrine	Precocious puberty
	Multiple hormonal hyperactivity may be seen (e.g. ovary, thyroid, adrenal glands, pituitary)
Bone	Polyostotic fibrous dysplasia (visible as radiolucent areas on X-ray)
Skin	Patchy hyperpigmentation and café-au-lait patches (of very irregular outline)

DELAYED PUBERTY

Girls	Failure of onset of any signs of puberty by 13 years
Boys	Failure of onset of any signs of puberty by 14 years

Mainly boys are affected, and the cause is usually **constitutional delay** (short child with delayed bone age and family history).

Causes

Gonadotrophin secretion low	Gonadotrophin secretion high
Constitutional • familial or sporadic	*Gonadal dysgenesis* • Turner syndrome
Hypothalamic–pituitary: • Panhypopituitarism • GnRH deficiency • Kallman syndrome • Intracranial tumour, e.g. prolactinoma	*Gonadal disease* • trauma, torsion, DXT *Steroid hormone enzyme deficiencies* • CAH 3β-deficiency (see below)
Systemic disease: • Any severe disease, e.g. renal failure, malnutrition • Hypothyroidism • Emotional, e.g. anorexia nervosa	*Chromosomal* • Klinefelter syndrome

Investigations

1. Pubertal staging and bone age
2. Routine FBC, biochemistry, ESR and coeliac screen

3. TFTs
4. Gonadotrophin and sex steroid hormone levels
5. Karyotype
6. Occasionally LHRH test and hCG test to check testicular responsiveness in terms of testosterone production
7. MRI brain and hypothalamic–pituitary area

Treatment

This depends on the cause. In males with constitutional delay, low-dose testosterone can be given to induce puberty. In females, ethinyl oestradiol can be used for the same purpose.

Kallman syndrome

Syndrome of isolated hypogonadotrophism, causing secondary hypogonadism. Other features are anosmia, cleft palate, colour blindness, ichthyosis and renal abnormalities. Inheritance usually X-linked.

SEXUAL DIFFERENTIATION DISORDERS – AMBIGUOUS GENITALIA

Disorders of sexual differentiation can be due to:

- Virilization of a female (female pseudohermaphrodite, 46, XX)
- Undervirilization of a male (male pseudohermaphrodite, 46, XY)
- True hermaphrodite (both ovarian and testicular tissue present)

Affected patients have a discrepancy between the morphology of the gonads and the morphology of the external genitalia.

CAUSES

Female pseudohermaphrodite (virilized) (46, XX + ovaries)

Fetal	CAH 21-hydroxylase deficiency
	11β-hydroxylase deficiency
Maternal	Virilizing tumours (adrenal, ovarian)
	Virilizing drugs

Male pseudohermaphrodite (undervirilized) (46, XY + testes)

Defect in testes differentiation	Gonadal dysgenesis/agenesis
Defect in testicular hormones	CAH-3β-hydroxysteroid dehydrogenase deficiency
Defect in androgen activity	5α-reductase deficiency
	Androgen insensitivity syndrome (complete or partial)

True hermaphrodite (ovarian + testicular tissue)

- 46, XX
- 46, XY
- Mosaic karyotypes, e.g. 46, XX/XY (chimera), XO/XY

INVESTIGATIONS

- Karyotype
- Pelvic and abdominal USS (to assess internal genitalia and adrenal glands)
- Adrenal steroid profile

- Testosterone and dihydrotestosterone (DHT)
- Other tests such as LHRH test, hCG test, Synacthen test
- Occasionally need to perform EUA or laparoscopy to determine external and internal genitourinary structures

NB: The basic pattern in development is female. The presence of testosterone causes the external male sexual characteristics to develop. The sex of rearing of a child should be determined in infancy to allow for the appropriate medical and social management before the child has a clear sexual identity; late changes may be very traumatic.

CONGENITAL ADRENAL HYPERPLASIA

Incidence 1:10 000. A group of autosomal recessive conditions resulting from various defects in the enzymes involved in the adrenal steroid synthetic pathways. The enzyme defect causes the steroid pathway to be deflected from cortisol synthesis down alternative mineralocorticoid and androgenic pathways, with resultant excess or deficiency of other steroids.

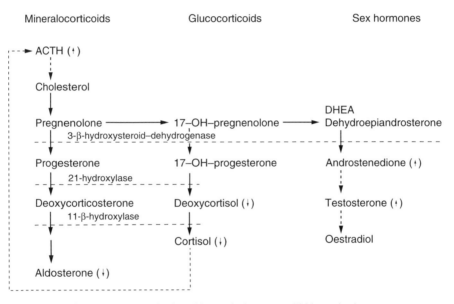

Figure 10.6 Effects of congenital adrenal hyperplasia on steroid biosynthesis

21-hydroxylase deficiency

The most common cause. Genetic defect on chromosome 6.

Clinical features

- Virilization of a female baby (cliteromegaly, etc.)
- Adrenal crisis may occur in first 1–2 weeks of life (NB: They lose salt)
- May present late with precocious puberty, advanced bone age, tall stature in childhood (eventual short stature), hypertension, hirsutism and skin pigmentation

Hormones

- ACTH (↑)
- Aldosterone ↓

- Testosterone ↑
- Cortisol ↓
- Androstenedione ↑

Investigations

- Plasma 17-OH-progesterone (↑)
- Urine steroid profile – urine pregnanetriol (↑)
- Serum electrolytes: Na ↓, K ↑, glucose ↓
- Karyotype
- Pelvic USS (looking for female organs in a virilized female)

NB: Boys with CAH are more likely to be diagnosed late because the androgen excess does not cause a clearly abnormal appearance in the newborn.

Treatment

Drugs	Hydrocortisone and fludrocortisone daily
Surgery	If necessary to improve female anatomy
Monitor	Monitor growth and skeletal maturity

NB: Antenatal diagnosis is possible. Dexamethasone is given to the mother in order to decrease fetal ACTH and hence reduce the chance of having a virilized female infant.

Other variants

11β-hydroxylase deficiency (5–8%)	Non salt-losing, Na ↑, K ↓, BP ↑ Virilization Diagnosis: 11-deoxycortisol ↑
3β-hydroxysteroid dehydrogenase deficiency (<5%)	Salt-losing, Na ↓, K ↑ Virilization of girls, incomplete virilization of boys Diagnosis: elevated pregnenolone, DHEA, 17-OH-pregnenolone

ENDOCRINE TESTS

NB: These are outlined for exam reference only. Tests performed in expert centres.

GH STIMULATION TEST

GH secretion is stimulated in a variety of ways, e.g. exercise, glucagon, clonidine or arginine. Hypoglycaemia with a blood glucose < 2.2 mmol/L is produced and samples collected as described below.

Time (min)	0	30	60	90	120	(180) for glucagon test only
Glucose	*	*	*	*	*	(*)
Cortisol	*	*	*	*	*	(*)
Growth hormone	*	*	*	*	(*)	
*Indicates sample should be taken. Normal response = GH > 20 mU/L						
= cortisol increase >200 nmol/L and/or peak >500 nmol/L						

COMBINED PITUITARY PROVOCATION TEST

Growth hormone stimulation test + TRH + LHRH stimulation tests.

TRH STIMULATION TEST

Give TRH and sample:

Time (min)	0	20	60
TSH	*	*	*
Prolactin	*	*	*

LHRH STIMULATION TEST

Give LHRH and sample:

Time (min)	0	20	60
LH	*	*	*
FSH	*	*	*
NB: Absent response does not establish pituitary deficiency.			

DEXAMETHASONE SUPPRESSION TESTS

Overnight suppression test

- Used to confirm normal suppression of adrenal cortex
- Dexamethasone 0.3 mg/m^2 given orally at 22:00 hours
- Plasma cortisol measured at 08:00 on the following day
- Normally plasma cortisol is suppressed to < 100 nmol/L
- In Cushing syndrome there is failure to suppress

Low-dose suppression 48-h test

- Confirmation of Cushing syndrome, where there is failure of suppression
- Dexamethasone given 0.5 mg/kg orally 6 hourly for 48 h

Time (h)	0	24	48	72
Plasma cortisol	*	*	*	
ACTH			*	
24-h urine free cortisol	*			*
Normal = 48-h plasma cortisol < 140 nmol/L, ACTH < 5 pmol/L, urine cortisol to less than half the baseline.				

High-dose suppression

- Used to differentiate pituitary-dependent Cushing syndrome (which will suppress in 90%) from ACTH-independent disease which will still not suppress. NB: This test can be hard to interpret
- Dexamethasone 2 mg given 6 hourly for eight doses from 09:00 on day 1
- Plasma cortisol and 24 h urine steroids measured at 09:00 on days 0 and 2
- Normally plasma cortisol is suppressed on day 2 to < 50% of the value on day 0

SYNACTHEN STIMULATION TESTS

Short Synacthen test (ACTH analogue)

- Purpose – used to detect primary adrenal failure, where the cortisol levels are below expected
- Dose of 0.25 mg (250 μg) Synacthen (tetracosactrin) given IM or IV and cortisol levels measured as follows

Time (min)	0	30	60
Cortisol	*	*	*

Normal = cortisol increase > 200 nmol/L, cortisol peak >500 nmol/L
Peak value may occur at 30 or 60 min

Long Synacthen test

- Purpose – differentiates primary from secondary adrenal failure (in secondary adrenal failure, cortisol production will be stimulated)
- Six 12-hourly tetracosactrin 0.5 μg/m² SA IM. Measure:

Time (min)	08:00h day 1	08:00h day 2	08:00h day 3
Cortisol	*	*	*

Normal = cortisol peak > 500 nmol/L
Depressed response with elevated ACTH levels confirms **primary** adrenal failure

GLUCOSE TOLERANCE TEST

A standard dose of glucose is given after an overnight fast. Blood glucose levels are taken at time 0 and 2 h, though usually serial measurements at 30 min intervals are also taken, i.e. 0, 30, 60, 90, 120.

Time (min)	0	120
Plasma glucose (normal)	< 7.1	< 11.1
Plasma glucose (diabetes)	> 7.1	> 11.1
Plasma glucose (IGT)	< 7.1	7.8–11.1

FURTHER READING

Brook CG, Clayton P, Brown R, eds *Brook's Pediatric Clinical Endocrinology*, 5th edn. Oxford: Blackwell Publishing, 2005

Brook CGD *A Guide to the Practice of Paediatric Endocrinology*. Cambridge University Press, Cambridge, 1993

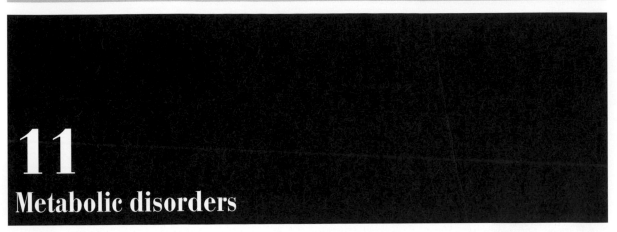

11
Metabolic disorders

- *Basic mechanism underlying metabolic disorders*
- *Classification*
- *Group 1: Rapid toxic accumulation of a small molecule*
- *Group 2: Lack of energy*
- *Group 3: Defects in the synthesis of large molecules resulting in a dysmorphic child*
- *Group 4: Defects in the metabolism of large complex molecules*
- *Group 5: Mitochondrial diseases*
- *Hyperlipidaemias*
- *Porphyrias*

Inborn errors of metabolism are inherited biochemical disorders and are generally autosomal recessive caused by **single gene disorders**. They are individually rare yet collectively not uncommon.

BASIC MECHANISM UNDERLYING METABOLIC DISORDERS

- The molecular anomaly leads to a defect in an **enzyme** (or cofactor), or less commonly a **structural protein** such as a transmembrane transporter
- Decreased enzyme activity results in an *accumulation* of the biochemical substrate or a *deficiency* of a product. This can be particularly harmful if the former is toxic or the latter is essential for cellular function
- The enzyme may require a particular **cofactor** such as a vitamin to function and deficiencies of this cofactor can lead to symptoms similar to those caused by deficiency of the enzyme

Metabolic diseases usually affect children although increasingly adult phenotypes are being described. Due to the rarity of the individual conditions, the multitude of possible presentations and the perceived complexity of the investigations required, metabolic diseases are likely to be frequently undiagnosed. This is unfortunate as once suspected they are, in general, relatively easy to diagnose and subsequent treatment is often inexpensive yet effective.

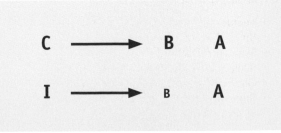

Figure 11.1 Decreased enzyme C function leading to an accumulation of A and/or a deficiency of B

CLASSIFICATION

> Most metabolic diseases can be classified into five main groups:
>
> **Small molecule diseases** resulting in:
>
> 1 **Rapid toxic accumulation** of a small molecule
> 2 A **lack of energy**
>
> **Large molecule diseases:**
>
> 3 A **defect in the synthesis** of a large molecule resulting in a **dysmorphic child**
> 4 A **slow accumulation** of a large complex molecule resulting in **slowly progressive symptoms**
>
> 5 **Mitochondrial diseases**

FEATURES SUGGESTIVE OF A METABOLIC DISORDER

The following are features to look for when considering a metabolic diagnosis.

Parental history

- Consanguinous parents
- Previous unexplained neonatal deaths
- Particular ethnic group (certain diseases only)

Clinical features

Neonatal presentation
Poor feeding
Vomiting
Lethargy
Seizures
Coma
Unusual odour
Metabolic imbalance – hypoglycaemia, acidosis, alkalosis (with some defects)
May appear normal at birth (some conditions associated with dysmorphism)

Post-neonatal presentation
Developmental regression, encephalopathy, seizures
Intermittent episodes of vomiting, acidosis, hypoglycaemia and/or coma triggered by stress, e.g. infections, surgery

Examination findings

- Neurological abnormalities, developmental delay
- Unusual odour
- Skin manifestations
- Ocular involvement, e.g. cherry red spot
- Cardiac disease, liver disease, renal disease
- Organomegaly, e.g. hepatomegaly
- Dysmorphism

Investigations that may be used in a metabolic screen

Serum	Ammonia	↑ Urea cycle defects, organic acidaemias
	Glucose	↓ FAODs and mitochondrial defects
	Ketones	↑ Organic acidaemias
		Inappropriately low in FAODs
	Lactate	↑ Mitochondrial disorders
	U&Es	May be deranged, features of dehydration
	LFTs	May be abnormal (tyrosinaemia, urea cycle defects, FAODs, mitochondrial defects and galactosaemia)
	Plasma amino acids	Aminoacidopathies
		Urea cycle defects
	Acylcarnitine profile	Organic acidaemias, FAODs
	VLFCAs	Peroxisomal biosynthesis disorders
Blood gas	pH	Acidosis (organic acidaemias, mitochondrial defects)
		Respiratory alkalosis (urea cycle defects)
Urine	Organic acids	Organic acidaemias, FAODs
	Orotic acid	Urea cycle defects
	Amino acids	Aminoacidopathies
	GAGs	Mucopolysaccharidoses
	Ketones	↑ Organic acidaemias
		Inappropriately low in FAODs
CSF	Lactate	↑ Mitochondrial disorders

Special investigations

Enzyme assays (lymphocytes, liver biopsy, fibroblasts)	GSD, lysosomal storage disorders
Molecular diagnosis (gene analysis)	Most conditions
Transferrin isoelectric analysis	CDG
CSF	Amino acids (NKH), glucose (GLUT1 transporter)
Muscle biopsy	Mitochondrial disease

GROUP 1: RAPID TOXIC ACCUMULATION OF A SMALL MOLECULE

This group includes:

- Organic acidaemias
- Urea cycle defects
- Aminoacidopathies

ORGANIC ACIDAEMIAS

Organic acids are produced though the removal of the amino group (nitrogen) from amino acids. They are metabolized in the cell to produce energy. **Enzyme defects** in these pathways lead to an accumulation of the *preceding* organic acids. This occurs particularly during periods of increased protein turnover from:

- Dietary sources, or
- Intercurrent illness (endogenous catabolism ↑)
- Early neonatal period (a natural physiological catabolism occurs making this a particularly vulnerable time)

Presentation

Neonate	Lethargy, poor feeding and vomiting, and severe ketoacidosis
Infancy	Intermittent acute attacks of above symptoms during illness or certain diets
	Episodes are often initially mistaken for sepsis
Long-term	(If untreated) Mental retardation, movement disorders, faltering growth, renal impairment

Investigations

Initial	Blood gas – acidosis
	Plasma ketones ↑, ammonia ↑, glucose ↓
Diagnosis	Urine **organic acids**, or
	Plasma or blood spot **acylcarnitine profile** (carnitine derivatives of organic acids)

Confirmation of diagnosis is with enzyme or molecular analysis.

Disease examples	Enzyme defect	Symptoms	Routine investigations	Special investigations	Treatment
Methylmalonic acidaemia Propionic acidaemia Isovaleric acidaemia	MM mutase or cobalamin (B$_{12}$) defect Propoinyl CoA dehydrogenase Isovaleric CoA dehydrogenase	Lethargy Encephalopathy Vomiting Poor feeding Seizures	Blood gas (acidosis) Ketones (↑) Ammonia (↑) Glucose (↓)	Urine organic acids Acylcarnitine profile	Low protein diet Vitamin co-factors, e.g. B$_{12}$ Carnitine Haemofiltration Avoid catabolism (see metabolic decompensation below)

Biotinadase deficiency

Classically presents in infantile period with a combination of seizures, lactic acidosis, developmental delay, an eczema-type rash, angular stomatitis, alopecia, hearing loss and ataxia. There is a characteristic urinary organic acid picture with confirmation of the diagnosis by measuring biotinadase activity.

UREA CYCLE DISORDERS

Similar acute episodes can occur in the **urea cycle disorders**, a group of conditions caused by enzymological defects in the conversion of ammonia and nitrogen waste into urea.

The **urea cycle** converts ammonia to non-toxic urea:

		Urea cycle
Protein feed (amino acids) ⟶	Ammonia ⟶	Urea
	Toxic	*Non-toxic*

The five enzymes involved in urea synthesis are:

- Carbamylphosphate synthetase (CPS)
- Ornithine transcarbamylase (OTC)
- Arginosuccinate synthetase (AS) (citrullinaemia)

- Arginosuccinate lyase (AL) (arginosuccinic acidaemia)
- Arginase (argininaemia)

N-acetylglutamate synthetase is required for the activation of the cycle. Deficiencies of all these enzymes occur, resulting in urea cycle defects.

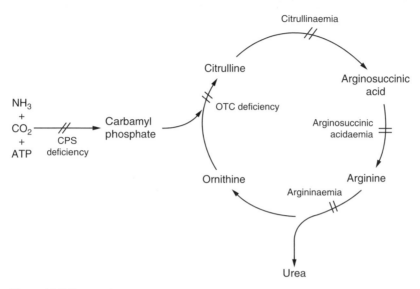

Figure 11.2 Urea cycle

Presentation

Neonate (common)	Severe **hyperammonaemia** and subsequent encephalopathy (lethargy, poor feeding, seizures and coma)
Childhood	Faltering growth, cyclical vomiting and encephalopathy
	Developmental delay (some types)

Investigations

Initial	Plasma **ammonia** ↑↑ (> 200 μmol/L) (key investigation)
	(urea cycle disorder or an organic acidaemia should be suspected)
	Blood gas (respiratory alkalosis – may be present)
Diagnosis	Plasma amino acids (particular profile will usually indicate type of urea cycle disorder)
	Urine orotic acid
	Confirmation with enzyme or molecular analysis

Management

Acute	Urgent haemofiltration to lower the toxic ammonia and related compounds
Long-term	Low protein diet
	Ammonia lowering medication, e.g. sodium phenylbutyrate, arginine

Episodes of metabolic decompensation

Despite treatment, children with organic acidaemias and urea cycle diseases may have frequent episodes of **metabolic decompensation**. These often occur during periods of intercurrent viral infections. Prompt instigation of a high carbohydrate–low protein diet (the emergency regimen) can prevent or at least curtail these, although hospital admission for IV glucose and medications is often required.

Disease	Symptoms	Routine investigations	Special investigations	Treatment
Ornithine transcarbamylase deficiency (OTC) (XL-recessive)	Lethargy Encephalopathy Vomiting Poor feeding	Ammonia ($\uparrow$) (> 200 µmol/L – key investigation) Blood gas (may have respiratory alkalosis)	Amino acids Orotic acid	Low protein diet Sodium phenylbutyrate Arginine Haemofiltration

AMINOACIDOPATHIES

Maple syrup urine disease (MSUD)

This is an inability to break down the branched chain amino acids isoleucine, leucine and valine. Usually present in the neonatal period with encephalopathy.

Defects in the metabolism of the other amino acids (aminoacidopathies) do not tend to present as suddenly or acutely as MSUD or the organic acidaemias.

Phenylketonuria (PKU)

Incidence 1:15 000 (the most common metabolic disorder)

A defect in the breakdown of phenylalanine:

Phenylalanine
hydroxylase

Pathway: Phenylalanine————X————→Tyrosine

Enzyme deficiency   Phenylalanine hydroxylase (low or absent)

Biochemical result   Phenylalanine and its alternative pathway metabolites accumulate in the tissues

Clinical features

NB: These only develop if condition is untreated.

- Slowly progressive mental retardation
- Musty odour (classic, though in reality simply smells unusual)
- Spastic cerebral palsy, athetosis, hyperactivity, acquired microcephaly
- Fair hair, fair skin and blue eyes (if not treated)

Neonatal screening is well established for PKU (Guthrie test – phenylalanine levels $\uparrow$) and the classical phenotype is now rarely seen.

Tyrosinaemia (Type 1)

Enzyme deficiency   Fumarylacetoacetase
Biochemical result   Tyrosinaemia and succinylacetonuria

Clinical features

Liver	Acute or chronic liver disease
Renal	Renal Fanconi syndrome, renal rickets
Odour	Cabbage/sweet
Other	Faltering growth, developmental delay

Homocystinuria

Prevalence 1:200 000, autosomal recessive.

Enzyme deficiency	Cystathionine synthase
Biochemical result	Homocysteine and methionine accumulation

Clinical features

General	Marfanoid habitus, fair hair, fair skin, blue eyes, malar flush
CNS	Learning difficulties (common), seizures (20%)
Skeletal	Osteoporosis, platyspondyly
CVS	Cerebral vascular events, arterial and venous thromboembolism
Eye	Lens subluxation

Diagnosis of the aminoacidopathies

- Amino acid profile (plasma or urine), e.g. PKU – phenylalanine ↑
- Enzyme or molecular test confirmation if necessary

Treatment of the aminoacidopathies

- Very low protein diet
- Specialized medications (BH4 for some forms of PKU, NTBC for tyrosinaemia, and pyridoxine or betaine for homocystinuria)
- Supplementary specialized formula (contains all the vitamins, minerals, carbohydrates and essential amino acids minus the one(s) the patient cannot metabolize, to make a complete diet). E.g. PKU – low-phenylalanine diet for life. *Some* phenylalanine must be given as it is not synthesized in the body. During pregnancy woman with PKU must strictly adhere to the diet because high phenylalanine levels result in fetal abnormalities, e.g. CHD, and mental retardation

Non-ketotic hyperglycinaemia

Autosomal recessive.

Enzyme defect   Defect in the glycine cleavage system involved in glycine degradation

Clinical features

- Neonatal illness with vomiting, lethargy, seizures, coma and death within hours if untreated
- If survival occurs, severe mental retardation, myoclonic seizures and spasticity are seen
- A late-onset mild form with developmental delay, ataxia and seizures is also described

Investigations

- Glycine levels – ↑ in plasma, urine and CSF. High CSF:plasma glycine ratio
- No demonstrable organic acidaemia

Management

Sodium benzoate lowers glycine levels but in typical severe cases there is no effective long-term treatment and management is palliative.

GROUP 2: LACK OF ENERGY

The small molecule diseases leading to a lack of energy include:

- Disorders of carbohydrate metabolism
- Fatty acid oxidation defects

DISORDERS OF CARBOHYDRATE METABOLISM

Glycogen storage diseases (GSDs)

To maintain blood glucose normal children, when fasted, rely initially on the breakdown of **hepatic glycogen** and later on the oxidation of fat. Children with GSDs can make glycogen but cannot effectively catabolize it. Glycogen is thus stored in huge quantities in the liver. During periods of **starvation**, e.g. during an intercurrent viral illness, the children become hypoglycaemic and lethargic. There are several different types of GSD involving different enzyme deficiencies.

Disease	Enzyme defect
GSD I	Glycogen-6-phosphatase
GSD III	Debrancher enzyme
GSD VI	Liver phosphorylase
GSD IX	Liver phosphorylase kinase

Presentation

GSD I and III	Hypoglycaemia and massive hepatomegaly in first few months of life
GSD VI and IX	Milder disease. Hypoglycaemia if significantly stressed, often only have mild moderate hepatomegaly and an otherwise excellent prognosis
Long-term complications	Short stature, developmental delay, seizures (from hypoglycaemia), hepatoma, osteoporosis and cardiac disease if untreated

Diagnosis

- Enzyme activity (blood or liver) and/or
- Molecular analysis of appropriate gene

Management

- Regular high carbohydrate meals during the day
- Continuous feeds during the night (or uncooked cornstarch, a slow release form of glucose, every 4–6 h)

Prognosis

Depends on the degree of metabolic control. It is hoped that with modern management the previously seen long-term complications can be mostly avoided.

Galactosaemia

Incidence 1:60 000. Autosomal recessive. Gene locus 9p13. Common mutation Q188R accounts for majority of cases although many mutations described.

Enzyme deficiency   Galactose-1-phosphate uridyl transferase (mnemonic = GAL-I-PUT). This results in inability to metabolize galactose or lactose (glucose + galactose)

Pathogenesis unclear but probably related to accumulation of metabolites

Clinical features

Newborn/infant   Vomiting, hypoglycaemia, feeding difficulties
Seizures, irritability, developmental delay
Jaundice, hepatomegaly, liver failure, DIC
Cataracts, splenomegaly, *E. coli* sepsis (typical)

Diagnostic investigations

Diagnosis   Enzyme assay in red blood cells
Urine   Non-glucose reducing substances present when milk fed, i.e. Clinitest positive, Clinistix negative (specific for glucose)

Management

Lactose and galactose-free diet. Speech and language problems (especially dysarthria), mild progressive cognitive problems and ovarian failure almost inevitable even with therapy.

Hereditary fructose intolerance

Incidence 1:40 000, autosomal recessive.

Enzyme deficiency   Aldolase B. This results in inability to metabolize fructose or sucrose (glucose + fructose)
Biochemical result   Fructose-1-phosphate accumulates in hepatocytes

Breast milk and most formulae do not contain fructose; thus symptoms occur upon introduction of fruits and vegetables.

Clinical features

- Abdominal pain, vomiting (often soon after ingesting fructose)
- Proteinuria
- Liver disease results from chronic fructose ingestion

Diagnostic investigations

- Urine-reducing substance that is not glucose
- Enzyme analysis (liver)
- Genetic marker

Management

Elimination of fructose from the diet.

FATTY ACID OXIDATION DEFECTS (FAODs)

During fasting **fats** or **fatty acids** are metabolized to **ketones**. These are used as an alternative energy source to glucose and are the main source of energy during starvation. FAODs are defects in this pathway and are more variable than the GSDs in their presentation.

Some children may not be exposed to significant catabolic stress during early life and therefore FAODs may not present until mid-childhood or even adulthood.

MCAD	Medium-chain acyl-CoA dehydrogenase deficiency
VLCAD	Very long-chain acyl-CoA dehydrogenase deficiency
LCHAD	Long-chain L-3-hydroxyacyl-CoA dehydrogenase deficiency
CPT1	Carnitine palmitoyl transferase 1 deficiency

Clinical features

Typical presentation   Hypoglycaemia and encephalopathy during fasting
Other initial symptoms   Rhabdomyolysis, cardiomyopathy and arrhythmia (as skeletal and cardiac muscle is particularly reliant on fatty acids for cellular metabolism)
During metabolic stress   Hypoglycaemia with inappropriately low ketones (hypoketotic hypoglycaemia)

Diagnosis

Relies on a strong clinical suspicion and specialized tests:

Measurement of fatty acids   Urine **organic acids**
Fatty acid carnitine derivatives   Blood **acylcarnitine profile** (can be done on Guthrie test)

Confirmation is by fibroblast FAOD enzyme studies and/or molecular analysis.

Treatment

Relatively easy, cheap and effective:

- Regular oral feeds
- Regular intake of a carbohydrate solution, either orally or IV, during periods of catabolic stress is essential

NB: Many of the small molecule metabolic diseases can now be screened for on Guthrie test with tandem mass spectrometry. Hopefully this will result in the classical presentations described above becoming much less common.

GROUP 3: DEFECTS IN THE SYNTHESIS OF LARGE MOLECULES RESULTING IN A DYSMORPHIC CHILD

This is a relatively new yet rapidly expanding group of metabolic disorders, including:

Enzyme defects in the **synthesis of cholesterol**, e.g. Smith–Lemni–Opitz syndrome

Peroxisomal biogenesis disorders. There is a defect in the transport of enzymes into the peroxisome and thus normal peroxisomal anabolic function is not possible. (Peroxisomes are intracellular organelles and are important in cell membrane formation, synthesis of bile acids and breakdown of very long chain fatty acids [VLCFAs]). Diagnosis is usually made by measurement of VLCFAs

Congenital disorders of glycosylation (CDG disorders, alternatively carbohydrate deficient glycoprotein disorders). Prior to a protein being exported from a cell carbohydrate moieties are attached by the endoplasmic reticulum and golgi apparatus in a process known as **glycosylation**. This requires a huge variety of enzymes and defects in any one of these lead to a CDG disorder. Preliminary diagnosis is made by studying the glycosylation pattern of **transferrin** (a glycoprotein)

These children tend to be *abnormal at birth* although recognition of this may not be until later. Treatment of all these conditions is generally disappointing.

Disease	Symptoms	Signs	Investigations
Smith–Lemli–Opitz	Failure to thrive Mental retardation	Upturned nares 2–3 toe syndactyly Small penis/ambiguous genitalia in males	Cholesterol (low) 7-dehydrocholesterol
Peroxisomal biogenesis disorders, e.g. Zellweger syndrome, neonatal adrenoleucodystrophy, infantile Refsum disease	Poor feeding Seizures Mental retardation	Hypotonia Large fontanelle Hepatomegaly Corneal clouding, cataracts, retinopathy Dysmorphism Chondrodysplasia punctata on X-ray (stippled appearance of epiphyses)	VLCFAs (high)
CDG1a	Mental retardation Abnormal eye movements	Abnormal fat pads, inverted nipples Cerebellar hypoplasia Hypotonia Multiorgan dysfunction	Abnormal transferrin isoelectric focusing
CDG1b	Failure to thrive Vomiting Diarrhoea	Hepatic and gastrointestinal abnormalities	Abnormal transferrin isoelectric focusing

NB: **Chondrodysplasia punctata** is seen in:

- Zellweger syndrome
- Rhizomelic chondrodysplasia punctata
- Warfarin teratogenicity
- Conradi–Hunermann syndrome

GROUP 4: DEFECTS IN THE METABOLISM OF LARGE COMPLEX MOLECULES

LYSOSOMAL STORAGE DISEASES (LSDS)

Lysosomes are cell organelles important in the recycling of sphingolipids, mucopolysaccharides and oligosaccharides. These large complex molecules are made up of fatty acid chains, carbohydrate moieties and amino groups and are important as structural components of cells and organelles. They are catabolized in a stepwise fashion by a series of enzyme reactions in the lysosome. A defect in any one of these enzymes leads to a **slow accumulation of the preceding compound** and a corresponding **slowly progressive clinical phenotype**.

These lysosomal diseases can show considerable locus and allelic heterogeneity. Different enzyme defects can result in a similar phenotype; alternatively, various lesions in the same gene can result in a severe infantile disease or a relatively mild adult onset, depending on the degree of residual enzyme activity. There are over 40 known LSDs.

Clinical features

CNS **Neurological regression** (most affect the CNS and thus they need to be strongly considered in children and young adults with neurological regression)

Other organs All organ systems can be affected by the accumulation of these compounds:

Hepatosplenomegaly
Cardiomyopathy, valvular lesions
Bone disease
Infiltrative lung disease
Renal impairment
Progressive dysmorphic facial features

> All frequently seen

Diagnosis

Blood white cell enzymes Measurement of individual enzyme activity in leucocytes

Management

- Traditionally treatment has been supportive only
- Organ transplantation (BMT) is successful in some conditions
- Recombinant enzyme replacement therapy is becoming increasingly available (expensive yet effective)

Disease	Symptoms – all progressive	Signs	Investigations
Neimann Pick disease	Cognitive regression Visual impairment	Cherry red spot at macula Hepatomegaly	White cell enzymes – Sphingomyelinase
Mucopolysaccharidosis I: Hurler disease	Cognitive regression Coarse facial features, progressive Dysostosis multiplex	Coarse facial features Dysostosis multiplex* Hepatomegaly Cardiomyopathy, valvular lesions Corneal clouding Skin thickening	Urine glycosaminoglycans (GAGs) White cell enzymes

Disease	Symptoms – all progressive	Signs	Investigations
Tay Sachs disease	Early neurological regression Visual impairment Seizures Decerebration	Truncal hypotonia Hyperreflexic Cherry red spot (retina)	White cell enzymes – Hexominidase A
Metachromatic leucodystophy	Ataxia Muscle spasms Speech, swallowing difficulties Neurological regression	Hypertonia Hyperreflexic	White cell enzymes – Arylsulphatase A
Gaucher disease (Type I)	Sore joints, fractures Malaise Abdominal distension	Hepatosplenomegaly Bone disease	White cell enzymes – Glucocerebrosidase
Neuronal ceroid lipofuscinosis	Neurological regression Seizures Visual impairment Decerebration	Truncal hypotonia Hyperreflexic	Skin/conjunctival/rectal biopsy White cell enzymes Molecular

*Skeletal deformity involving: gibbus deformity, oval-shaped vertebrae, oar-shaped ribs, thickened skull, coax valga, cortical thinning of long bones, tapered phalanges.

Mucopolysaccharidoses

Type 1	Hurler	AR	See above. Vision impaired
Type 2	Hunter	XLR	Similar to Hurler. Vision good (hunters can see to hunt)
Type 3	Sanfilippo	AR	Less severe skeletal/facial features. Neurological regression
Type 4	Morquio	AR	Severe skeletal deformity, normal IQ

GROUP 5: MITOCHONDRIAL DISEASES

Mitochondrial disease usually refers to defects in the **respiratory chain**. This electron transport chain is responsible for the production of ATP via the transport of electrons from NADH and FADH obtained primarily from the Krebs cycle. Defects in this pathway lead to a failure of ATP production and/or an accumulation of oxidative stress and thus cell death.

Tissues that have high-energy demands appear to be particularly vulnerable to mitochondrial cytopathies. The **CNS**, especially the brainstem and basal ganglia, is often affected. The **eye**, **heart**, **liver** and **renal tubules** are also vulnerable, and multiorgan involvement is common.

Inheritance

The respiratory chain involves five enzyme complexes each composed of a number of subunits. These subunits can be encoded for by the nuclear DNA in the traditional manner or alternatively by the 16 kb circular DNA present in each mitochondria. As mitochondria are inherited from the mother, this leads to the possibility of the unique concept of inheritance of disease through **maternal lines**. Without a molecular diagnosis genetic counselling can thus be difficult.

Clinical features

Features suggestive of mitochondrial dysfunction include (especially when in combination):

Muscle	Abnormal tone, weakness, exercise intolerance
Eyes	Ophthalmoplegia, optic atrophy, cataract, retinitis pigmentosa, cortical blindness
CNS	Developmental delay, seizures, movement disorders, coma, stroke
Cardiac	Cardiomyopathy, conduction defects
Hepatobiliary	Liver failure, pancreatic dysfunction
Haematological	Anaemia (sideroblastic in Pearson), pancytopenia
Renal	Tubulopathy
Gastrointestinal	Dysfunction
Other	Growth retardation

Examples of mitochondrial diseases

Congenital lactic acidosis	Floppy neonate, often with cardiomyopathy, liver dysfunction and renal tubular dysfunction. Lactate very high. Death in infancy
Leigh syndrome	Initially normal child, progressive basal ganglia and brainstem dysfunction
MELAS	**M**itochondrial **E**ncephalomyopathy, **L**actic **A**cidosis and **S**troke-like episodes. Short stature, lactic acidosis, mitochondrial point mutations (maternal inheritance). Onset usually in late childhood or adulthood
Pearson syndrome	Transfusion-dependent sideroblastic anaemia, pancreatic dysfunction, short stature, myopathy, developmental delay, mitochondrial DNA deletions

Diagnosis

Plasma lactate	↑ (and especially an elevated CSF lactate) is strongly suggestive of mitochondrial disease (if characteristic signs and symptoms)
Muscle biopsy	The next investigation in most childhood cases. Should be sent to a recognized laboratory for specific histochemistry and enzymology
Molecular diagnosis	May then be sought based on the results of the muscle biopsy. Recent rapid advances in mitochondrial genomics and DNA technology suggest that a molecular approach may be more rewarding and could be regarded as the first-line investigation in the near future

Management

Current treatment is unfortunately generally disappointing. A variety of vitamins, antioxidants and special diets are used and while there is theoretical, laboratory and anecdotal support for these treatments there is, as yet, little objective evidence of clinical benefit.

HYPERLIPIDAEMIAS

These are a range of inherited disorders that result in raised serum lipoproteins. Investigation is with a fasting blood lipid profile.

Classification

Name	Cause	Lab. findings	Clinical
1. Hypertriglyceridaemias			
Lipoprotein lipase (LPL) deficiency	LPL mutations resulting in inability to hydrolyse triglycerides in chylomicrons and VLDLs	↑ Triglycerides (mainly chylomicrons)	Recurrent pancreatitis Xanthomata
Familial hypertriglyceridaemia	Heterogeneous	↑ Triglycerides	Asymptomatic in children Associated with IDDM, obesity, hypertension and coronary heart disease
2. Hypercholesterolaemia			
Familial hypercholesterolaemia	LDL receptor deficiency	↑ Cholesterol (mainly LDL)	Usually asymptomatic in childhood Xanthomata and early atherosclerosis in adulthood
Polygenic hypercholesterolaemia	Heterogeneous	Moderate ↑ cholesterol	Increased risk of CHD in adulthood
3. Combined hyperlipidaemia			
Familial combined hyperlipidaemia	Heterogeneous	↑ Cholesterol and triglycerides (LDL and VLDL)	Increased risk of CHD in adulthood Xanthomata

PORPHYRIAS

These are disorders of the enzymes involved in haem biosynthesis. They may cause cutaneous symptoms, acute symptoms or a mixture of both. The excess porphyrins may be stored in the liver (**hepatic**) or the bone marrow (**erythropoietic**). Certain porphyrins react on exposure to sunlight to produce oxygen free radicals and cause photodamage.

Clinical classification

Cutaneous	Erythropoietic protoporphyria (EPP) AD
	Porphyria cutanea tarda (PCT) AD
	Congenital erythropoietic porphyria (CEP) AR
	Hepatoerythropoietic porphyria (HEP)
Mixed	Porphyria variegata (PV) AD
	Hereditary coproporphyria (HCP) AD } Usually present after puberty
Acute	Acute intermittent porphyria (AIP) AD
	5-Aminolaevulinate dehydratase deficiency porphyria (ADP) } Present after puberty

Haem biosynthesis pathway

Pathway intermediates	Enzyme	Porphyria
Glycine and succinyl CoA		
↓	ALA synthase	
δ-aminolaevulinic acid (ALA)		
↓	**ALA dehydratase**	ADP
Porphobilinogen (PBG)		
↓	**PBG deaminase**	AIP
Hydroxymethylbilane		
↓	**Urogen III synthase**	CEP
Uroporphyrinogen I + Uroporphyrinogen III		
	↓ **Urogendecarboxylase**	PCT/HEP
	Coproporphyrinogen III	
	↓ **Copro-oxidase**	HCP
	Protoporphyrinogen IX	
	↓ **Proto-oxidase**	PV
	Protoporphyrin IX	
	↓ **Ferrochelatase**	EPP
	Haem	

Clinical features

Cutaneous porphyrias	Mostly present in childhood (not sporadic PCT)
	Acute photosensitivity (severe sunburn, bullae, scarring) (EPP, CEP, HEP)
	Subacute symptoms (skin fragility, vesicobullous lesions with minor trauma) (PCT, CEP, HEP)

	Hypertrichosis (PCT, CEP)
	Red teeth, nail dystrophy, photophobia, corneal scarring, blindness and splenomegaly (CEP)
	Chronic liver disease (EPP and PCT)
Acute porphyrias	Present after puberty
	Acute attacks (abdominal and neurological symptoms induced by metabolic stress, e.g. illness, and certain drugs)
Mixed porphyrias	Usually present after puberty, may develop earlier
	Acute attacks and **subacute skin symptoms** (PV and HCP)

Diagnosis

- Measurement of porphyrin metabolites in urine, stool and RBCs (during attack in acute porphyrias)
- Enzyme assay (tissues/RBCs)

Management

- Photoprotection – avoid sun exposure, sunscreen, β-carotene (EEP) (a scavenger of singlet oxygen)
- Chloroquine – PCT
- Acute attacks – emergency porphyrin removal. Avoidance of future attacks
- Stem cell transplant may be indicated, e.g. CEP

FURTHER READING

Fernandes J, Saudubray JM, Van den Berghe G, eds. *Inborn Errors of Metabolism*, 3rd edn. Berlin: Springer-Verlag, 2000

Nyhan WL, Ozand PT *Atlas of Metabolic Disease*. London: Chapman and Hall Medical, 1998

Scriver CR, Beaudet AL, Valle D, Sly WS, ed. *Metabolic and Molecular Basis of Inherited Disease*, 8th edn. New York: McGraw-Hill, 2001

12 Dermatology

- *Dermatological examination*
- *Terminology of common lesions*
- *Neonatal conditions*
- *Nappy rash*
- *Atopic eczema (atopic dermatitis)*
- *Acne vulgaris*
- *Psoriasis*
- *Keratosis pilaris*
- *Pityriasis rosea*
- *Infections*
- *Cutaneous reactions*

- *Vascular birthmarks*
- *Naevi*
- *Alopecia*
- *Disorders of pigmentation*
- *Congenital ichthyoses*
- *Vesiculobullous disorders*
- *DNA fragility syndromes*
- *Ectodermal dysplasias*
- *Ehlers–Danlos syndromes*
- *Cutis laxa*

DERMATOLOGICAL EXAMINATION

Includes:

- Examination of *all* the skin (do not miss bits)
- Hair
- Nails
- Mucous membranes
- Teeth

Describing/illustrating rashes

Include:

Individual lesions	Type (see below), shape, colour, margination, consistency
Arrangement	Linear, annular, localized, diffuse, confluent, symmetrical
Distribution	Areas affected, mucous membrane involvement

TERMINOLOGY OF COMMON LESIONS

Lesion	Description	Examples
Macule	Flat lesion with alteration in colour or texture	Vitiligo, freckle
Papule	Elevated lesion < 0.5 cm diameter	Molluscum contagiosum
Nodule	Elevated lesion > 0.5 cm diameter	Viral wart
Plaque	Elevated area > 2 cm diameter	Psoriasis
Wheal	Transient dermal oedema	Urticaria
Vesicle	Small fluid-filled lesion < 0.5 cm diameter	Herpes simplex
Bulla	Larger fluid-filled lesion > 0.5 cm diameter	Bullous impetigo
Pustule	Pus-filled lesion	Folliculitis
Scales	Flakes of stratum corneum	Ichthyosis, psoriasis
Excoriation	Damage to skin due to scratching	Any pruritic condition
Lichenification	Thickening due to rubbing	Chronic atopic dermatitis
Erosion	Loss of epidermis, heals without scarring	Seen in eczema
Ulcer	Loss of both dermis and epidermis	Aphthous ulcer
Maculopapular	Rash containing both flat and raised lesions	Measles

NEONATAL CONDITIONS

ERYTHEMA TOXICUM NEONATORUM

Benign condition occurring in first few days of life in half of term infants. Eruptions of red papules ± pustules (containing eosinophils) with surrounding erythematous flare. Affects whole body except palms and soles. Self-limiting condition (2–4 days).

MILIA AND SEBACEOUS GLAND HYPERPLASIA

Milia are epidermal follicular keratin-filled cysts, seen in around half of neonates. Small white papules common on the face, gingiva (Epstein's pearls), labia minora, arolae + scrotum. Resolve within a few weeks.

Sebaceous gland hyperplasia (secondary to maternal androgens). Seen in most neonates. Similar appearance to milia – small white papules over the nose, forehead, cheeks and upper lip.

SUCKING PAD

Area of hyperkeratosis on the central lower ± upper lip.

NB: **Sucking blister** is a bulla on the finger, lips or forearm caused by *in utero* sucking of the affected area.

MONGOLIAN BLUE SPOT

Blue macule(s) on trunk ± limbs. Common in dark-skinned races. Due to melanocytes arrested in the dermis on their way to the basal layer of the epidermis. Generally fade during first few years (though they may persist).

SEBACEOUS NAEVUS

Yellow oval plaque with no hair, on the head or neck. Composed of sebaceous glands and may become malignant (basal cell carcinoma) around adolescence, therefore should be removed before adolescence.

APLASIA CUTIS CONGENITA

Developmental absence of skin, usually solitary or multiple small ulcers on the scalp. May be associated with malformation syndromes, embryological defects or intrauterine infection.

NAPPY RASH

The main causes of nappy rash are:

Cause	Phenotype appearance	Treatment
Irritant dermatitis	Due to irritant effect of urine and faeces Skin creases spared	Barrier ointment Regular nappy change Combined antifungal and hydrocortisone ointment
Candida infection	No sparing of skin creases Satellite lesions	Topical antifungal, or Combined antifungal and hydrocortisone ointment Occasionally requires oral antifungal
Seborrhoeic dermatitis	Red moist rash with fine yellow scales Non-pruritic ± Cradle cap	Topical antifungal and hydrocortisone ointment and emollients
Atopic eczema	May present as nappy rash due to increased local irritability	Emollients and combined antifungal and hydrocortisone ointment
Psoriasis	Intractable well-demarcated nappy rash Rare	Emollients and topical steroids initially

ATOPIC ECZEMA (ATOPIC DERMATITIS)

An itchy recurrent or chronic inflammatory skin disease, often associated with other atopic diseases.

Incidence 10–20% of children.

Associations   Family/personal history of atopy, i.e. asthma, hayfever, eczema, raised total IgE (80%)

Generally begins from 3 months–2 years and improves with age.

Features

- Pruritis (itchiness)
- Dry skin, lichenification post-inflammatory pigmentation changes (chronic eczema)
- Hyperlinearity palms and soles
- Dry irritated swollen eyelids, Denni–Morgan fold (fold under eyes, not specific to eczema)
- Lymphadenopathy in widespread disease
- **Acute and subacute eczema** – erythema, vesicles, weeping and crusting of excoriated areas
- **Chronic eczema** – lichenification (thickening) and post-inflammatory hyper- and hypo-pigmentation
- Other forms include **discoid** (annular lesions) and **pompholyx** (tiny vesicles, very pruritic, palms and soles)

Distribution varies with age:

Infants   Face and extensor surfaces
Older children   Elbow and knee flexures, wrists, ankles, neck ± lichenification

Complications

Secondary bacterial infection   With Staphylococcus aureus or Streptococcus pyogenes usually
Viral infection   Several viral infections are more widespread and severe in children with eczema:
- **Eczema herpeticum** – HSV infection in a child with atopic eczema. Can be widespread, potentially serious infection. Must be treated with antivirals (aciclovir given IV if concern)
- Molluscum contagiosum
- Viral warts
- Varicella

Growth impairment   An intrinsic feature of atopic children. More common in severe eczema. Can also be secondary to overzealous dietary restrictions, associated enteropathy with malabsorption, prolonged course of systemic steroids or, rarely, if too much potent topical steroids are given

Management

Several therapies are available. In order of increasing disease severity:

General advice   Detailed advice about eczema, environmental factors and how to use topical steroids. Keep nails short
Avoid triggers

Allergens:	House dust mite reduction (regular hoovering, no carpets, mattress, duvet and pillow covers)	
	Pets (cats, dogs and horses)	
Irritants:	Soap and biological detergents	
	Hot and cold conditions	
	Wool (only loose cotton clothing)	

Emollients   In the bath and instead of soap, e.g. emulsifying ointment BP
                         After baths on skin, e.g. white soft paraffin BP
Topical corticosteroids   Use *minimum* strength effective to minimize side-effects

Topical steroid groups	
Potency	**Example**
Mild	Hydrocortisone
Moderate	Eumovate
Potent	Betnovate
Very potent	Dermovate

Antihistamines   Regular oral antihistamines reduce eczema severity
Antibiotics   If infected
Topical immunomodulators   E.g. tacrolimus
Food allergy management   In some children certain foods worsen their eczema. A trial avoiding them may be undertaken with the dietician's help
Wet wraps and bandages   Wet wraps are double layer cotton wraps, the inner layer is applied wet and under this topical emollients ± steroids are applied. They are changed 12–24 hourly. They pro-

vide (1) physical protection, (2) prolong the effect of emollients and (3) increase the penetration of steroids. NB: These increase the steroid potency by 10 times
Paste bandages with icthamol impregnated into them help reduce lichenification

Oral steroids	May be given as short oral beclomethasone course
Phototherapy	A 6–8-week course of narrow-band ultraviolet-B phototherapy
Chinese herbs	E.g. tea (NB: renal and liver toxicity reported)
Immunosuppressives	For severe eczema courses of these drugs may be needed, e.g. cyclosporin

ACNE VULGARIS

A common inflammatory disorder of the pilosebaceous unit. Incidence high during puberty and generally improves by early–mid 20s. Primarily due to androgen-induced sebum production. Lipophilic bacteria (especially *Propionibacterium acnes*) colonize the hair follicles.

Androgen levels are high directly after birth (due to maternal androgens) and can cause **infantile acne.**

Clinical features

Face, chest and upper back (sebaceous glands most numerous) most commonly affected.

Lesions of acne	Comedo (plug of sebaceous material within the hair follicle)
	(Open comedo = blackhead; closed comedo = whitehead)
	Papules, pustules, cysts, nodules, scars

Treatment

Topical therapy	Antibacterial and keratolytic agents, e.g. benzoyl peroxide
	Antibiotics, e.g. erythromycin, clindamycin
	Retinoic acid lotion or gel (prevents comedones by reducing follicular hyperkeratosis)
Systemic therapy	Antibiotics, e.g. erythromycin for 6–12 months
	Antiandrogens, e.g. oral contraceptive pill containing cyproterone acetate
	Isotretinoin (oral therapy 1 mg/kg dose over 4–6 months):

- Actions – decreases size of sebaceous glands, reduces sebum production and reduces follicular hyperkeratosis
- Side-effects – dry skin and lips, muscular aches, depression, elevated serum lipids, hepatitis, teratogenicity

PSORIASIS

An inflammatory disease of rapid epidermal proliferation (increased skin turnover) causing patches of red thickened skin.

Unusual in childhood (affects 2% population, but < 10% present in childhood). Childhood onset most commonly 7–8 years. Often positive family history.

Clinical features

Two common forms in childhood:

Chronic plaque psoriasis	Well-demarcated silvery-scaled red plaques
	In children the face and scalp are often first affected
	Classically over extensor surfaces (elbows, knees)
	May present as intractable nappy rash in infancy
	Nail pitting and onycholysis rare in children

| *Guttate psoriasis* | Many scattered small plaques on trunk |
| | Often precipitated by streptococcal sore throat (therefore perform throat swab and ASOT titre) |

Treatment

Emollients	(In baths, as soap and after baths)
	Topical treatments applied once or twice daily:
	• Mild or moderate topical steroids
	• Steroid and tar mixtures (ointments, shampoo, soap)
	• Vitamin D$_3$ analogue, e.g. calcipitriol
	• Dithranol (a tree bark extract, applied in day treatment centre)
Phototherapy	Often used in guttate psoriasis as plaques too small to apply topical therapies
	A 6–8-week course of narrow-band ultraviolet-B phototherapy
Systemic treatment	In severe refractory cases, e.g. acitretin, methotrexate

KERATOSIS PILARIS

- Common autosomal dominant condition
- Small rough keratin plugs develop in the hair follicles
- Affects outer arms, thighs and cheeks
- Associated with atopic dermatitis and Down syndrome
- Treatments limited (emollients containing keratolytics give temporary improvement)

PITYRIASIS ROSEA

Common rash in children and adolescents.

Clinical features

Prodrome (unusual)	Mild fever, malaise, arthralgia
Skin	**Herald patch** – a large (1–10 cm) pink annular lesion with raised border
	5–10 days later many smaller pink lesions with a peripheral collarette of scale. Sometimes pruritic
	Rash follows cutaneous cleavage lines and hence makes a '*Christmas tree*' pattern on the back.
	Resolves spontaneously in 2–12 weeks

Management

Emollients only. Mild topical steroids if necessary to speed resolution.

INFECTIONS

IMPETIGO

Common contagious bacterial epidermal infection seen in two forms:

| *Impetigo contagiosa* | Honey-coloured crusts usually around the mouth and nose, may be widespread. Highly contagious |
| *Bullous impetigo* | Fragile vesicles and bullae, i.e. localized SSSS |

Causes

- *Staphylococcus aureus* (bullous impetigo usually due to phage group II)
- Group A β-haemolytic streptococcus (*Streptococcus pyogenes*)

Treatment

- Topical antibiotics if minor
- Systemic antibiotics if widespread

STAPHYLOCOCCAL SCALDED SKIN SYNDROME (SSSS)

Rare exfoliative dermatitis caused by epidermolytic toxin (ET) producing strains of *Staphylococcus aureus* (usually phage group II types 3A, 3C, 55 and 71).

Generally affects children < 5 years.

Clinical features

Skin	Brightly erythematous skin, fissuring and crusting around eyes, nose and lips, blistering and skin tenderness
	Superficial desquamation (peeling sheets of epidermis) 2–3 days later
	Nikolsky sign positive, i.e. epidermis separates with gentle pressure
Systemic	Severe malaise, fever, dehydration, irritability, sepsis, electrolyte imbalance
Other	Pharyngitis, conjunctivitis

Investigations

Cultures	Skin swabs of potential causative sites, e.g. nose, umbilicus, and blood cultures
Blood	FBC (features of sepsis), electrolytes (features of dehydration)
Skin biopsy	Intraepidermal splitting (between granular and spinous layers)
(If diagnostic doubt)	Frozen section of peeled skin can give a rapid diagnosis if necessary

Management

Antibiotics	Systemic antistaphylococcal antibiotic therapy
Skin	Emollient application, non-adherent dressings, low pressure mattress
General	Care of systemic state. Monitor closely vital signs and fluid balance
	(Problems – fluid and electrolyte balance, protein loss, temperature control)
	Keep in warm side-room. IV fluids may be necessary

MOLLUSCUM CONTAGIOSUM

Common infection in school children with DNA pox virus. Spread by contact and scratching lesions. Widespread infection in immnuosuppression and atopic dermatitis.

Clinical features

Pearly papules with a central umbilicus. If squeezed, the central cheesy core of cells infected with viruses is extruded.

Clinical diagnosis, though central plug material may be identified on microscopy.

Management

Spontaneous resolution within 6–9 months (can last years). Advise to use separate towel and baths. No treatment is usually necessary. If necessary can be treated with cryotherapy.

VIRAL WARTS

Extremely common in childhood; spread by contact with people or objects. The various wart viruses (human papillomaviruses [HPV]) are associated with different forms of wart:

Common warts   Papules typically on fingers, hands, face, knees and elbows. HPV type 2
Plantar warts   Flat painful warts on soles. 'Verrucas'. HPV type 1
Filiform warts   Protruberant warts, around lips and nostrils. Refractory to topical therapy
Plane warts   Small flat warts on face and dorsum of hands. Resistant to treatment. Koebnerize. HPV type 3
Anogenital warts *Condylomata accuminata* (occur on mucous membranes)
                   Papillomatous in perianal area, labia, vaginal introitus and penis
                   Also occur on the lips, tongue and conjunctivae
                   NB: May indicate sexual abuse
                   If < 3 years, may be transferred from the birth canal

Management

Warts eventually disappear spontaneously (months–years). Treatments to speed up resolution:

- Wart paints (keratolytics) together with paring of the wart (common, plantar)
- Cryotherapy (freezing). NB: This is painful, therefore best avoided
- Imiquimod 5% cream (anogenital warts)

RINGWORM (TINEA)

Ringworm is caused by superficial fungal infection with dermatophytes which invade the keratin layer. The three species of superficial dermatophyte are: trichophyton, epidermophyton and microsporum.

'Tinea' means moth-eaten.

The areas affected are:

- Tinea capitis   = scalp
- Tinea corporis   = body (trunk and limbs) } Common in children
- Tinea pedis   = feet (mainly soles and toe webs)
- Tinea ungium   = nails – rare in children

Clinical features

A ringworm lesion is typically red, scaly and annular with an active raised border and central clearing.

In tinea capitis hairs may be broken just above the scalp, producing a black dot appearance. A **kerion** is an inflamed, pustular scalp lesion.

Investigations

Fungal identification   (Skin scrapings, nail clippings, hair) Fungal hyphae may be seen on microscopy but fungal culture is essential for confirmation and identification of the fungus

Treatment

Tinea corporis   Topical antifungal for 2–4 weeks
Tinea capitis, T. ungium   Systemic antifungal course for at least 6 weeks
and widespread *T. corporis*

NB: Check if siblings/parents are affected.

PITYRIASIS VERSICOLOR

Common superficial yeast infection of adolescence with *Pityrosporum orale* (*Malassezia furfur*) (a skin commensal). Presents as pink–brown (hypopigmented if sun-tanned) macules, usually on the neck, upper chest, upper arms and back.

Investigations

Woods light view   Lesions become more apparent
Skin scrapings   Microscopy and culture

Management

Topical anti-yeast cream, e.g. ketoconazole.

HEAD LICE

Very common infestation usually confined to the scalp. *Pediculus humanus capitis* (head louse).

Clinical features

- Itchy scalp
- Eggs stuck to hair shaft
- Lice crawling around scalp

Treatment

- Comb hair with lice comb to remove both eggs and lice
- Chemical applications, e.g. malathion, superior to shampoos (resistance is a problem)

SCABIES

An irritative skin reaction to the female mite *Sarcoptes scabiei*.

Transmission by direct contact.

Clinical features

Scabies burrows   Curved red tracts with the mite in a vesicle at one end. Usually very few (< 10) mites
Most likely to be found:
- Infants: palms, soles and side of feet. Often widespread papules
- Older children: finger webs, wrists, elbows, ankles, axillae, scrotum and penis
Rash   Widespread intensely itchy *allergic* reaction to mites, their eggs and excretia after 4–6 weeks – erythematous papules, pustules and excoriations

Investigations

- Clinical diagnosis
- Removal of the mite or its eggs by applying KOH solution over a burrow, scraping with a needle and identification under the microscope

Treatment

- Treat patient and all close contacts
- Topical scabicide, e.g. permethrin cream, after a bath to whole body (and head in infants < 2 years)
- All bed linen and immediate clothes hot washed

NB: The itching usually improves rapidly but may take a few weeks to resolve completely.

CUTANEOUS REACTIONS

ERYTHEMA NODOSUM

Females > males. Usually > age 6 years.

Clinical features

- Painful, shiny, hot, red elevated oval nodules (1–3 cm) over the shins (sometimes thighs and upper limbs)
- Become purple and then fade over 2–4 weeks
- Systemic symptoms: fever, malaise, arthralgia and hilar lymphadenopathy

Causes

Infections	Bacterial – streptococcus, mycoplasma, TB
	Enteric infections – salmonella, yersinia
	Viral – EBV, HBV, chlamydia
	Fungal – histoplasma, coccidiomycosis
Inflammatory bowel disease	Crohn disease, ulcerative colitis
Autoimmune disease	Sarcoidosis, SLE, Behçet disease
Drugs	Sulphonamides, oral contraceptive pill

Management

Bed rest and NSAIDs. Treat the cause.

ERYTHEMA MULTIFORME

A cutaneous reaction pattern of variable appearance.

Clinical features

- **Target lesions –** erythematous border, dusky centre and middle paler ring. May become bullous. Anywhere on the body (classically hands and feet initially)
- Typical target lesions not always seen

No treatment is required. Spontaneous resolution in 2–3 weeks.

Causes

- Herpes simplex virus infection (most common cause)
- Post-infection
- Drugs, e.g. sulphonamides

Stevens–Johnson syndrome

A severe form of EM (considered on a spectrum with TEN) involving:

- Cutaneous erythema multiforme rash
- Systemic upset with fever
- Profound mucous membrane involvement: Conjunctivitis, uveitis, corneal ulceration, corneal scarring may occur
  Oral and genital ulcers

Causes

Infections	Bacterial – Group A streptococcus, mycoplasma
	Viral – HSV, EBV
	Fungal – histoplasmosis
Drugs	Penicillin, sulphonamides, aspirin, anticonvulsants, barbiturates
Connective tissue disease	SLE, sarcoidosis
Malignancy	Leukaemia, lymphoma
Other	Vaccinations, radiotherapy

Treatment

- Supportive, e.g. IV fluids and intensive therapy, as needed
- Steroids controversial
- Ophthalmological consultation essential

TOXIC EPIDERMAL NECROLYSIS (TEN)

A more severe disease (usually a drug reaction) causing damage to the basal cell layer of the epidermis with generalized bullae and loss of sheets of epidermis. Extensive mucous membrane involvement and systemic upset. More common in adults.

Management

- Remove cause
- Intensive care with attention to fluid and electrolyte balance, analgesia, secondary infection, specialist skin and eye care, nutrition, ventilation if necessary and monitoring of other systems (renal, liver, gut, cardiovascular, respiratory)

Most cases survive but there is significant mortality.

NB: Toxic shock syndrome (TSS) is a condition seen most commonly in menstruating women, involving erythema and desquamation, but there are no bullae and no skin tenderness (see p. 58).

MASTOCYTOSIS

Disorder involving proliferation of mast cells, mostly in the skin. The clinical picture is variable with urticaria pigmentosa most commonly seen in children.

Clinical features

Urticaria pigmentosa	Small red–brown macules and papules containing the mast cells widely dispersed on the skin; may blister
	Develops during first 2 years of life
	Darier's sign = if lesions rubbed, wheal and flare occurs due to local histamine release
Solitary mastocytoma	Solitary skin lesion 1–2 cm diameter. Involutes spontaneously
Diffuse cutaneous mastocytosis	Rare. Diffuse skin involvement causing yellow thickened cracked skin, intense pruritis ± systemic involvement

Systemic features of histamine release (tachycardia, hypotension, syncope, wheezing) may rarely occur.

Prognosis

Spontaneous resolution over a number of years.

VASCULAR BIRTHMARKS

PORT-WINE STAIN (PWS, NAEVUS FLAMMEUS)

Permanent vascular malformation due to ectasia of superficial dermal capillaries. Always present at birth. Appear as a macular erythema that gradually darkens with age.

Treatments

- Pulsed dye laser therapy (destroys the ecstatic capillaries)
- Cosmetic camouflage

Associations

Glaucoma	PWS of the face with eyelid involvement may be associated with glaucoma of the affected eye
Sturge–Weber syndrome	1. PWS of the face roughly in the distribution of V1 and V2 branch of the trigeminal nerve, almost always involving the forehead and upper eyelid, and 2. Ipsilateral leptomeningeal vascular abnormality with neurological symptoms: • Focal seizures, and/or • Hemiparesis (slowly progressive) • Mental retardation Glaucoma of the ipsilateral eye may be present (30–60%)

Investigations

(Necessary if glaucoma or Sturge–Weber syndrome suspected)

Skull X-ray	Intracranial calcification, 'railroad track' appearance
CT brain scan	Intracranial calcification, cortical atrophy
MRI brain scan	Vascular anomaly outlined (with gadolinium enhancement)
Ophthalmology	Intraocular pressure measurement

Management

Seizures	Anticonvulsants Surgery (hemispherectomy or lobectomy) may be considered
Glaucoma	Regular intraocular pressure checks and any necessary treatment
Port-wine stain	Laser therapy and camouflage, as above

KLIPPEL–TRENAUNAY SYNDROME

A syndrome involving:

- Port-wine stain on a limb
- Soft tissue and bony hypertrophy

There may also be:

- Venous varicosities, thromboses, ulceration
- A-V fistulae (described by Weber, i.e. Klippel Trenaunay Weber syndrome)

Complications

Cardiac failure, DVT, pain, haematuria (bladder lesions), rectal bleeding (bowel lesions).

Investigations

- Angiograms, if needed
- MRI scan, if needed

Management

- Port-wine treatment, as above
- Cardiac failure treatment
- Orthopaedic procedures (leg length discrepancies)
- Surgical treatment if necessary

SALMON PATCH

A common pale pink vascular malformation (due to dilated superficial dermal capillaries) present at birth on the face (eyelids, glabella, forehead). They tend to fade during first few months of life.

Those on the nape of the neck are known as '**stork bites**' and usually remain for life.

INFANTILE HAEMANGIOMAS

Incidence 1:20 infants.

Association   Premature birth

- Benign vascular tumours
- Rarely present at birth, but appear during the first few weeks
- Enlarge over 6–12 months, then slowly regress. Most have involuted by 5 years. Residual cosmetic defect in a few
- May be *superficial* (bright red, **strawberry haemangiomas**), *deep* (bluish, **cavernous haemangiomas**) or *mixed*

No treatment necessary unless:

- Large disfiguring lesion
- Complications

Complications

- Ulceration/infection
- Haemorrhage
- Interfering with vision
- Interfering with breathing
- Interfering with feeding
- Platelet consumption coagulopathy (Kasabach–Merritt)
- Heart failure (multiple haemangiomas with internal lesions)

Treatment

- Systemic steroid course
- Intralesional steroid injection
- Laser therapy (early, ulcerated lesions)
- Surgical excision

KASABACH–MERRITT SYNDROME

A syndrome of:

- Rapidly enlarging haemangioma
- Consumption coagulopathy (acute or chronic) – thrombocytopenia, consumption of clotting factors, petechiae, haemorrhage, anaemia

High-output cardiac failure may result from A-V shunting in large lesions.

Management

- Platelet, blood and FFP transfusions
- Cardiac failure treatment
- Haemangioma therapy (as above); embolization may be necessary

NEONATAL HAEMANGIOMATOSIS

- Multiple small haemangiomas of the skin, with internal haemangiomas of two or more organs, e.g. liver, CNS, gastrointestinal tract and lung
- USS and CT/MRI scans needed to detect extent of disease
- High-output cardiac failure may occur from A-V shunting, particularly if liver haemangiomas are present

NAEVI

Naevi are skin lesions with a collection of particular cells that are normally found in the skin. Melanocytic naevi (moles) are benign tumours of melanocytes. They may be congenital or acquired.

CONGENITAL MELANOCYTIC NAEVI (CMN)

- Present at birth. May be small or very extensive (giant)
- Incidence approximately 1% of infants
- Giant CMNs (> 20 cm diameter) incidence 1:10 000. Generally on the trunk or lower limbs, e.g. '**bathing trunk naevus**'
- Associated with **intracranial** and **intraspinal melanosis** (diagnosed on MRI scan)
- Small increased risk of malignant transformation (melanoma) with larger CMNs
- Treatment to improve cosmetic appearance is possible but case-specific. Treatment options include dermabrasion, laser therapy and full depth excision. Often left untreated

ACQUIRED MELANOCYTIC NAEVI (MOLES)

- These develop during childhood and new moles continue to appear well into adult life. Average number is 25–50 per adult
- Classified as **junctional** (within the epidermis – flat and pigmented), **compound** (junctional and dermal components – raised and pigmented), **intradermal** (within the dermis – raised and flesh-coloured) or **blue naevus** (deep dermal – dark bluish colour) according to their depth
- Increased melanoma risk related to number of naevi, family history, sun exposure and sunburn during childhood, and immunosuppression

SPITZ NAEVUS

Rapidly growing reddish naevus of childhood, most commonly on the face. It is benign, however histological features can resemble a melanoma and therefore it is removed if there is diagnostic doubt.

INFLAMMATORY LINEAR VERRUCOUS EPIDERMAL NAEVUS (ILVEN)

An uncommon condition usually appearing in the first 6 months of life. A linear epidermal naevus that has a warty appearance and may be pruritic. It is generally refractory to treatments. Treatment options include steroids, cryotherapy, surgical excision and laser therapy. ILVEN may improve spontaneously.

ALOPECIA

This is hair loss to the extent that the scalp becomes abnormally visible.

DIFFUSE HAIR LOSS

Telogen effluvium	Hair loss in the telogen (resting) phase
	Seen 3–4 months after an event or illness, e.g. severe illness, pregnancy, stress, sudden weight loss, recovers 6 months later
Anagen effluvium	Hair loss in the anagen (growing) phase, e.g. chemotherapy

PATCHY HAIR LOSS

Alopecia areata	Gradual patches of hair loss develop
	Lower occipital hairline may be lost
	Cause unknown
	Scalp is normal, and short broken '**exclamation mark**' hairs seen (short new hairs the shape of exclamation marks under the microscope)
	Eyebrows, eyelashes and body hair may be affected
	Nail pitting is common
	Alopecia totalis – total scalp hair loss
	Alopecia universalis – total scalp and body hair loss
	Associations: autoimmune disease, atopy, Down syndrome
	Variable prognosis. Usually hair re-grows spontaneously within weeks/months. 90% recovery if only one patch, worse prognosis if extensive
Trichotillomania	Hair loss (usually patchy) due to child pulling hairs
	Common in a mild form in young children, in whom it may reflect anxiety. Extensive disease (generally seen in adolescents) can be a sign of severe emotional disturbance, and associated with other psychopathology

DISORDERS OF PIGMENTATION

ALBINISM

This is due to a partial or complete failure of melanin synthesis of which there are many types, mostly autosomal recessive.

The degree of hypopigmentation varies depending on whether there is reduced or absent melanin synthesis.

Ocular albinism	Affects only the eyes. Four types. Sensorineural deafness may be associated
Oculocutaneous albinism	Affects eyes and skin. Nine types

Melanin production:

$$Phenylalanine \rightarrow Tyrosine \rightarrow Melanin$$

Tyrosinase catalyses three steps in this process.

Clinical features

Skin	Depigmentation of skin (white or pale) and hair (white or blonde)
Eyes	Blue–grey iris, nystagmus, photophobia, decreased acuity, prominent red reflex
	Depigmentation of retina
Complications	Blindness, skin cancers

Oculocutaneous albinism

There are nine types of oculocutaneous albinism, including:

Type IA (tyrosinase negative)	Pale skin, white hair, red iris. Tyrosinase gene mutations
Type II (tyrosinase positive)	Most common, some pigmentation. Gene defect on chromosome 15q11–13 (p gene, catalyses steps in melanin synthesis)
	Seen in 1% of Prader–Willi and Angelman syndrome
Hermansky–Pudlack syndrome	A tyrosinase-positive albinism associated with:
	• Platelet storage pool deficiency and coagulation problem
	• ± Pulmonary fibrosis, granulomatous colitis
Chediak–Higashi syndrome	Tyrosinase-positive oculocutaneous albinism with abnormal leucocyte granules and increased infections (see p. 34)

Management

There is no specific management. Complete sun protection and regular ophthalmology follow-up are important.

INCONTINENTIA PIGMENTI

X-linked dominant (mostly lethal in males, functional mosaic in females). Gene locus has been demonstrated on Xq28 and Xp11.2.

Clinical features

There are three stages but the sequence is irregular and stages may overlap.

Skin	Stage 1	Vesicles in linear patterns on limbs, occur in crops (first weeks of life)
	Stage 2	Red plaques, papular, warty lesions in linear patterns (from 4 months)
	Stage 3	Classic picture, from 1–16 years. Hyperpigmentation in linear streaks and whorls (following lines of Blashko) in a 'splashed' or 'Chinese figure' distribution. This may be the only stage seen. These slowly fade to become hypopigmented, atrophic lesions
Teeth	Conical teeth, hypodontia	
Hair (25%)	Cicatricial alopecia	
Eye (30%)	Microphthalmos, optic atrophy, strabismus, cataracts, blindness	
CNS (25%)	Seizures, microcephaly, mental retardation, spasticity, paralysis	
Nails	Usually normal, may be dystrophic and small	

HYPOMELANOSIS OF ITO

A clinical picture of hypopigmented lines and whorls following lines of Blashko, usually present from birth, resembling (though unrelated to) the late stages of incontinentia pigmentii.

Clinical features

CNS	Mental retardation, seizures, microcephaly, hypotonia
Musculoskeletal	Scoliosis, limb deformities

| *Eyes* | Strabismus, nystagmus |
| CVS | CHD |

PIEBALDISM (WHITE SPOTTING)

Autosomal dominant. Localized patches of depigmentation due to absence of melanocytes, mostly on the upper chest, abdomen and limbs, and a white forelock. Bilateral involvement, though not symmetrical. The patches are present from birth and remain unchanged throughout life.

WAARDENBURG SYNDROME

Autosomal dominant, variable penetrance. Type I caused by mutations in PAX3 gene (Ch2q), type II by mutations in Ch3p.

A syndrome of:

- Lateral displacement of inner canthi (type I only), inner third of the eyebrow is hyperplastic, brows may be confluent, broad nasal bridge
- White forelock, premature greying in the third decade
- Deafness (25% type I, 50% type II)
- Heterochromic iris (25%), hypopigmented fundus
- Cutaneous depigmentation lesions resembling piebaldism

VITILIGO

A common acquired condition in which the melanocytes are destroyed, resulting in depigmented patches, which may be extensive.

Thought to be autoimmune. Associations with other autoimmune disorders:

- Thyroid disease, hypoparathyroidism
- IDDM, pernicious anaemia, Addison disease
- Myaesthenia gravis, alopecia areata, morphoea
- Halo naevus
- Raised autoantibodies
- Positive family history (40%)

Clinical features

- Usually symmetrical completely depigmented macules, especially around the eyes and mouth, nipples, genitalia, knees and elbows (areas that are usually hyperpigmented), and trauma sites
- Premature greying of hair associated
- Presentation < 20 years in half of cases
- Segmental childhood form (in which only one area is affected) has a good prognosis

Management

May repigment spontaneously (10–20%) but usually progresses. Treatment is disappointing and includes:

- Drug treatments: Topical steroids to affected areas for a few weeks, topical immunomodulators
  Oral psoralens with UV light
- Camouflage make-up
- Sun protection for affected areas

CONGENITAL ICHTHYOSES

These are a heterogeneous group of conditions with rough, dry skin and scaling.

ICHTHYOSIS VULGARIS

- Autosomal dominant. Incidence 1:300
- Mild dry rough skin and hyperlinear palms
- Increased incidence of atopic eczema. Treated with regular emollients

COLLOIDIAN BABY

A distinct appearance at birth of a tight, glistening membrane (like a sausage skin), which slowly sheds to reveal the skin beneath. Everted lips and eyes may be present. These features result in limited chest expansion, temperature instability, potential dehydration and electrolyte imbalance, feeding difficulties and susceptibility to infections.

Initial management

- Intensive care in a warm humidified incubator
- Regular application of paraffin oil
- High fluid intake (may need NG or IV) with careful electrolyte monitoring
- Early recognition and treatment of sepsis

Usually due to rare forms of ichthyosis (lamellar or ichthyosiform erythroderma), and occasionally to a mild ichthyosis.

HARLEQUIN ICHTHYOSIS

A severe type of ichthyosis with a distinct appearance at birth. Features include the following:

- Prematurity (occasionally stillborn)
- A rigid, hyperkeratotic covering of thick, yellow plaques at birth
- Cracks occur soon after birth leaving deep red fissures (like a harlequin)
- Ears are tethered, hands and feet encased, mouth open
- Severe ectropion (everted eyes) and eclabion (everted lips)

Treatment is as for colloidian baby, and in addition oral retinoid therapy may be used. With good general care and early retinoid therapy these babies now survive. They have a distinct severe ichthyosis however.

X-LINKED RECESSIVE ICHTHYOSIS (XLRI)

- X-linked, female carriers may have some features
- A mild ichthyosis with dark skin scaling, corneal opacities
- There is an underlying lipid defect of steroid sulphatase deficiency
- **Prolonged labour** in carrier mothers (due to placental steroid sulphatase deficiency)

Kallman syndrome

XLRI associated with anosmia, hypogonadotrophic hypogonadism and neurological defects.

LAMELLAR ICHTHYOSIS

- Autosomal recessive, very rare condition
- Brown, scaly skin ('lizard skin'), with thick soles and palms

NON-BULLOUS ICHTHYOSIFORM ERYTHRODERMA (NBIE)

Autosomal recessive, rare condition. Fine white scales and erythroderma.

Management of Ichthyoses

- Emollients (bath oils, frequent application of paraffin oil)
- Oral retinoid therapy in severe types

VESICULOBULLOUS DISORDERS

EPIDERMOLYSIS BULLOSA

A group of inherited skin disorders characterized by **skin fragility** and **blister formation**.

The three main types (of which various subtypes exist):

Epidermolysis bullosa simplex

The most common form. Autosomal dominant. Non-scarring intraepidermal blisters of the arms, legs, hands, feet and scalp. Palms and soles mainly affected in some types. Limits walking. Improves with age. Mutations in keratin genes.

Junctional epidermolysis bullosa

A more severe form involving blisters within the lamina lucida of the epidermis. All areas of skin affected, nails are shed. Internal blistering of the respiratory and gastrointestinal tracts, mid-facial erosions, hoarse voice, stridor.

Dystrophic epidermolysis bullosa

A variably severe form involving blisters below the lamina densa of the epidermis. The blisters leave atrophic scars and milia. Two types, both caused by mutations in the COL7A1 gene that encodes for the anchoring fibril protein, type VII collagen.

Autosomal dominant form	Scarring blisters mostly of the hands, feet and sacrum Nail loss. Generally less severe than recessive form
Autosomal recessive form	Severe disease with widespread atrophic scarring blisters with milia formation, **mitten hand** deformity (digital fusion) Oesophageal strictures affect nutrition. Sparse hair, dystrophic nails, corneal ulceration

CHRONIC BULLOUS DERMATOSIS OF CHILDHOOD (LINEAR IgA DERMATOSIS)

Usually occurs < 10 years.

Associations	HLA-B8, DR3

Clinical features

Bullae	Multiple tense bullae on buttocks, genitals, trunk, perioral area, face and limbs Urticated plaques with blisters around the edge (**string of pearls** sign) Mucosal involvement. Blisters may form rosettes Pruritis sometimes present Usually of 3–4 years' duration

Investigations

Skin biopsy	Subepidermal blister, linear IgA BMZ antibodies

Management

Dapsone (steroids if no response).

DNA FRAGILITY SYNDROMES

XERODERMA PIGMENTOSUM (XP)

Autosomal recessive. Disorder of defective DNA repair. Light in the wavelengths 280–340 nm results in DNA damage. Seven complementation groups (on different chromosomes) known.

Clinical features

Skin	Freckling, erythema, scaling, crusting and telangiectasia in sun-exposed areas (premature ageing)
	Skin cancers develop (BCC, SCC, malignant melanoma)
Eyes	Corneal opacities, blepharitis, photophobia, eventual blindness
CNS (20%)	Mental retardation, deafness

Management

- Total sun protection (glasses, clothes, total sunblock)
- Antenatal diagnosis possible with amniocentesis

Prognosis

Early death from developing cancers and neurological problems.

ECTODERMAL DYSPLASIAS

A group of many disorders involving a defect of teeth, hair, nails and skin. There are many subtypes.

EEC SYNDROME (ECTRODACTYLY-ECTODERMAL DYSPLASIA CLEFTING SYNDROME)

Autosomal dominant.

- Ectodermal dysplasia (dry skin, wispy hair, no eyelashes)
- Cleft lip palate
- Lacrimal duct stenosis
- Ectrodactyly (split hands and feet, 'lobster claw' deformity)
- Peg-shaped teeth

HYPOHIDROTIC ECTODERMAL DYSPLASIA

X-linked recessive. A syndrome of:

- Decreased/absent sweat glands – discomfort in hot temperatures, unexplained fevers
- Hypotrichosis
- Hypodontia, conical teeth

Other features include:

Facial dysmorphism	Large ears, flat nasal bridge, frontal bossing, thick everted lips
Hair	Sparse, dry, short scalp hair
Skin	Dry, hypopigmented, prematurely aged, brittle nails
CNS	Learning difficulties in approximately 30%

Investigations

Sweat pores	Absent or decreased in palmar ridges
Sweat test	Reduced or absent (pilocarpine iontophoresis)
Skin biopsy (palm)	Eccrine gland hypo/aplasia

HIDROTIC ECTODERMAL DYSPLASIA

Autosomal dominant.

- Small/absent dystrophic nails
- Hyperkeratosis of palms and soles
- Thin, pale, brittle hair

NB: Normal sweating and teeth.

EHLERS–DANLOS SYNDROMES

A group of connective tissue disorders of different genetic origin, involving deficiencies of collagen.

Clinical features

Normal at birth

Skin	Hyperelasticity, fragility, easy bruising, atrophic 'cigarette paper scars'
Joints	Hypermobile, tendency to dislocate

There are several different types (10 at present), each possessing specific clinical features which include:

- Premature birth (with PROM)
- Mitral valve prolapse, dissecting aortic aneurysm
- Bowel rupture, uterine rupture

Mutations have been found in collagen III and other genes.

CUTIS LAXA

Autosomal recessive, autosomal dominant or acquired. Pathogenesis is due to defect(s) in elastin (exact mechanism unknown). **Acquired cutis laxa** appears during childhood and may follow a febrile illness; connective tissue disease, e.g. SLE, amyloidosis; inflammatory skin condition, e.g. erythema multiforme; or occur in babies from women on penicillamine.

Clinical features

Skin	Folds of lax skin from birth or later in childhood. Premature ageing, **'bloodhound'** facial appearance
Other features	(Seen in recessive types) Hernias, rectal prolapse, diverticular disease, pneumothoraces, emphysema, peripheral pulmonary stenosis, aortic dilatation, skeletal abnormalities, dental caries and growth retardation

FURTHER READING

Harper J, Oranje A, Prose N *Textbook of Paediatric Dermatology*. Oxford: Blackwell Science, 2000

Higgins E, duVivier A *Skin Disease in Childhood and Adolescence*. Oxford: Blackwell Science, 1996

13

Rheumatic and musculoskeletal disorders

- Autoantibodies
- Juvenile idiopathic arthritis
- Systemic lupus erythematosus
- Antiphospholipid syndrome
- Idiopathic inflammatory myopathies
- Scleroderma disorders
- Mixed connective tissue disease
- Sjögren syndrome

- Vasculitis
- Amyloidosis
- Osteogenesis imperfecta
- Osteopetrosis (marble bone disease)
- Osteochondrodysplasias
- Non-inflammatory pain syndromes
- Syndromes involving absent radii

AUTOANTIBODIES

Non-organ specific autoantibodies associated with rheumatic disease are outlined. None is absolutely diagnostic but many are quite sensitive and specific.

Rheumatoid factor (RhF)

Antibody to the Fc portion of IgG (usually IgM detected, also IgG, IgA and IgE).

Positive in   JIA (some types)
               Adult RA (commonest group)
               Connective tissue disease, e.g. SLE, Sjögren syndrome
               Chronic infections, e.g. HIV, hepatitis, TB, endocarditis
               Leukaemia, lymphoid malignancies
               Pulmonary fibrosis
               General population ($\leq 4\%$)

Antinuclear antibodies (ANA)

These are antibodies to nuclear components and include:

Anti-ds DNA   SLE (80%, specific)
Anti-ss DNA   SLE (90%, non-specific), drug-induced lupus, other connective tissue disease

| Anticentromere | Limited cutaneous systemic sclerosis (formerly CREST syndrome) |
| Antihistone | SLE, drug-induced lupus particularly |

Antiextractable nuclear antigens (ENAs)

Anti-Sm (Smith)	SLE (20%, quite specific), normal population
Anti-nRNP	MCTD (100%), SLE
Anti-SSA (Ro)	SLE, neonatal lupus, Sjögren syndrome, rarely normal population
Anti-SSB (La)	SLE, neonatal lupus, Sjögren syndrome, rarely normal population
Anti Jo-1	JDM some forms, rarely juvenile

Antineutrophil cytoplasmic antibodies (ANCAs)

Antibodies to antigens within the cytoplasm of neutrophils.

| c-ANCA (cytoplasmic) | Wegener granulomatosis (specific usually to proteinase 3 antigen), microscopic polyangiitis (renal) |
| p-ANCA (perinuclear) | Non-specific usually to myeloperoxidase (infection, many autoimmune diseases, e.g. Churg–Strauss, Kawasaki disease) |

Antiphospholipid antibodies

Antibodies to phospholipid antigens. Associated with thrombosis *in vivo* but coagulation prolongation *in vitro* (lupus anticoagulant test positive).

Seen in SLE and antiphospholipid syndrome, e.g. anti-β_2-glycoprotein and anticardiolipin antibodies.

JUVENILE IDIOPATHIC ARTHRITIS (JIA)

A group of disorders defined as:

- **Chronic synovitis** ($\geq$ 6 weeks) $\pm$ extra-articular features
- Occurring *before* 16 years of age

Some are reclassified at 6 months due to evolution.

Cause unknown, though autoimmune genetic and environmental factors probably interact.

Features of involved joints

- Early morning stiffness
- Swelling, warm (not hot), occasionally red and tender
- Limited painful movement
- Contractures may develop rapidly
- Bony deformity may develop rapidly

X-ray changes

Early Soft tissue swelling, osteopenia, periosteal new bone formation
Late Bony overgrowth, osteoporosis, subchondral bone erosions, joint space narrowing, collapse, deformity, fusion, subluxation

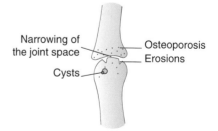

Figure 13.1 X-ray changes in JIA

JIA subclassification
Oligoarticular JIA ≤ 4 joints
Polyarticuar JIA > 4 joints
Systemic-onset JIA
Enthesitis-related arthropathy (ERA; formerly juvenile spondyloarthropathy)
Psoriatic arthropathy
Other

OLIGOARTICULAR JIA

Involvement of ≤ 4 usually large lower limb joints in the first 6 months of disease.

- Female > male, onset 2–4 years of age
- Knees, ankles, elbows – bony overgrowth, leg length discrepancy and valgus deformity are important features
- $^1/_5$ will go on to have > 4 joints affected beyond 6 months (extended oligoarticular JIA)
- Chronic iridocyclitis (uveitis) ($^1/_3$)
  No early symptoms, detectable with slit-lamp only. Untreated causes synechiae, glaucoma, cataracts and blindness
  Slit-lamp examination *imperative* 3 monthly
  Treatment with topical steroids and mydriatics
- ANA positive (90%) – increased risk of eye disease
- HLA-DR5, 8, DP0201 positive
- RhF and HLA-B27 negative
- ESR (↑ or N)

POLYARTICULAR JIA

Involvement of > 4 joints by 6 months of onset (usually many more). Female > male.

Two sub-types:

RhF negative (30% of JIA)	Moderate to severe disease, < 8 years, HLA-DR1
	Asymmetrical, small and large joints, especially the TMJ and cervical spine
	Occasional iridocyclitis (5%)
RhF positive (10% of JIA)	Equivalent to adult RA
	More severe, ≥ 8 years, HLA-DR4
	Symmetrical, hands and feet, and hips
	Rheumatoid nodules, tenosynovitis and vasculitis may develop

Particular joint problems seen due to distorted growth:

Cervical spine	Fusion or subluxation, anaesthetic difficulties
Temporomandibular joint (TMJ)	Micrognathia, dental hygiene and anaesthetic difficulties
Hips	Destruction, limb shortening
Knee	Overgrowth causing valgus deformity

Investigations

- ESR often marked ↑
- ANA may be positive in 30–40%

SYSTEMIC-ONSET JIA (SOJIA)

All ages, but peak 3–6 years. Females = males.

A clinical **diagnosis of exclusion**. Differential diagnoses:

- Infection
- Malignancy, e.g. leukaemia, neuroblastoma
- Vasculitis, other connective tissue disease

Clinical features

Defined by:

- **Arthritis** and characteristic **fever** – quotidian fever (39–40°C × 1–2 per day returning to baseline); usually appears very unwell while febrile
- Plus one of: **Evanescent rash** – classically heat/fever-induced salmon pink macular but may be urticarial and red in some
  Lymphadenopathy
  Hepatosplenomegaly
  Serositis (typically pericarditis)
- Also: myalgia, arthralgia, abdominal pain, pleuritis
- **Joints** – polyarthritis may be delayed some months in onset and is severely destructive in 50%. The other half have relatively remittive or mild disease
- **Late features** – short stature, micrognathia, amyloidosis (now rare)

Investigations

FBC	Anaemia of chronic disease, WCC ↑ (neutrophilia), platelets ↑
Acute phase proteins	ESR usually very marked↑, CRP ↑
Autoantibodies	ANA and RhF negative

ENTHESITIS-RELATED ARTHOPATHY (ERA)

These children typically have an enthesitis (swelling at tendon and ligament insertions, including Achilles tendon and plantar fascia). ERA is part of a general group called spondyloarthropathies. Predominantly males, ≥ 8 years.

- Arthritis and enthesitis, or
- Arthritis or enthesitis plus at least two of: Sacroiliac or inflammatory spinal pain
  Acute anterior uveitis (10%)
  HLA-B27 positive
  Positive family history of B27 positive disease
- Typically lower limb, great toe, tarsus, hip and enthesitis (especially heel), sacroiliac and axial arthritis in only ≤ 20% over time
- May progress to ankylosis
- HLA-B27 (90%)
- RhF and ANA negative, ESR (↑ or N), anaemia of chronic disease

X-ray changes

As for oligo/polyarthritis, and with spinal disease:

- Erosion of sacroiliac joints
- Loss of lumbar lordosis
- Tramline appearance (due to calcification of interspinous ligaments)
- Bamboo spine

Spondyloarthropathies	
ERA	See above
Reactive arthritis/Reiter syndrome	Sterile arthritis following infection, e.g. gastrointestinal, influenza, mycoplasma, EBV, streptococcal
	Affects a few joints only, may be migratory and is self-limiting. Some children develop a chronic spondylarthropathy later
	NB: Rheumatic fever is a reactive arthritis (see p. 314)
Arthritis of IBD	Arthritis associated with Crohn disease or ulcerative colitis. Usually varies with bowel disease activity, though some cases (spondylitic) progress regardless of control of underlying bowel disease
	Not considered really a spondylarthropathy by most but a 'seronegative arthropathy'
Juvenile psoriatic arthropathy	Arthritis associated with psoriasis. Rare in childhood. Usually oligoarticular, dactylitis typical with skin and nail changes which may predate or follow

REACTIVE ARTHRITIS

Reactive arthritis is **viral and post-infectious arthritides**, including acute rheumatic fever and arthritis following respiratory, genitourinary tract and gastrointestinal tract infections.

(Reiter syndrome is a special subtype with a classical triad – arthritis, conjunctivitis, urethritis/cervicitis – usually coexisting. Very rare in childhood.)

Clinical features

- Predominantly lower limb, asymmetric, oligoarthritis
- Clear history of infection during preceding 4 weeks (esp. diarrhoea)
- No clear clinical infection of the joint and no other known cause of arthritis present
- Yersinia, shigella, salmonella, campylobacter (adolescent – venereal infection)
- Mycoplasma and streptococcal infections may precipitate
- May last weeks–months with recurrences over several years

Investigations

- Throat and stool culture
- Serology and PCR
- ANA and RhF negative. Sometimes HLA-B27 positive (if arthritis ERA-like)
- Synovial and urethral tests where appropriate

MANAGEMENT OF JIA

- Early intervention improves prognosis and may delay/prevent irreversible bony changes and loss of function
- Physiotherapy, occupational therapy, podiatry – for stretching, increasing strength, improving function, joint splinting, foot orthoses
- NSAIDs for initial symptom control
- Intra-articular crystalline steroid injections are mainstay of all mild to moderate disease
- Disease-modifying drugs (DMARDs) if polyarticular or uncontrolled oligoarticular or systemic, e.g. methotrexate, leflunomide, cyclosporine
- Biological anticytokine therapies for severe resistant disease – etanercept or infliximab (anti-TNF therapy), or anakinra (anti-IL-1)

- Sulphasalazine for FRA
- Steroids – oral prednisolone or IV pulsed methylprednisolone if rapid control required, but aim to withdraw as soon as possible

SYSTEMIC LUPUS ERYTHEMATOSUS (SLE)

A multisystem autoimmune disease associated with serum antibodies against nuclear components. Females > males, usually > 10 years at onset.

Associations	HLA-B8, -DR2, -DR3
	African/oriental > Caucasians

Clinical features

General (v. common)	Faltering growth, malaise, weight loss, fever
Skin (v. common)	**Butterfly rash** (80%) – over nose and cheeks
	Photosensitivity (33%)
	Discoid lupus: plaques causing scarring and scarring alopecia. Skin *only* involved in some
	Also papular, vesicular, purpuric, vasculitic lesions or periungual erythema
	Raynaud phenomena, alopecia, mucosal ulcers
Kidneys (common)	Proteinuria, glomerulonephritis, BP ↑, renal failure (see p. 229)
Musculoskeletal (common)	Arthralgia (80%), arthritis, aseptic necrosis hip and knee, myalgia, myositis
Blood (common)	Platelets ↓, haemolytic anaemia, neutrophils ↓
CNS	Headache, behavioural change, depression, epilepsy, blurred vision
Eyes	Iritis, episcleritis, retinitis, Sjögren syndrome
Lungs	Effusions, pleurisy, interstitial fibrosis, haemorrhage
Heart	Pericarditis, myocarditis, Libman–Sachs endocarditis, cardiomyopathy
Gastrointestinal	Hepatosplenomegaly, mesenteric arteritis, IBD

Investigations

FBC	Anaemia (chronic disease or haemolytic), platelets ↓, lymphopaenia characteristic
Acute phase proteins	ESR ↑ (with disease activity), CRP typically low or normal
Autoantibodies	**dsDNA** (50%), anti-Sm (20%) *specific* for SLE
	ANA (usually strongly positive)
	Anticardiolipin (antiphospholipid), RhF (50%)
Immunology	Complement (C3 ↓ in active disease), IgG and IgM (↑)
Histology	Haematoxylin bodies (amorphous extracellular material staining with haematoxylin), vasculitis, granulomas. Immune complex, immunoglobulin and complement deposition

Management

- NSAIDs for mild joint disease
- Hydroxychloroquine (for skin, arthralgia and lethargy, and prevention of dyslipidaemia)
- Systemic steroids (oral or pulsed IV)
- Immunosuppressants, e.g. cyclophosphamide, azathioprine, mycophenolate mofetil. Biologics for severe resistant disease.
- For skin disease: topical steroids and hydroxychloroquine

NEONATAL LUPUS

Usually occurs in infants of mothers with SSA(Ro) ± SSB(La) antibodies (SLE or Sjögren syndrome), and is acquired transplacentally.

Clinical features

This presents with different combinations of clinical features.

1. Congenital heart block (permanent), or
2. Neonatal lupus rash, often with
3. Haematological abnormalities (Hb ↓, platelets ↓,WCC ↓) ⎫
4. Hepatic involvement – mild ⎭ Self-limiting

Investigations

Autoantibodies	ANA, anti-SSA (Ro), anti-platelet, Coombs' positive
FBC	Platelets ↓, Hb ↓,WCC ↓
ECG	Complete heart block, may be partial and progress

Management

Pacing for cardiac disease.

ANTIPHOSPHOLIPID SYNDROME

A syndrome characterized by antiphospholipid antibodies which are involved in thrombosis. May be associated with SLE. The lupus anticoagulant is a specific laboratory test which usually correlates with the presence of APL antibodies.

Clinical features

Thrombosis	Arterial and venous, strokes, Budd–Chiari syndrome
CNS disease	Epilepsy, migraine, strokes
Skin	**Livedo reticularis**, thrombophlebitis, splinter haemorrhages, fingertip ulcers
Other	Valvular heart disease, recurrent spontaneous abortions

Investigations

Serum antibodies	Antiphospholipid antibodies
	Lupus anticoagulant
Coagulation	APTT prolonged and does *not* correct with added serum *in vitro*

Management

- Anticoagulation – aspirin if antibody strongly positive, warfarin if serious thrombotic event
- Treatment of SLE

IDIOPATHIC INFLAMMATORY MYOPATHIES

These include:

- Dermatomyositis (commonest)
- Polymyositis (no skin involvement)
- Other myositis: Infectious, e.g. cryptococcus
                     Postinfectious, e.g. influenza A, streptococcus
                     Inclusion body
                     Focal

JUVENILE-ONSET DERMATOMYOSITIS

A multisystem disease involving **inflammation of striated muscle and skin.**

Associations	HLA-B8, -DR3, DQA1*0501
	Female > male

Clinical features

Muscle	Symmetrical proximal muscle weakness and pain (Gower sign and waddling gait)
	Respiratory muscle weakness
	Dysphagia, dysphonia, palatal regurgitation
Skin	Classic **heliotrope violaceous rash** over upper eyelids
	Gottron's papules – red rash overlying DIP, PIP joints and knees
	Nail fold capillaritis
	Photosensitive rash, butterfly rash
	Subcutaneous calcium deposits (20–50%) which may extrude
Joints	Arthralgia and arthritis with contractures
Gastrointestinal	Vasculopathy (ulcerations, bleeding), hepatosplenomegaly
Cardiac	Myocarditis (arrhythmias)
Other	Nephritis, interstitial lung disease, pulmonary haemorrhage, retinitis, CNS involvement

Investigations

Diagnosis based on clinical picture plus:

MRI	Confirms typical inflammation of thigh muscles
Muscle enzymes	LDH ↑, CK ↑, AST ↑, ALT ↑ (may be deceptively normal)
EMG	Myopathic. Rarely required
Muscle biopsy	(Vasculopathy, inflammatory infiltrate and consequent muscle fibre necrosis) in equivocal cases.
Autoantibodies	ANA may be positive, RhF usually negative, anti-Jo-1 when overlap with other CTD

Management

- Early active physiotherapy and splinting
- Systemic steroids (oral or pulsed IV)
- Immunosuppressives – methotrexate or cyclosporin. Cyclophosphamide in severe disease. Biologics in resistant disease.
- Other treatments, e.g. IV immunoglobulins, plasmapheresis, autologous stem cell transplantation in rare cases

Prognosis

Untreated, the mortality is up to 40%, otherwise 2–5%. 30–40% will remain disabled

SCLERODERMA DISORDERS

LOCALIZED SCLERODERMA (MORPHOEA)

Clinical features

Skin	Discrete firm plaques (**morphoea**) or linear lesions following Blashko's lines (**linear scleroderma**). The lesions are initially erythematous, becoming atrophic and shiny with raised violaceous borders. They are hyper- or hypo-pigmented
	Scarring and fibrosis beneath affected skin may lead to **severe contractures and limb shortening en Coup de Sabre** (lesion involving half of upper face, forehead and scalp, and may involve underlying vasculitis in the brain and uveitis)
Other	Tendon nodules, joint stiffness, arthritis

The natural history is usually for the disease to 'burn out' after a number of years. Methotrexate and biologics are used to limit damage during the active phase.

SYSTEMIC SCLEROSIS

This is a multisystem disease characterized by **occlusive vasculitis** and **fibrosis**. Two forms are recognized:

- Diffuse cutaneous
- Limited cutaneous (formerly CREST syndrome)

Females > males. Rare in children, systemic manifestations cause significant morbidity and mortality.

Clinical features

Hands	Raynaud phenomenon, digital ulcers, sclerodactyly (sausage fingers)
Skin	Diffuse thickening and tightening, beak nose, small mouth, telangiectasia
Musculoskeletal	Synovitis, tenosynovitis, myopathy
Gastrointestinal	Dysphagia (oesophageal involvement), malabsorption
Lungs	Fibrosis, pulmonary hypertension
Cardiac	Pericarditis, cardiac failure
Renal	Obliterative endarteritis, hypertension, chronic renal failure

Investigations

ESR	Normal
Autoantibodies	ANA (positive), RhF (may be positive), Scl70 (positive in some in systemic forms)
Skin biopsy	Typical features of morphoea
Muscle biopsy	Perivascular infiltration and fibre necrosis may be present

Management

- Physiotherapy
- Systemic steroids, immunosuppressants
- Antiprostacyclin agents for gangrene
- Bosentan (endothelin receptor blocker) or sidenafil for pulmonary hypertension
- Autologous stem cell transplantation

MIXED CONNECTIVE TISSUE DISEASE (MCTD)

One of the **overlap syndromes**. This may not be a distinct entity and includes features of SLE, rheumatoid arthritis, dermatomyositis and scleroderma. Mostly girls >6 years are affected. High titres of anti-RNP (ribonucleoprotein) autoantibodies and speckled ANA. Predominantly a moderate polyarthritis and features of peripheral scleroderma (sclerodactyly).

Prognosis is variable; renal involvement may occur and it may progress to classic SLE or scleroderma.

SJÖGREN SYNDROME

Very rare in children, this disease typically involves:

- Dry eyes (keratoconjunctivitis sicca)
- Dry mouth (xerostomia)
- Parotitis
- Other vasculitis complications
- Dryness of the vagina and skin may also occur

Mothers who are anti-Ro positive may have infants with congenital heart block.

Associations	HLA-B8, -DR3
	Other connective tissue disease, e.g. SLE, vasculitis, Raynaud phenomenon
	Autoimmune disease, e.g. thyroid disease, chronic active hepatitis
	Renal tubule defects, e.g. nephrogenic DI, renal tubular acidosis

Clinical features

Eyes	Photophobia, burning eyes
Glands	Parotid and salivary gland enlargement
Mouth	Decreased taste, dysphagia, angular cheilitis, fissured tongue
Nose	Decreased sense of smell, epistaxis
Respiratory	Bronchitis, otitis, hoarseness
Malignancy	Lymphoma risk

Investigations

Autoantibodies	Anti-Ro (SSA) (70%), anti-La (SSB)
	ANA (positive 70%)
Schirmer test	Filter paper placed inside eyelid. Wetting of < 10 mm in 5 min indicates decreased tear production
Biopsy	Lip or salivary gland (focal lymphocytic infiltration)

Management

- Symptomatic (artificial tears and lozenges)
- Systemic steroids or immunosuppression may be needed

VASCULITIS

Vasculitis is inflammation of the blood vessel wall. It may be a primary or secondary phenomenon.

Suggestive features

General	Weight loss, fever, fatigue of unknown origin
Skin	Levido reticularis, palpable purpura, vasculitis urticaria, nodules, ulcers
CNS	Focal CNS lesions, mononeuritis multiplex
Musculoskeletal	Intense arthralgia ± myalgia, arthritis, myositis
Vascular	BP ↑, pulmonary haemorrhage
Laboratory	ESR ↑, CRP ↑, eosinophilia, anaemia, ANCA, factor VIII related AG (VWF), haematuria, cryoglobulinaemia

CLINICAL CLASSIFICATION	
Polyarteritis	Macroscopic, e.g. polyarteritis nodosa (PAN)
	Microscopic polyangitis
	Kawasaki disease
Granulomatous vasculitis	Churg–Strauss syndrome, Wegener granulomatosis
Leucocytocytoclastic vasculitis	Henoch–Schönlein purpura (HSP)
Hypersensitivity arteritis	
Cutaneous polyarteritis	Post-streptococcal angitis
Giant cell arteritis	Takayasau disease
Secondary to connective tissue disease or periodic fever syndrome	SLE, dermatomyositis, scleroderma, JIA, MCTD, FMF
Miscellaneous vasculitides	Behçet, sarcoidosis, Cogan syndrome

MJ Dillon, 5:11:8, p. 1402. Oxford Textbook of Rheumatology, Second edition, Maddison PJ, Isenberg D, Woo P, Glass DN. Oxford Medical Publications 1998.

KAWASAKI DISEASE

A predominantly infantile polyarteritis postulated to be secondary to an as yet unidentified infectious agent in an immunologically or genetically susceptible individual.

Diagnostic criteria

Fever	38.5°C for > 5 days and four of:
	Conjunctivitis – bilateral non-purulent
	Cervical lymphadenopathy – with one node > 1.5 cm
	Rash – polymorphous, no vesicles or crusts
	Changes of lips or oral mucosa – red cracked lips; 'strawberry tongue'; or diffuse erythema of oropharynx
	Extremities (feet and hands) – initially erythema and oedema of palms and soles. In convalescent stage peeling skin from fingertips
	(May be diagnosed with fewer than four of the above if coronary artery aneurysms are detected)
Other features	**Extreme irritability** (almost universal)
	Arthritis, asceptic meningitis, pneumonitis, uveitis, gastroenteritis, meatitis, dysuria and otitis

Cardiac complications

- 20–40% of untreated children will develop **coronary artery aneurysms**, a major cause of morbidity
- Cardiac tamponade
- Cardiac failure
- Myocarditis, myocardial infarction
- Pericarditis

Investigations

Bloods	Neutrophils ↑
	Marked thrombocythaemia (2nd–3rd week)
	ESR, CRP ↑
	LFTs (may be deranged)
Urine	Sterile pyuria
Cardiac	ECG and 2D echocardiogram. Consider CXR

Management

- High dose IVIG (2 g/kg) over 10 h, within 10 days of disease
- Aspirin for 6 weeks or until coronary aneurysms gone
- Steroids may be used in resistant disease
- 2D echocardiogram at presentation, regularly during acute disease and at follow-up

Early treatment with aspirin and IVIG reduces the occurrence of coronary artery aneurysms.

POLYARTERITIS NODOSA (PAN)

A necrotizing vasculitis of medium and small arteries. Males > females, uncommon in children.

Clinical features

General	Malaise, fever, weight loss, myalgia
Joints	Migratory arthralgia, arthritis
Renal	Haematuria, proteinuria, chronic renal failure (major cause of death), hypertension
Neurological	Mononeuritis multiplex, symmetrical peripheral neuropathy, seizures, stroke

Cardiac	Aneurysms, myocardial infarction, cardiac failure
Lungs	Cough, wheeze, pleuritis
Abdominal	GI bleeding, infarction, abdominal pain, liver pain (splenic and coeliac vessels)
Gonads	Orchitis, epididymitis
Skin	Nodules, ulcers, erythematous rashes, purpura

Investigations

FBC	Anaemia, WCC ↑
ESR	Marked ↑
Autoantibodies	p-ANCA (may be positive)
Biopsy	Muscle, nerve or skin may show characteristic features
Angiography	Mesenteric or renal microaneurysms

Management

Steroids and imunosuppressants or biological agents.

TAKAYASAU DISEASE

An arteritis of the aorta and major branches ('pulseless disease'), autoimmune inflammatory disease. Most common in young women. Poor prognosis in children.

Associations	Orientals, blacks

Clinical features

CVS	Claudication in arms and legs, absent peripheral pulses, BP ↑
General	Fever, malaise, myalgia
Other	Arthritis, pericarditis, rashes, CNS disturbance

Investigations

ESR	↑
FBC	Anaemia, neutrophilia
Doppler and angiography	(Occlusion, stenosis and aneurysms)

Management

- Systemic steroids and cytotoxic agents may be considered
- Surgery as necessary

WEGENER GRANULOMATOSIS

A systemic necrotizing vasculitis most prominent in the lungs and kidneys, and destructive granulomas of the respiratory tract. Rare in childhood.

Clinical features

Upper respiratory tract	Rhinorrhoea, nasal ulceration, granulomas, progressive destruction of nasal septum, pharynx, larynx and trachea
Lungs	Cough, haemoptysis, pleurisy, granulomas
Kidneys	Proliferative glomerulonephritis, renal failure
Other	Malaise, fever, weight loss, arthritis, arthralgia, splenomegaly, rash

Investigations

Autoantibodies	c-ANCA, good correlation (90%)
CXR	Pulmonary infiltrates
Sinus X-ray	Bony destruction nose and sinuses
Renal function	Microhaematuria, red cell casts
Biopsy	Granulomatous inflammation respiratory tract, and nephritis

Management

Steroids and cyclophosphamide or biological agents.

BEHÇET SYNDROME

Rare in children.

Associations   Turkish, Arabic, Japanese, HLA-B51

A vasculitis of small and medium-sized arteries involving:

- Oral ulcers
- Genital ulcers
- Eye inflammation (anterior or posterior uveitis, retinal vasculitis may lead to blindness)

The course is variable with recurrent exacerbations and disease-free intervals. Additional features include:

Skin	Mucous membrane ulcers, erythema multiforme, erythema nodosum
Joints	Arthritis (asymmetrical, recurrent, knees, wrists, ankles)
Vascular	Thrombophlebitis, arterial aneurysms, pericarditis
CNS	Cranial nerve palsies, psychosis, meningo-encephalitis
Other	Fevers, colitis

Diagnosis

- Clinical diagnosis
- Skin **pathergy** may be present (pustule developing at site of skin needle prick after 24–48 h)

Management

Systemic steroids, colchicine, thalidomide and other immunosuppressive therapy have been effective in some patients.

AMYLOIDOSIS

This is characterized by deposition of amyloid in the extracellular matrix around blood vessels and in parenchymal organs. It may be primary or secondary.

Type	Amyloid characteristics	Associated disease	Clinical features
Primary	AL (homologous with immunoglobulin K or L light chains)	Myeloma Macroglobulinaemia	Arthritis, macroglossia, carpal tunnel syndrome, neuropathy, cardiac failure, malabsorption, gastrointestinal bleeding

Type	Amyloid characteristics	Associated disease	Clinical features
Secondary	AA (unique protein)	Systemic-onset JIA	Nephrotic syndrome
		Familial Mediterranean fever	Diarrhoea
			Hepatosplenomegaly
		Inflammatory bowel disease	Anaemia
			Hypergammaglobulinaemia

Diagnosis

Biopsy　Staining with Congo red dye, green under polarizing light.

Treatment

Treat underlying disorder; alkylating agents, e.g. chlorambucil, may be used in secondary amyloid.

OSTEOGENESIS IMPERFECTA

A group of disorders of fragile bones due to defective and/or reduced type 1 collagen. They are most commonly due to mutations in the genes *COL1A1* and *COL1A2*. The severity of the clinical features depends on the type.

Type	Inheritance and incidence	Relative Severity	Clinical features
I	AD (¾), new mutation 1:15 000–20 000	Mildest	Multiple bony fractures pre-puberty Near normal stature See below
II	New mutation 1:60 000	Most severe	Frequently fatal. Neonates severely affected Severe deformity, multiple fractures Very small stature, small chest and lungs
III	New mutation 1:60 000	Second most severe	Features as for type I but more severe Fractures common at birth Very short stature Severe early hearing loss
IV	AD, new mutation 1:20 000–30 000	Second mildest	Features as type I but more severe Near normal coloured sclera Multiple fractures before puberty Brittle discoloured teeth

Clinical features of type I

Skeletal　Multiple fractures pre-puberty
Kyphoscoliosis, barrel-shaped chest, soft skull
Short bowed legs and arms, joint hypermobility
Triangular face, small nose
Soft brittle discoloured teeth (dentinogenesis imperfecta)

	Short stature
Skin	Loose, thin and smooth, easy bruising
Eyes	Blue–grey sclera
ENT	Deafness in 50% from age 20 years (most commonly conductive)
Other	Compromised cardiovascular and respiratory function secondary to skeletal deformity

Causes of blue sclera

- Marfan syndrome,
- Ehlers–Danlos syndrome
- Pseudoxanthoma elasticum
- Osteogenesis imperfecta

Investigations

Blood   Alkaline phosphatase (N or ↑), acid phosphatase (↑)
Urine   24-h hydroxyproline (↑)
X-rays Wormian bones (skull), fractures, osteopenia, deformity

Management

Supportive	Physiotherapy, splints, physical aids, psychological support
Drug therapy	Bisphosphonates (increase bony density), growth hormone
Surgical	Fracture management. Corrective surgery (scoliosis, bowing of bones)

OSTEOPETROSIS (MARBLE BONE DISEASE)

A disease of increased skeletal density and brittle bones. There are several forms; the type presenting in the new-born period with early death, **osteopetrosis with precocious manifestations**, an autosomal recessive condition, is described.

Clinical features

General	Faltering growth
Marrow failure	Anaemia, thrombocytopenia, infections, hepatosplenomegaly
Hyperostosis	Optic atrophy, blindness, deafness, cranial nerve palsies, hydrocephalus

Investigations

Blood	Ca ↓, PO4 ↓, alkaline phosphatase ↑
	Hb ↓, platelets ↓,WCC ↓
X-rays	Bone density ↑
	'Bone in bone' appearance of vertebral bodies
	Clubbed metaphyses, 'rugby jersey' pattern of spine
	Osteosclerosis

Management

- Low-calcium diet, phosphate supplements
- Drugs – oral steroids, interferon-α
- Stem cell transplant
- Neurosurgery to the orbital roof

OSTEOCHONDRODYSPLASIAS

ACHONDROPLASIA

A pure skeletal dysplasia. Incidence: 1:15 000–27 000. New mutations (mostly), autosomal dominant.

Clinical features

Proportions	Short limbs and trunk, large head
Other skeletal	Exaggerated lumbar lordosis, genu varum, 'trident' hands and brachydactyly
	Mid-facial hypoplasia, relative prognathism, narrow nasal airways
Neurological	Hydrocephalus (1–2%)
	Obstructive sleep apnoea
	Spinal canal stenosis
	Intelligence normal
	Hypotonia in infancy and delayed motor milestones
ENT	Serous otitis media

NB: Specific growth charts have been designed for these children. Lifespan is normal.

THANATOPHORIC DWARFISM

A 'lethal' dwarfism, though a few survive > 1 year.

Clinical features

- Similar proportions to achondroplasia (large head, small body)
- Severe thoracic dysplasia with respiratory distress
- Bow limbs, flat nasal bridge, brachydactyly
- X-rays – thin vertebral bodies, femoral head banana-shaped, metaphyseal flaring and cupping

ELLIS–VAN CREVELD SYNDROME

Autosomal recessive syndrome featuring:

- Skeletal dysplasia including mild thoracic involvement
- Four limb postaxial polydactyly
- Conical teeth, oligodontia, dysplastic nails
- CHD (40%)

STICKLER DYSPLASIA

A group of autosomal dominant disorders with a defect in the *COL2A1* gene for type II collagen on chromosome 12q.

Clinical features

- Marfanoid habitus, hyperextensible joints, enlargement of large joints
- Retinal detachment, myopia, deafness, cleft palate
- X-ray – 'dumbbell'-shaped long bones
- Early severe degenerative OA of hips and knees

SPONDYLOEPIPHYSEAL DYSPLASIAS

These diseases are characterized by disproportionate short stature (short trunk). They include three main forms.

Type	Inheritance	Clinical features
Congenita	AD	Cleft palate, hypertelorism, myopia, retinal detachment
	COL2A1 gene (type II collagen)	Hip and shoulder epiphyseal dysplasia
	Chromosome 12	Short limbs, platyspondyly, pectus carinatum, talipes talipes equinovarus
Pseudochondrodysplasia	AD, AR	Progressive scoliosis, normal head, long bone epiphyseal irregularities
Tarda	Variable	**Pseudorheumatoid** subgroup involves progressive joint deformity, arthritis in some, short stature, platyspondyly, hip and back pain and stiffness

MULTIPLE EPIPHYSEAL DYSPLASIAS

These are similar to spondyloepiphyseal dysplasias, with mild spinal disease, short phalanges and fragmentation of the epiphyses of hips, knees and other joints.

NON-INFLAMMATORY PAIN SYNDROMES

These pains have characteristic patterns, are often distressing and may lead to significant loss of function. Aetiologies are not well understood. Diagnoses are best made through a full history and examination, which will exclude other pathologies and may identify the features below. May be acute soft tissue rheumatism disorders such as 'anterior knee pain syndromes', 'bursitis' or 'housemaid's knee', all of which are rare in children.

CHRONIC IDIOPATHIC PAIN SYNDROME

Includes reflex sympathetic dystrophy, fibromyalgia, chronic widespread pain disorders syndrome.

- Onset often associated with minor trauma and immobilization
- If diffuse pain, onset is vague with gradual deterioration
- Pain generated by normally non-painful stimuli (**allodynia**)
- Generally heightened sensation (**hyperaesthesia**)
- Skin changes – colour (blue, pallor), hair loss, shiny
- Symptoms and loss of function in excess of clinical signs
- Possible pseudoparalysis if limb involved
- Psychosocial features may have precipitated and maintain pain

Management

Two goals:

Restore function	Multidisciplinary team approach focusing on rehabilitation
	Intense physiotherapy
	Psychological support
Relief of pain	Acknowledgement of pain and explanation of management
	Simple analgesia
	Teaching skills to cope with pain

GROWING PAINS

- Typically shin pain in evening and may wake from sleep
- Mostly affect young children
- Settle with gentle rubbing of the area

BENIGN HYPERMOBILITY SYNDROME

- Pain associated with hypermobility of joints
- A probable mild **form fruste** of Ehlers–Danlos syndrome
- Typically pain in evening or after increased activity
- Usually minimal functional loss unless unfit or unwell for long periods

Management

- Education
- Supportive footwear
- Physiotherapy – correct imbalance and improve muscle support

---

SYNDROMES INVOLVING ABSENT RADII

- Absent thumbs
- Holt–Oram syndrome
- Fanconi anaemia
- VATER syndrome
- TAR syndrome (thrombocytopenia with absent radii), 100% have cow's milk protein sensitivity

---

FURTHER READING

Cassidy JT, Petty RE *Textbook of Paediatric Rheumatology*, 5th edn. Philadelphia: WB Saunders, 2003

Maddison PJ, Senberg DA, Woo P, Glass DN, eds *The Oxford Textbook of Rheumatology*, 3rd edn. Oxford: Oxford University Press, 2004

14

Neurological and neuromuscular disorders

- *Physiology and anatomy*
- *Investigations*
- *Development*
- *Structural brain anomalies*
- *Seizures*
- *Headaches*
- *Neuroectodermal syndromes*

- *Ataxia*
- *Cerebral palsy*
- *Neurodegenerative disorders*
- *Stroke*
- *Spinal cord disorders*
- *Neuromuscular disorders*
- *Psychiatric disorders*

PHYSIOLOGY AND ANATOMY

The nervous system can be divided into:

1. **Central nervous system (CNS)** – brain and spinal cord
2. **Peripheral nervous system (PNS)** – somatic and autonomic nervous systems conveying information into (afferent, sensory) and away from (efferent, motor) the CNS

For a detailed review, anatomy and physiology texts must be consulted.

BRAIN

Some major areas of function within the cerebral cortex are shown in Figure 14.1 and the ventricular system is outlined in Figure 14.2.

The internal carotids and the basilar artery supply the circle of Willis, from which the three cerebral arteries (anterior, middle and posterior) branch. The vertebro-basilar system supplies the cerebellum and brainstem and the cerebral arteries supply the cerebrum (see Figure 14.3).

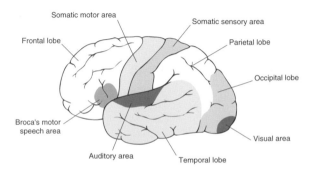

Figure 14.1 Major functional areas of the cortex

328

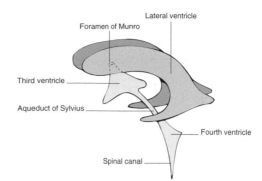

Figure 14.2 The ventricular system

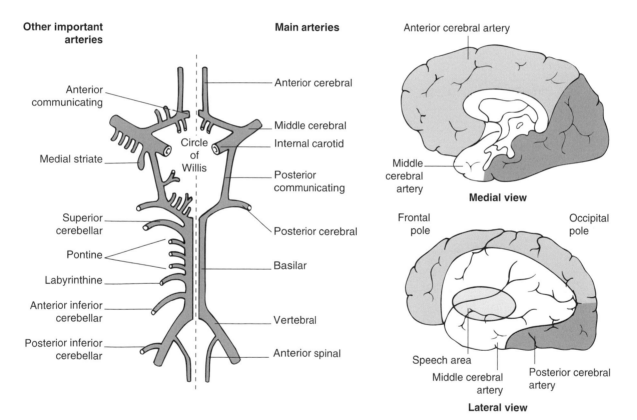

Figure 14.3 Blood supply to the brain

CRANIAL NERVES

For a detailed outline see an anatomy text.

Number	Name	Motor component	Sensory component
I	Olfactory	None	Smell
II	Optic	None	Vision
III	Oculomotor	Eye movements (all EOM except lateral rectus and superior oblique)	None
IV	Trochlear	Superior oblique muscle (intorsion)	None
V	Trigeminal	Masseter muscles	Facial, buccal mucosa and anterior $2/3$ tongue via: • V1 (ophthalmic branch) • V2 (maxillary branch) • V3 (mandibular branch)
VI	Abducens	Lateral rectus muscle (outward lateral gaze)	None
VII	Facial	Facial muscles Stapedius muscle Secretomotor to submandibular, sublingual and lacrimal glands	Taste (anterior $2/3$ tongue via chorda tympani)
VIII	Vestibulocochlear	None	Hearing (cochlear nerve) Balance (vestibular nerve)
IX	Glossopharyngeal	Tongue (stylopharyngeus) Secretomotor to parotid gland	Taste (posterior $1/3$) Gag afferents Sensation from tonsils, pharynx, posterior $1/3$ tongue
X	Vagus	Gag efferent Larynx, bronchial muscles, alimentary tract, epiglottis Secretomotor to alimentary tract, bronchial muscle glands	Dura, external auditory meatus Respiratory tract, alimentary tract, heart
XI	Accessory	Sternomastoid, trapezius	None
XII	Hypoglossal	Tongue muscles	None

MOTOR AND SENSORY SYSTEMS

Motor system

Corticospinal tracts (pyramidal system)

These originate in the cortex (layer V) and terminate on the motor nuclei (cranial nerves) or anterior horn cells (spinal cord).

The nerve fibres *decussate* (cross over) in the medulla.

Disease of the pyramidal system causes an upper motor neuron (UMN) lesion and disease of the anterior horn cells and peripheral nervous system results in a lower motor neuron (LMN) lesion.

Extrapyramidal system

Basal ganglia, involved in movement. Lesions result in a reduction in movement, involuntary movements and rigidity.

Cerebellum

Involved in posture and balance, lesions producing classic cerebellar signs.

Peripheral nerves run from the anterior horn cell via α motor nerve fibres to the motor endplate (the **LMN pathway**).

UMN lesion	Sign	LMN lesion
↑ (spastic)	Tone	↓ (hypotonia)
Weakness	Strength	Weakness
No wasting	Muscles	Wasting, fasciculation
↑	Reflexes	↓
Upgoing	Plantar response	Downgoing/equivocal

Reflexes	Level
Supinator	C5–6
Biceps	C5–6
Triceps	C7
Knee	L3–4
Ankle	S1

Clinical signs of cerebellar disease

Gait	Ataxic, broad based. Patient falls to the side of the lesion
Movements	Dysmetria (imprecise movements in force and distance)
	Dysdiadokinesis, past-pointing on finger–nose testing
Tremor	Intention tremor
	Titubation (head tremor)
Nystagmus	Towards the affected side
	Coarse, horizontal
Speech	Dysarthria, 'scanning' speech
Reflexes	Pendular

Lesions within a lateral lobe produce symptoms in the same side of the body. Midline lesions produce truncal ataxia.

Sensory system

Peripheral nerves run from free or specialized nerve endings to the dorsal root ganglia and along the spinal cord (see Figure 14.4) via:

- Posterior columns (vibration, proprioception, light touch). Decussate in the medulla
- Spinothalamic tracts (crude touch, temperature, pain). Cross in the cord at entry

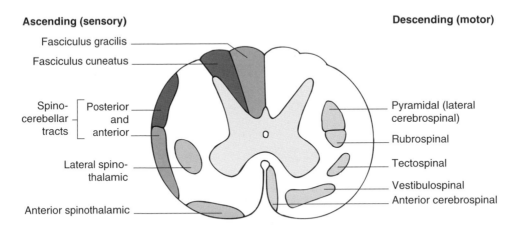

Figure 14.4 Motor and sensory tracts

RAISED INTRACRANIAL PRESSURE

This may be an acute emergency or a chronic disorder.

Causes

Infection	Meningitis, encephalitis
Trauma	Intracranial haemorrhage, stroke
Intracranial mass	Brain tumour, haematoma, cyst, abscess
Cerebral oedema	Stroke, hepatic encephalopathy, infection
CSF disorder	Hydrocephalus, blocked VP or VA shunt
Benign intracranial hypertension (BIH)	

Acute ↑ ICP

Clinical features

Vital signs	BP ↑ and pulse ↓ (**Cushing reflex**) – due to medullary ischaemia **Pupillary dilatation**
False localizing signs	III and VI cranial nerve palsies (these nerves become squashed as they have a long pathway in the CSF)
Coning	(i.e. herniation of brain contents) Bradycardia, hypertension, respiratory depression, bilateral pupillary dilatation, decerebrate posturing and then death

Emergency management

1. *Mannitol*   0.25 g/kg over 30 min on 2–3 occasions
2. *Hyperventilation*   Aim for PCO_2 25–35 mmHg (low end of normal range causes cerebral vasoconstriction)

3. *Minimize cerebral metabolism*   Sedation, analgesia, muscle paralysis, low:normal temperature
4. *Treat cause*   E.g. steroids for cerebral oedema, surgery for blocked shunt or acute bleed

Chronic ↑ ICP

Clinical features

- Headache (early morning, worse on lying down and with coughing and crying)
- Drowsiness, diplopia, vomiting
- Papilloedema (see p. 378)
- Infant – bulging fontanelle, macrocephaly, faltering growth

Management

Drugs   Acetazolamide
          Steroids (may make BIH worse)
Surgery   Shunt insertion

Treat underlying cause.

Benign intracranial hypertension (BIH)

This is a condition of raised intracranial pressure in the absence of an obstruction to CSF flow. It may be seen in:

- Idiopathic in adolescent girls
- Steroid withdrawal, oral contraceptive pill, isotretinoin, tetracycline
- Head injury

Clinical features

Those of chronic ↑ ICP, in particular:

- Diplopia
- Marked papilloedema
- Infarction of the optic nerve may occur with subsequent blindness

Investigations

- Lumbar puncture – diagnostic (very high CSF pressures)
- CT brain – normal (normal ventricles)

Management

- Lumbar puncture (CSF drainage) and thiazide diuretics
- Dexamethasone if prolonged (ICP ↑)
- Surgical shunting may be necessary

INVESTIGATIONS

ELECTROMYOGRAPHY (EMG) AND PERIPHERAL NERVE CONDUCTION

EMG

A needle electrode is inserted into voluntary muscle and an amplified recording is made.

Changes seen   Myopathic, myotonic, myaesthaenic, denervation, reinnervation

Peripheral nerve conduction

Measurements are taken of conduction velocity, distal motor latency, sensory and muscle action potentials.

ELECTROENCEPHALOGRAM (EEG)

Notes on EEG interpretation

1. Obvious pattern present, e.g. hypsarrythmia, 3/s spike and wave
2. No obvious pattern, check: Scale (amplitude)

Montage (map)

Time marker

- Nature of the feature, e.g. spikes, slow waves
- Whether it is generalized (in all channels)
- Or focal (in certain channels only)

Some basic EEG patterns

1. **Absence seizures**. 3 per second spike and wave activity

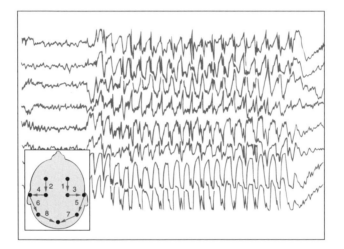

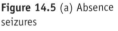

Figure 14.5 (a) Absence seizures

2. **Myoclonic epilepsy**. Bursts of generalized spikes and slow waves

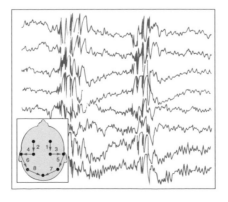

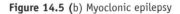

Figure 14.5 (b) Myoclonic epilepsy

3. Focal activity left temporal area, e.g. caused by a left temporal infarct. High-amplitude slow activity over the left temporal and posterior temporal areas

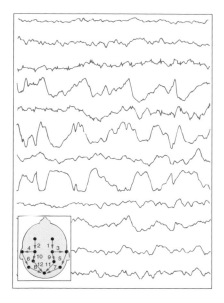

Figure 14.5 (c) Focal activity in left temporal area

4. **Hypsarrhythmia.** A mixture of high-amplitude irregular slow activity and some discharges, following no pattern

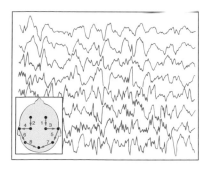

Figure 14.5 (d) Hypsarrhythmia

5. **Acute encephalopathy.** Typical pattern of irregular slow activity caused by encephalopathy of any cause

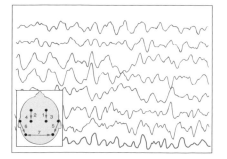

Figure 14.5 (e) Acute encephalopathy

6. **Burst suppression pattern**. Isoelectric EEG with bursts of spikes and other activity. These findings indicate a hopeless prognosis for recovery in a child.

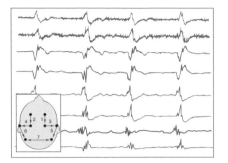

Figure 14.5 (f) Burst suppression pattern

DEVELOPMENT

AREAS OF CHILD DEVELOPMENT

- Gross motor (includes primitive reflexes and postural responses)
- Fine motor (and vision)
- Communication (speech and language, non-verbal communication and hearing)
- Social, emotional and behavioural

KEY DEVELOPMENTAL MILESTONES

Age	Fine motor	Gross motor	Language	Social
Newborn	Follows face and light to midline	Head lag Fetal position, symmetrical	Cries	Follows face
6 weeks	Follows face and objects to midline	Head control on tummy (raises head)	Responds to mother's voice	Smiles
3 months	Fixes and follows face through midline Hand regard Reaches	Pushes up with arms on tummy Head control good	Cries, laughs May babble	Smiles
6 months	Palmar grasp (transfers from hand to hand)	Sits unsupported (just, back bent)	Babbles	Eats finger foods Turns towards quiet sounds
9 months	Pincer grasp (9–14 months)	Sits well Pulls to stand Crawls	Daddy (non-specifically)	Stranger awareness Understands 'no' Plays peek-a-boo
1 year	Releases object	May walk (unsteady) or bottom shuffle	Mummy and daddy (specific)	Waves bye-bye (from 10 months) Mimics Cup drinking

Age	Fine motor	Gross motor	Language	Social
15 months	Scribbles	Walks well (most)		
18 months	Scribbles 3-cube tower	Walks upstairs	5–10 words Names six body parts	Feeds with spoon Symbolic play
2 years	Circular scribbles 6-cube tower	Kicks, runs Kicks a ball	2–3 word sentences	Undresses
3 years	Draws circle Bridge 3 cubes	Jumps	Says first name Colours 3–4 word sentences	Dresses Has friend Interactive play Buttons (50%)
4 years	Draws cross	Stands on one leg Hops	Good speech Says surname	Buttons (all)
5 years	Draws triangle	Bicycle	Good speech	Shoe laces

NB: The above ages are the *latest* that these skills should be acquired by.

REFLEXES

Primitive reflexes

These are all present from birth and asymmetry or persistence for longer suggests neurological deficit.

Reflex	Usual age to disappear (All variable)	Description
Sucking reflex	} 6–8 weeks	Automatic suck if object placed in mouth
Rooting reflex		Stroke cheek and mouth opens and moves towards hand
Placing reflex		
Palmar grasp	3–4 months	Stroke palm and it closes
Plantar grasp	12–18 months	Stroke sole and it closes
Stepping reflex	2 months	When held and 'walked' with the feet touching the ground, the feet move in a stepping sequence
Moro reflex	4–5 months	Sudden neck extension causes extension, abduction and adduction of upper extremities and flexion of fingers, wrists and elbows
Asymmetric tonic neck reflex	6 months	In a supine infant, turning the head laterally causes extension of the arm and leg on the side to the turn and flexion of both on the side away from the turn (the fencer position)

Postural responses

Reflex	Appears	Disappears	Description
Forward parachute	5–6 months	Stays for life	When held prone by the waist and lowered, the arms and legs extend
Landau reflex	3–6 months	1 year	When held prone, the legs, spine and head extend
Lateral propping reflex	7 months	Stays for life	When sitting and pushed sideways, the arms extend to prevent a fall

The **Babinsky reflex** is upgoing initially and downgoing from around 1 year.

STRUCTURAL BRAIN ANOMALIES

ABNORMAL HEAD SHAPE AND SIZE

Large (macrocephaly)	Familial, i.e. normal
	Neurofibromatosis
	↑ ICP, e.g. hydrocephalus, subdural haematoma
	Sotos syndrome
	Metabolic storage disorder, e.g. Hunter syndrome
Small (microcephaly)	Familial, i.e. normal
	AR
	Craniosynostosis (see below)
	Prenatal/delivery cerebral insult, e.g. cerebral palsy, congenital infection
	Postnatal cerebral insult, e.g. meningitis
Abnormal shape (symmetrical or asymmetrical)	Positional moulding, e.g. premature infants lying head side a lot (dolicocephaly)
	Floppy babies head remains stationary for prolonged time
	Normal infants always put on back (brachycephaly)
	Premature suture closure
	Differential growth rate at the sutures

Abnormal head shapes

Brachycephaly	Flat occiput, e.g. Down syndrome
Scaphocephaly (dolichocephaly)	Long, narrow, e.g. premature babies, Hurler syndrome
Turricephaly	Tall head
Trigonocephaly	Keel-shaped forehead, hypotelorism
Kleeblattschädel deformity	Cloverleaf shape
Plagiocephaly	Asymmetrical, parallelogram (as if skull pushed one side and pulled the other)

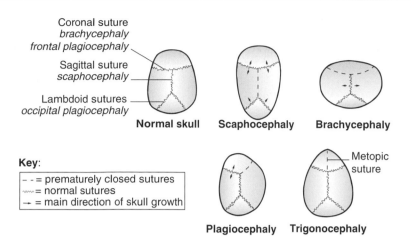

Figure 14.6 Cranial sutures and abnormal head shapes

CRANIOSYNOSTOSES

This is premature closure of the cranial suture, with resultant cranial deformities dependent on the suture(s) involved. It can be only one suture, some or all sutures (causing microcephaly). It may be associated with a syndrome (see below).

Children with craniosynostosis may develop:

- Hydrocephalus, ↑ ICP, optic atrophy
- Deviated nasal septum, choanal atresia, speech disorders and deafness

Craniofacial surgery may be necessary

Some craniosynostoses have been found to have mutations in the FGFR2 (fibroblast growth factor receptor 2) gene, e.g. Apert, Crouzon.

Syndrome	Inheritance	Features
Crouzon	AD	Usually causes brachycephaly from coronal suture closure Proptosis Hypertelorism, frontal bossing Small maxilla
Apert	Sporadic, AD	Multiple suture closure, results in asymmetrical head and face Syndactyly of 2nd, 3rd, 4th fingers and toes Mental retardation (66%) Progressive calcification and fusion of cervical spine, hands and foot bones
Carpenter	AR	Multiple sutures affected, brachycephaly, Kleeblattschädel skull Syndactyly and brachydactyly hands and feet Mental retardation CHD, genu valgum, coxa valga, preaxial polydactyly of feet

Syndrome	Inheritance	Features
Chotzen	AD	Asymmetrical fusions, plagiocephaly Ptosis, hypertelorism Brachydactyly Syndactyly 2nd and 3rd fingers
Pfieffer	Sporadic, AD	Turricephaly, brachycephaly Prominent eyes, hypertelorism Short, broad thumbs Syndactyly

FONTANELLE CLOSURE

Normally the anterior fontanelle (2–3 cm at birth) closes between 9 and 18 months, and the posterior (< 1 cm at birth) at 6–8 weeks.

Delayed closure	Premature closure
Hypothyroidism	Hyperthyroidism
Malnutrition	Microcephaly
Rickets	Craniosynostosis
Hydrocephalus	
Chromosomal abnormality, e.g. Down	
Syndrome, Rubinstein–Taybii syndrome, trisomy 13	
Alpert syndrome	
Osteogenesis imperfecta	

NEURAL TUBE DEFECTS (NTDS)

These result from failure of the neural tube to close on day 21–26 of intrauterine life and may involve spinal cord and/or brain. If compatible with survival, may be closed surgically soon after birth.

Associations   Folate deficiency, sodium valproate, previous NTD
Antenatal detection   Direct view on USS, raised amniotic fluid α-FP
Recurrence risk   1 previous NTD 4%
                        2 previous NTD 10%

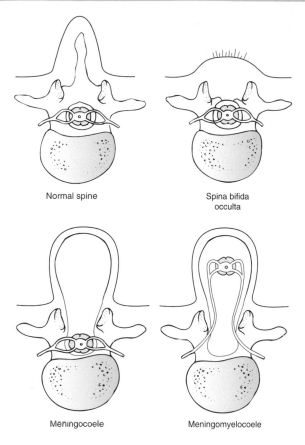

Figure 14.7 Neural tube defects

Spina bifida occulta

- **Failure of vertebral arch fusion (L5, S1).** Up to 5% population affected. (NB: This is normal < 10 years).
- Overlying skin lesion (hair tuft, sinus, lipoma, pigmented lesion)
- Mostly asymptomatic
- Neural tethering may cause bladder & lower limb problems (**cauda equina syndrome**)

Meningocoele

- **Protrusion of meninges only** through vertebral defect
- May be normal with surgical repair

Meningomyelocoele

- **Protrusion of meninges and spinal cord/nerves**
- Incidence 1:1000 live births
- Paralysis (UMN) and sensory loss in legs
- Neuropathic bladder and bowel (involvement < S1)
- Talipes, hip dislocation, scoliosis
- ± Hydrocephalus (Arnold–Chiari malformation)

Raschisis

- **Open meningomyelocoele**
- Failure of fusion of the neural tube with CSF leakage
- Incompatible with postnatal survival

Encephalocoele

- **Midline defect of the skull with brain protrusion**. Usually occipital, may be frontal or nasofrontal
- Developmental delay, visual defects, hydrocephalus, seizures, microcephaly
- Operative excision and repair of defect may be possible

Meckel–Gruber syndrome

- Autosomal recessive
- Occipital encephalocoele
- Cleft palate
- Microphthalmus, microcephaly
- Abnormal genitalia, polycystic kidneys
- Polydactyly

Anencephaly

- **Failure of closure of the rostral neuropore** results in rudimentary brain and large defect of the meninges and skull
- Incidence 1:1000 live births
- Other anomalies in 10–20%
- Incompatible with survival

HYDROCEPHALUS

This is dilatation of the CSF spaces.

Causes

Obstruction to CSF

Intraventricular block	Meningitis
	Congenital aqueductal stenosis (aqueduct of Sylvius)
	Dandy–Walker syndrome:
	• Occlusion of the exit of the fourth ventricle
	• Large 4th ventricle and cerebellar hypoplasia
	Arnold–Chiari malformation:
	• Downward displacement of cerebellar tonsils and brainstem
	• ± Spina bifida
	Neoplasm or vascular malformation
Extraventricular block	Posthaemorrhagic, e.g. SAH in premature infant
	Infection, e.g. TB meningitis
	Leukaemic infiltrates

Decreased CSF reabsorption

Venous hypertension from dural venous sinus thrombosis (severe dehydration).

Increased CSF production

Choroid plexus papilloma (very rare).

Clinical manifestations

These are variable depending on the *duration* and *rate of increase* of the CSF pressure, and age of the child.

Infant	Head circumference crossing centiles
	Bulging fontanelle, distended scalp veins
	'Setting-sun' eye sign
	Developmental delay
	Ataxia
Older child	Signs of raised intracranial pressure (see p. 332)

Investigations

Neuroimaging (USS/CT/MRI)   Dilated ventricles, structural malformations

Management

- Treat the underlying cause if possible
- Surgical shunt is inserted to drain the excess CSF either to the peritoneum (V-P shunt) or less commonly the right atrium (A-P shunt). Shunt complications: blockage, infection

NEURONAL MIGRATION DISORDERS

These occur during fetal development and may be very minor or have major sequelae. They are diagnosed on MRI brain scans. Important types include the following.

Lissencephaly (smooth brain)

- Absent cerebral convolutions and rudimentary Sylvian fissure
- Large lateral ventricles, microcephaly, microphthalmia
- Manifest as severe developmental delay, failure to thrive and seizures

Miller–Deiker syndrome

- Lissencephaly, characteristic facial dysmorphism
- Chromosome deletions of 17p 13.3

Schizencephaly

- Clefts in the cerebral hemispheres from the cortex to the ventricles, the entire cleft being coated with cortex
- Presents with epilepsy and/or focal neurology

Porencephaly

- Cysts within the brain
- Presents with focal neurology

AGENESIS OF THE CORPUS CALLOSUM

X-linked recessive, autosomal dominant, sporadic. This may be completely asymptomatic (if isolated) or produce severe intellectual impairment when associated with other defects.

Associations   Cell migration defects, e.g. pachygyria, microgyria; trisomy 18

Aicardi syndrome

- Agenesis of the corpus callosum
- Retinal abnormalities, e.g. coloboma, pits
- Seizures refractive to treatment
- Severe mental retardation
- Vertebral abnormalities

SEIZURES

A **seizure (convulsion)** is an abnormal burst of electrical activity in the brain, which may manifest in various ways. **Epilepsy** is recurrent seizures unrelated to fever or acute cerebral insult.

Generalized seizures   Whole cortex involved diffusely, always impaired consciousness
Partial seizures   One area of the cortex involved; may become generalized

INTERNATIONAL CLASSIFICATION OF EPILEPTIC SEIZURES

Generalized seizures

Absence:
  Typical
  Atypical
Myoclonic, e.g. juvenile myoclonic epilepsy, infantile spasms
Tonic
Tonic–clonic
Atonic

Partial seizures

Simple partial (remain conscious):
  Motor
  Sensory
  Autonomic
  Psychic
Complex partial (impaired consciousness):
  Simple partial extended
  Initial complex partial, e.g. temporal lobe epilepsy
Partial with secondary generalization

INVESTIGATING EPILEPSY

It is always necessary to do a full history and clinical examination, including developmental check. For first convulsion, investigate only if <1 year of age or unwell child, or abnormal findings on examination.

EEG   Demonstrate baseline activity and seizure if occurs during recording
Blood   Glucose (peri-ictal)
                Electrolytes, metabolic screen, congenital infection screen
Neuroimaging USS (infants with patent fontanelle)
                Skull X-ray (intracranial calcification, trauma)
                CT scan (urgent if unwell)
                MRI scan

Lumbar puncture In an unwell child. Low threshold in febrile convulsion if child < 18 months. NB: Not if raised ICP signs

COMMON SEIZURE TYPES

Absence seizures

Typical	Sudden loss of awareness with eyelid fluttering, no motor activity
	No postictal phase
	Last < 30 s
Complex	Motor component (myotonic movements, loss of body tone)
EEG	Typical 3/s generalized spike and wave
Treatment	Ethosuximide
	Sodium valproate (NB: Potential for precipitating fulminant liver failure)
	Lamotrigine

Generalized tonic–clonic seizures

These may follow a partial seizure. May be idiopathic or induced by infection, stress or drugs. An 'aura' suggests a focal origin.

Features

Tonic phase	Sudden loss of consciousness with a tonic contraction, apnoea, cyanosis, eyes roll backwards
Clonic phase	Rhythmic contractions of all muscle groups
	Tongue-biting, sphincter control lost
Postictal phase	Semiconscious for 30 min–2 h

Treatment

- Sodium valproate, carbamazepine
- Lamotrigine
- Clobazam

Simple partial seizures

These are usually motor, involving asynchronous tonic or clonic movements and the child is conscious. Aura may occur. May be confused with tics (which can be suppressed temporarily).

Complex partial seizures

These involve altered consciousness and may follow on from a simple partial seizure. Temporal lobe epilepsy (a form of complex partial seizure) may produce outbursts of emotions. Automatisms are a common feature (lip smacking, chewing, drooling).

EEG	Focal spikes or sharp waves
	Brought on by sleep deprivation
MRI scan	Looking for structural brain abnormalities

EPILEPSY SYNDROMES

Childhood absence epilepsy

Usually age 3–10 years, girls > boys, family history in 40%.

Seizure types   Typical or atypical absence seizures
Induced by   Hyperventilation, emotion, hunger
Treatment   As for absence seizures

Juvenile myoclonic epilepsy

5% of all epilepsy. Onset 12–16 years.

Associations   25% family history
                  90% develop generalized tonic–clonic seizures
                  25% develop absences
Features   Myoclonic jerks, worse in the morning (cannot brush their teeth, spill their tea)
                  No impairment of consciousness
EEG   Normal background, 4–6/s irregular polyspike and wave discharge pattern
                  Photosensitivity
Treatment   Sodium valproate
                  Lamotrigine

Infantile spasms

Incidence 1:3000. Onset age 4–6 months, boys > girls. Associated with arrested development.

Features   Symmetrical contractions of whole body, occur in bursts
              May be extensor, flexor (Salaam spasms, jack-knife) or mixed
EEG   **Hypsarrhythmia** (chaotic EEG with high-amplitude activity)

Cause

Aetiology not identified (20%)   Normal prior development, examination and CT scan
Aetiology identified (80%)   Structural, e.g. tuberous sclerosis, lissencephaly
                                    Metabolic disease
                                    Birth injury, e.g. hypoxic–ischaemic encephalopathy, IVH
                                    Postnatal injury, e.g. trauma, meningitis

Investigations of cause

- MRI brain
- Metabolic screen
- Chromosome analysis
- If tuberous sclerosis (TS) is suspected, do renal US and echocardiogram

Treatment options

- Vigabatrin
- ACTH (second line)

West syndrome

A triad of:

1. Infantile spasms
2. Hypsarrhythmia
3. Mental retardation

Temporal lobe epilepsy

Complex partial seizures originating in the temporal lobe area.

Features	Aura, e.g. dysphoria, fear or gastrointestinal symptoms
	May manifest as outbursts of emotions
EEG	Anterior temporal lobe focal spikes or sharp waves
MRI	To look for temporal lobe abnormalities

Benign Rolandic epilepsy (benign partial epilepsy with centrotemporal spikes)

Common partial epilepsy with good prognosis. Onset 2–14 years (peak 9–10 years).

Features	Drooling, abnormal sensations in mouth
	Secondary generalization
	75% occur in sleep, 25% occur on waking
EEG	Repetitive spike focus in the Rolandic area (centrotemporal)
Treatment	Carbamazapine
	Spontaneous resolution usually occurs by mid-teenage years

Landau–Kleffner syndrome (LKS)

- Onset 5 years, male > female
- Loss of language skills associated with seizures of several types in 70%
- EEG abnormalities more common during sleep

Rasmussen encephalitis

- Subacute inflammatory encephalitis with frequent focal seizures
- Associated with progressive hemiplegia

Pyridoxine deficiency

- Neonatal, infancy or adult onset generalized tonic–clonic seizures
- Autosomal recessive
- Treat with pyridoxine supplements

Lennox–Gastaut syndrome

This is an electroclinical syndrome comprising:

- Multiple seizure types (myoclonic, atypical absences, atonic 'drop' attacks, tonic nocturnal seizures, generalized tonic–clonic seizures)
- EEG shows slow spike and wave (2–3/s)

Onset mostly 4–5 years. Pre-existing severe seizures in 60%. Mental handicap initially 75% and regression. Epilepsy often intractable.

FEBRILE CONVULSIONS

These are convulsions secondary to a fever (often during a rapid temperature rise) caused by an infection (not directly involving the CNS). Often due to an URTI. Incidence 2–4% children under 5 years. Males > females. Family history in 30%.

Typical	Complex
6 months–5 years	< 6 months or > 5 years
Generalized tonic or tonic clonic	Focal
< 15 min	> 15 min
	Recurrent episodes within same febrile illness

Investigations

These depend on the clinical examination, searching for a source of infection, and age of the child. Urine specimen for infection should be done. Further investigations depend on clinical evaluation (FBC, CRP, blood cultures, CXR and LP if < 1 year or unwell and not contraindicated).

Management

- Admit if first fit, complex or child unwell
- Management of ABC and seizure control if still fitting
- Fever control with paracetamol or ibuprofen and tepid sponging
- If infectious bacterial focus or septicaemia or meningitis suspected give appropriate antibiotics
- If herpetic lesions or contact give aciclovir
- Parental advice on fever control and management of a fit

Risk of later development of epilepsy

General population   0.5%
Febrile convulsions   1% if typical
5–10% if risk factors (complex, family history epilepsy, febrile seizure < age 9 months, delayed milestones)

NON-EPILEPTIC 'FUNNY TURNS'

Syncope

Due to cerebral hypoperfusion and hypoxia causing bradycardia, pallor and then collapse. Different forms:

Vasovagal syncope   Precipitated by stress, emotions and confined spaces
Reflex anoxic seizures   Due to sensitive vago-cardiac reflex. Seen in toddlers after trauma
Orthostatic hypotension   Seen in adolescents on standing a long time
Cardiac syncope   Secondary to arrhythmias, e.g. prolonged QT syndrome. Rare in children

Breath-holding attacks

Age 6 months–3 years. Precipitated by fear, anger and pain. The child holds their breath in expiration causing cyanosis, then limpness, unconsciousness, and then tonic stiffening if severe. Rapid recovery.

Benign paroxysmal vertigo

1–5 years. Sudden onset of unsteadiness, pallor, horizontal nystagmus and vomiting. Consciousness maintained. Ear infections and migraine associated.

Night terrors

18 months–7 years. Partially wake from sleep during REM stage IV. Screaming, thrashing, tachycardia, does not recognize parents. Normal sleep afterwards.

Narcolepsy

Usually commences in adolescence. Attacks of REM sleep during the day, cataplexy (sudden inhibition of tone of a muscle group), frightening visual hallucinations, daytime sleepness and sleep paralysis (paralysis of voluntary muscles while falling asleep).

EMERGENCY MANAGEMENT OF STATUS EPILEPTICUS

NB: Status epilepticus is said to occur when a seizure lasts for 30 min.

- Stabilize the child (airway, breathing, circulation) and give high flow oxygen
- Establish IV access. Give IV fluids if signs of shock. Give antibiotics if sepsis or meningitis suspected.
- Bloods: BMStix (give IV glucose if hypoglycaemia)
            Glucose, U&E, Ca, Mg, FBC, cultures, ABG, drug screen
- Drug therapy (protocols vary, see latest APLS guidelines):
  IV lorazepam if IV access quickly established. If no IV access give rectal diazepam
  If convulsion continues after 10 min repeat lorazepam. Rectal paraldehyde in olive oil if no IV access
  If seizure continues get senior help (and liaise with anaesthetist/ITU). Give rectal paraldehyde if not already given
  IV phenytoin infusion over 20 min with ECG attached (phenobarbitone if already on phenytoin)
  If fitting continues: Re-check ABC
                          Have anaesthetist present
                          Take blood, correct any metabolic abnormality and treat pyrexia. Consider mannitol
                          Rapid sequence induction of anaesthesia with thiopentone and short-acting paralysing agent

ANTIEPILEPTIC DRUGS

Drug	Mode of action	Use	Side-effects
Sodium valproate (Epilim)	Unknown	Generalized seizures Atypical absences	Hyperphagia (weight gain) Sedation, tremor, excitation
		Partial seizures	Hepatotoxicity (irreversible) GIT disturbance Thrombocytopenia Alopecia (reversible)
Carbamazepine (Tegretol)	Sodium channel blocker	Partial seizures Generalized tonic–clonic	Enzyme inducer Ataxia, dizziness, drowsiness Blurred vision, diplopia Allergic skin rashes Transient lymphopenia
Lamotrigine	Presynaptic sodium channel blocker	Generalized seizures	Severe allergic reactions Arousing effect

Drug	Mode of action	Use	Side-effects
Phenytoin	Sodium channel blocker	Status Partial seizures	Enzyme inducer Hirsutism, acne Gum hyperplasia Rickets Aplastic anaemia Toxicity: ataxia, tremor, nystagmus, dysarthria
(NB: Phenytoin displays zero-order kinetics and therefore there is a rapid serum rise when the hepatic enzymes are saturated, causing toxicity with no therapeutic benefit. Serum levels must be monitored at some point.)			
Phenobarbitone	GABA inhibition	Neonatal seizures	Enzyme inducer Concentration impairment Memory loss, rickets Hyperactivity in children Learning difficulties Dependence
Vigabatrin	GABA transaminase inhibitor	Infantile spasms Intractable epilepsy Partial seizures	Drowsiness, agitation Excitation in children Peripheral retinal atrophy (visual field testing may be necessary) Psychosis
Gabapentin	Unknown	Partial seizures	Drowsiness, headache Tremor, ataxia, weight gain
Topiramate	Unknown	Severe epilepsy	Cognitive and psychological changes, weight loss

HEADACHES

These are a common problem and are rarely due to a severe underlying organic disorder. A full history and examination (including neurological) should be performed and further investigations only if worrying findings on history, e.g. increase in frequency or severity of headaches, developmental deterioration, behavioural change, features of ↑ ICP, or abnormal examination.

Examination should include:

- Full neurological, especially visual fields (intracranial mass), squint and pupil examination and cranial bruit examination (A-V malformation)
- Fundoscopy (BP ↑) and visual acuity
- Head size (crossing centiles)
- Blood pressure
- Teeth (dental caries)
- Face (sinus pain)

TENSION HEADACHE

Clinical features

- Common
- Dull ache or sharp pain at the vertex or unclear location
- May occur daily for weeks or be continuous
- Medication often ineffective
- No aura, no precipitants, no neurological signs
- Associated with difficulty sleeping, dizziness, family or school problems

MIGRAINE

These are recurrent headaches of uncertain pathology thought to involve both neurogenic and cerebrovascular mechanisms.

Clinical features

- Throbbing, bifrontal, unilateral, photophobia, phonophobia
- May wake child from sleep
- Transient hemiplegia or ataxia
- Lasts 1–72 h

Must be accompanied by at least two of: nausea, vomiting, abdominal pain, visual aura, family history.

Management

General measures	Regular mealtimes, regular bedtime, sufficient sleep, relaxation after a stressful situation
Avoid stimuli	E.g. stress, insufficient food, certain foods (chocolate, cheese, colourings), sun, lack of or excess sleep, dehydration
Acute episode	Bed rest/sleep in a dark quiet room
	Drugs: analgesics (paracetamol), antiemetic if nausea
	Selective 5-HT agonist if severe and > 12 years old
Prophylaxis	Pizotifen (histamine [H1] and serotonin receptor antagonist) is licensed in children > 2 years old

HEADACHES OF OTHER UNDERLYING PATHOLOGY

Features

- Those of underlying local pathology, e.g. sinusitis, toothache, fever
- Those of ↑ ICP – diffuse, frontal, worse on coughing, sneezing or lying down and in the mornings

Causes

Neurological	Postictal, post-concussion, meningitis, encephalitis, hydrocephalus (V-P shunt blockage), intracranial haemorrhage, BIH, brain tumour
Other	Infective illness (commonly URTI or viral illness), dental malocclusion, dental caries, myopia, hypermetropia, sinusitis, lead poisoning

NEUROECTODERMAL SYNDROME

These involve a defect in the differentiation of the primitive ectoderm and include:

- Neurofibromatosis

- Tuberous sclerosis
- Sturge–Weber syndrome (see p. 385)
- Von Hippel–Lindau disease
- Ataxia telangiectasia (see p. 32)
- Incontinentia pigmenti (see p. 304)

NEUROFIBROMATOSIS (NF, VON RECKLINGHAUSEN DISEASE)

Autosomal dominant, 50% new mutation rate. Incidence 1:4000. Extremely variable in severity.

NF1 (90%)

Gene on chromosome 17q. Diagnosis if *two or more* of the following occur:

1. ≥ 6 Café-au-lait patches (prepubertal > 5 mm, postpubertal > 15 mm)
2. Axillary freckles
3. ≥ 2 neurofibromas or one plexiform neurofibroma
4. ≥ 2 Lisch nodules (hamartomas) in iris
5. Bone lesion – sphenoid dysplasia (pulsating exophthalmos), or dysplasia of cortex of a long bone
6. Optic glioma
7. First-degree relative with NF

Other features

CNS	Macrocephaly, seizures, learning difficulties, speech defects, attention deficit disorder, aqueduct stenosis
Endocrine	Precocious puberty
Tumours	CNS tumours, Wilms tumour, phaeochromocytoma, leukaemia, sarcomas
Other	Renal artery stenosis, cardiomyopathy, lung fibrosis, kyphoscoliosis

NF2 (10%)

Gene on chromosome 22q. Diagnosis if one of the following present:

1. Bilateral VIII nerve acoustic neuromas
2. Unilateral VIII nerve mass in association with any two of: meningioma, neurofibroma, schwannoma, juvenile posterior subcapsular cataracts, glioma
3. Unilateral VIII nerve acoustic neuroma or other brain or spinal tumour as above and first-degree relative with NF2

Clinical features include: cerebellar ataxia, hearing loss, facial nerve palsy, headache. Skin lesions are less common than in NF1.

Management

- Investigations (led by examination) – MRI brain and optic nerves, ophthalmological assessment, skeletal survey, EEG, audiogram, brainstem auditory and visual evoked potentials, psychometric testing
- Genetic counselling
- Yearly assessment, including neurological examination, auditory and visual screening, and BP

TUBEROUS SCLEROSIS

Autosomal dominant, 80% new mutations. Gene on chromosome 9q and 16p. Wide variation in severity.

Clinical features

Skin	**Adenoma sebaceum (angiofibromas)** 85%, over cheeks and nose (> 3 years age)
	Hypomelanotic macules (Ash leaf macules) (80%, > 3)
	Shagreen patches (connective tissue naevi – 'orange peel skin' over lumbar spine)
	Ungual or **periungual fibromas** (> teenage)
	Fibrous plaque on forehead or scalp
	Gingival fibroma
CNS	Epilepsy (infantile spasms, partial)
	Autism
	Cortical tuber (hard nodules with bizarre giant cells), may calcify
	Subependymal glial nodules, project into ventricles, calcify, 'candle-dripping' appearance on CT scan (> 3 years age)
	Subependymal giant cell astrocytoma
	Gliomas
	White matter radial migration lines
Eye	**Multiple retinal nodular hamartomas (phakoma)** (optic nerve astrocytoma), Mulberry tumour
	Retinal achromic patch
CVS	**Cardiac rhabdomyoma(s)** (40–50%)
Renal	**Multiple angiomyolipomas**, hamartomas, polycystic kidneys
Lung	**Lymphangioleiomyomatosis**
Dental	Multiple pits in dental enamel
GIT	Hamartomatous rectal polyps
Bone	Cysts

Those in bold are major features. Two major features are required for diagnosis.

Management

This includes baseline investigations to look for associated features, seizure control, genotype, genetic counselling and regular follow-up (general and skin examination, neurodevelopmental assessments, renal USS, BP, echocardiogram, MRI brain scan, CXR and eye examination).

VON HIPPEL–LINDAU DISEASE

Autosomal dominant. Gene locus on chromosome 3p25.

Features

- Retinal angiomata
- Cerebellar haemangioblastomas
- Cystic lesions – renal, pancreas, liver, epididymis, spinal cord
- Tumours – phaeochromocytoma, renal carcinoma (most common cause of death)

ATAXIA

This may be due to **cerebellar disease** (most common cause in children) or to **sensory loss**.

Causes

Acute	Chronic
Cerebral infections (encephalitis)	*Congenital anomalies:*
Acute cerebellar ataxia:	Agenesis of cerebellar vermis
During infection (coxsackie, echovirus, EBV)	Joubert disease
Postinfectious (varicella)	Dandy–Walker malformation
Toxic – phenytoin, alcohol, piperazine	*Cerebral palsy (ataxic)*
Tumour – posterior fossa/brainstem	

Acute	Progressive
Seizures	Cerebellar tumour
Migraine	Cerebellar abscess
Hartnup disease	Subdural haematoma
MLD	Friedreich ataxia
	Ataxia telangiectasia
	Batten disease
	Abetalipoproteinaemia

LATE INFANTILE BATTEN DISEASE (CEROID LIPOFUSCINOSIS)

Autosomal recessive.

Clinical features

- Normal early development, then developmental regression from 2–5 years
- Ataxia, choreoathetosis
- Seizures
- Retinitis pigmentosa

Diagnosis

- Eye examination
- EEG
- Rectal biopsy (typical neurological features)

FRIEDREICH ATAXIA

Autosomal recessive. Gene on chromosome 9q13–21.1, encoding fraxatin. A progressive degeneration of cerebellar tracts and dorsal columns. Presentation usually around 10–12 years (always < 20 years) with difficulty walking, with progression of disease and death around 40 years.

Clinical features

- Progressive ataxia and dysarthria
- Lower limb weakness and amyotrophy

- Loss of position and vibration sense
- Pes cavus, scoliosis
- Loss of deep tendon reflexes with upgoing plantars
- Optic atrophy, nystagmus
- Dilated or restrictive cardiomyopathy, diabetes mellitus

Investigations

- Sensory (± motor) conduction velocities slightly decreased
- Sensory evoked potential absent or reduced
- Visual evoked potential diminished

CEREBRAL PALSY

Cerebral palsy is a disorder of movement and posture due to a *non-progressive* lesion in the developing brain. It is a static encephalopathy. Prevalence 2:1000 population.

Additional impairments

- Learning impairment
- Visual impairment and strabismus
- Hearing loss
- Speech and language difficulties
- Behavioural problems
- Epilepsy

Causes

Antenatal (80%)	Cerebral dysgenesis, cerebral malformation, congenital infection
Intrapartum (10%)	Hypoxic–ischaemic encephalopathy
Postnatal (10%)	Cerebral ischaemia, IVH, hydrocephalus, head trauma, non-accidental injury (NAI), severe neonatal hyperbilirubinaemia

Types

Spastic	Initial hypotonia progressing to spasticity with UMN signs. It may be: • **Hemiplegia** – unilateral involvement (arm > leg usually), e.g. IVH, meningitis • **Diplegia** – legs > arms (arms may be normal), e.g. PVL • **Quadriplegia** – all limbs involved (arms > legs), e.g. birth asphyxia
Ataxic hypotonic	Hypotonia, poor balance, tremor, incoordinate movements, e.g. hydrocephalus
Dyskinetic	Involuntary movements (athetosis, dystonia), fluctuating muscle tone (dyskinesia) and poor postural tone, e.g. hyperbilirubinaemia

Presentations

- Delayed motor milestones
- Abnormal tone in infancy
- Abnormal gait, e.g. toe walking, wide based
- Feeding difficulties
- Other developmental delay, e.g. language, social
- Persistence of primitive reflexes

Investigations

- Brain imaging – USS in neonates, CT or MRI scan
- Metabolic screen

Management

Cerebral palsy may be mild, requiring little input, or severe, necessitating an interdisciplinary approach to optimize the development of the child. Specialities involved include occupational therapist, physiotherapist, speech therapist, social worker, teacher and developmental psychologist. Physicians involved include the paediatrician, orthopaedic surgeon, neurologist, ophthalmologist and audiologist.

NEURODEGENERATIVE DISORDERS

Neurodegenerative disorders are diseases with a **progressive deterioration in neurological function**, with loss of speech, vision, hearing or locomotion. Often associated seizures, feeding difficulties and intellectual impairment.

- These diseases are usually rare neurometabolic, autosomal recessive disorders due to a specific enzyme defect, but may be due to chronic viral infection, e.g. SSPE, prion infection, e.g. Creutfeldt–Jakob disease (CJD) or other unknown cause
- In the metabolic conditions the neuronal degeneration occurs as a result of a build-up of the product preceding the missing enzyme, which is toxic to the nervous system, or lack of an essential metabolite. The excess product will also cause other effects and result in the characteristic disease findings. Some of these diseases are termed 'storage disorders', referring to the storage of the accumulated substance
- Can be subdivided into predominantly grey matter or white matter disorders:
  White matter disease   UMN signs early on
  Grey matter disease   Convulsions, intellectual impairment and visual impairment
- May present congenitally or in early or late childhood, adolescence or adulthood
- Generally progress relentlessly until death occurs months or years from onset

INVESTIGATIONS

These should be led by the clinical features, especially MRI findings. Often there will be strongly suggestive features suggesting a certain group of diagnoses.

All patients	
Radiology	MRI brain
Blood	TFTs Lipids, vitamin E Uric acid White cell enzymes (**lysosomal storage disorders**) Very long chain fatty acids Lactate Amino acids Copper and caeruloplasmin HIV status Karyotype
Urine	Organic acids GAGs

Consider	
DNA	Retts Fragile X Neuronal ceroid lipofuscinosis Other molecular? (Molecular tests are becoming more first line in the investigation of neurodegenerative conditions)
CSF	Protein, cells Measles antibody (**SSPE**) Lactate
Neurophysiology	EMG, EEG, nerve conduction studies ERG and VEP
Histology	Muscle biopsy Bone marrow (**Gaucher, Niemann–Pick**)
Hair analysis	**Menke kinky hair disease**
Blood	Neuronal ceroid lipofuscinosis enzymology (NCL1 and NCL2) Transferrin isoelectric focusing

TYPES OF NEURODEGENERATIVE DISORDERS

Neurometabolic disorders	
Lysosomal storage disorders	Leukodystrophies, e.g. metachromatic leukodystrophy Sphingolipidosis, e.g. Tay Sachs disease (see p. 284) Mucopolysaccharidosis, e.g. Hurler disease (see p. 283) Neuronal ceroid lipofuscinosis, e.g. Batten
Other leukodystrophies	Alexander, Pelizaeus–Merzbacher, vanishing white matter disease
Mitochondrial disorders	MELAS, MERRF
Peroxisomal disorders	Peroxisomal biogenesis disorders, Refsum
Organic acidaemias	Glutaric aciduria, methylmalonic aciduria
Amino acidopathies	Homocystinuria (see p. 278)
Metal overload disorders	Wilsons, Hallovorden–Spartz
Other biochemical	Neurotransmitters, creatine disorders
Infections	
Slow virus	SSPE, Lyme disease, HIV dementia
Prion infection	Creutzfeldt–Jakob disease
Other	
	Rett syndrome, Huntington dementia

RETT SYNDROME

A rare neurodegenerative disease. The gene is McCP2 on chromosome Xq28. Only females are affected.

Presentation is generally after 1 year of age with:

- Developmental regression (language and motor milestones)
- Characteristic 'hand wringing' repetitive movements and loss of hand function
- Ataxic gait
- Acquired microcephaly
- Autistic features
- Apnoeas, sighing respirations
- Seizures (generalized tonic–clonic)
- Death between 10 and 30 years (often from cardiac arrhythmias)

SUBACUTE SCLEROSING PANENCEPHALITIS (SSPE)

A neurodegenerative disease secondary to an altered host response to the measles virus.

- Incidence 1:100 000
- Usually develops 5–7 years after measles infection
- Insidious onset of intellectual deterioration, abnormal behaviour
- Rapid progression with intractable myoclonus, choreoathetosis, dementia and death
- EEG shows characteristic periodic complexes (normal background with high-voltage slow wave bursts)
- CSF may contain intrathecal anti-measles antibody
- MRI brain scan may be normal early on, then white matter abnormalities, cortical atrophy and ventricular dilatation develop
- No effective treatment

MENKE KINKY HAIR DISEASE

X-linked recessive, gene on chromosome Xq13. Underlying defect in copper transport.

Clinical features

Presentation in early months of life with:

- Progressive neurodegeneration, severe mental retardation
- Seizures, hypotonia, feeding difficulties, optic atrophy
- Hair colourless, kinky and fragile
- Chubby red cheeks
- Death < 3 years

Investigations

Hair shaft	Trichorrhexis nodosa (fractures along hair shaft)
	Pili torti (twisted hair)
	Monilethrix (brittle hair)
Serum	Copper ($\downarrow$), caeruloplasmin ($\downarrow$)

Management

Copper-histidine subcutaneously slows deterioration in some patients.

MULTIPLE SCLEROSIS

A disease of multiple central demyelinating lesions with plaque formation, separated by space and time. Characteristic remissions and relapses occur. It is mostly slowly progressive, though may have a rapid course.

Usual onset 20–35 years, though can occur in children (0.2–2% of cases).

Associations   Female > male, lower incidence closer to the equator
                      First-degree relative with multiple sclerosis, HLA-A3, B7 and DR2

Clinical features

Neurological symptoms depending on where the demyelination occurs. Some common symptoms are:

- Ataxia, weakness, headache, paresthaesias
- Optic neuropathy (blurred vision), optic neuritis (swelling of optic disc), optic atrophy

Unusual features include epilepsy, trigeminal neuralgia.

Investigations

MRI brain   Plaques
CSF   Cells ↑ (5–60/mm³, mononuclear)
              Protein ↑ (0.4–1 g/L) (in 60%)
              IgG ↑ (in 60%)
              Oligoclonal bands (in 80%)
VER   Delay (if optic nerve involvement)

Management

- Mostly supportive
- Steroids may help in acute attacks

STROKE

A focal neurological deficit with an underlying vascular pathology is defined as:

- **Stroke** – lasting > 24 h
- **Transient ischaemic attack (TIA)** – lasting < 24 h
- **Reversible ischaemic neurological deficit (RIND)** – lasting > 24 h but with full recovery

'**Stroke-like episode**' – focal neurological deficit lasting > 24 h with no obvious vascular pathology, e.g. brain tumour, brain abscess.

Causes

Stroke may be due to haemorrhage or ischaemia. Ischaemia may be caused by vessel spasm, stenosis or dissection or vessel occlusion (by thrombosis or embolism).

Ischaemia

Thrombosis   Sickle cell disease
                  Severe dehydration (venous sinus thrombosis)
                  Meningitis
                  Clotting disorder, e.g. protein S or C deficiency, antithrombin III deficiency, lupus
                  antibodies, factor V Leiden
                  Thrombocytosis
                  Homocystinuria
                  Leukaemia
Embolism   Cyanotic CHD, endocarditis
Vessel spasm   Meningitis

Large vessel stenosis	Sickle cell disease
	Varicella, AIDS, homocystinuria
Vessel dissection	Trauma, e.g. fall on a pencil in child's mouth
	Congenital heart disease
Moya moya disease	Moya moya (basal artery occlusion with telangiectasia)
	Also seen in Williams syndrome, Down syndrome

Haemorrhage

Low platelets	ITP
Bleeding disorder	Haemophilia
Vessel disorder	A-V malformation, cerebral aneurysm
Trauma	

Clinical features

- Deterioration in level of consciousness (seen in progression of bleed)
- Seizures (common in neonates)
- Hemiparesis, hemisensory signs, visual field defects

Investigations

These will be led by any underlying disease, and history and examination are essential to help elucidate the cause.

MRI brain scan	Outline area affected (thrombosis, bleed, abscess, tumour, etc.)
CT scan	If MRI unavailable (to exclude haemorrhage)
Magnetic resonance angiography (MRA scan)	Vascular outline
Transcranial Doppler USS	Large vessel disease
Cerebral angiogram	For more detailed outline. If MRA normal in ischaemia
	Later, after haemorrhage for, e.g. A-V malformation, aneurysm
ECG and echocardiogram	Cardiac anomaly or arrhythmia
Infection screen	
Haematological screen	Including sickle screen, FBC and clotting defects
Metabolic screen	If metabolic disease suspected

Management

This is dependent on the cause, e.g. exchange transfusion acutely in sickle cell disease, anticoagulants may be required in prothrombotic coagulopathy and surgery in A-V malformation and cerebral aneurysm. Extensive rehabilitation, depending on stroke severity, from multidisciplinary team.

SPINAL CORD DISORDERS

SPINAL CORD COMPRESSION

Causes

- Tumour – spinal cord intradural or extradural tumour, secondary deposit
- Trauma
- Infection – epidural abscess, TB
- Disc protrusion
- Vascular malformation

Clinical features

These depend on whether the transection is partial or involves the whole cord. Basic features are:

- Pain – back pain and pain at the level of compression (radicular pain)
- Paralysis – spastic para- or tetra-paresis from the level of compression
- Sensory loss – loss to the level of compression

Complete transection

Paralysis	Initial flaccid muscle paralysis (spinal shock), then spastic paralysis from the level of compression
	Loss of voluntary sphincter control (reflex emptying returns)
Sensory loss	Total loss of sensation in the regions supplied below the level of injury

NB: Fatal if above 4th cervical cord segment due to paralysis of the diaphragm.

Hemisection (Brown–Séquard syndrome)

Paralysis	Paralysis of muscles on the same side as injury below the level of transection
Sensory loss	Same side (paralysed limb) – loss of position sense, proprioception and tactile discrimination in the same side (dorsal columns)
	Opposite, unparalysed limb – loss of pain and temperature sensation (spinothalamic)

Investigations

X ray spine	(Bony destruction?)
MRI spine	Outline of lesion
Myelogram	(May be considered)

SYRINGOMYELIA AND SYRINGOBULBIA

A cystic degeneration of the centre of the cord (myelia) or brainstem (bulbia).

Clinical features

Destruction of spinothalamic tracts	Bilateral loss of temperature and pain in a bizarre distribution
Destruction of corticospinal tracts	Spastic paraparesis, absent tendon reflexes upper limbs, wasting of the small muscles of the hand
Brainstem (syringobulbia)	Nystagmus, hearing loss, Horner syndrome, loss of facial sensation, tongue atrophy and fasciculation

Investigations

- MRI
- Myelogram

Management

Surgical aspiration may be attempted.

TRANSVERSE MYELITIS

This is acute inflammation of the cord and paraplegia.

Causes

- Viral infection – EBV, HSV, mumps, rubella, influenza
- Multiple sclerosis, radiotherapy, anterior spinal artery occlusion

Clinical features

Abrupt onset of:

- Weakness – initially flaccid, becoming spastic, legs
- Sensory loss – pain, temperature and light touch, legs
- Back pain
- Sphincter disturbance
- Fever and nuchal rigidity

Investigations

LP   CSF shows lymphocytes ↑, (protein ↑, N)
MRI spine   Lesion outlined

Management

Supportive, complete spontaneous recovery may occur.

Differential diagnosis

- Guillain–Barré syndrome
- Acute poliomyelitis
- Cord compression

NEUROMUSCULAR DISORDERS

The neuromuscular disorders are diseases in which the main pathology is peripheral:

Anterior horn cells   Spinal muscular atrophies
Peripheral nerve   Peripheral neuropathies
Neuromuscular junction   Myaesthenic syndromes
Muscles   Myopathies and muscular dystrophies

They can be remembered and classified according to where along the motor pathway the pathology exists. They result in muscular weakness, often progressive.

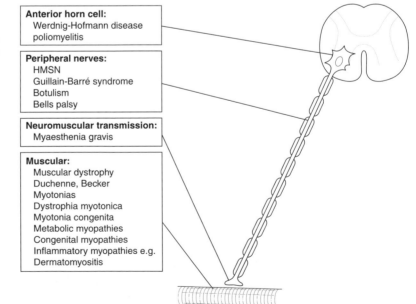

Anterior horn cell:
Werdnig-Hofmann disease
poliomyelitis

Peripheral nerves:
HMSN
Guillain-Barré syndrome
Botulism
Bells palsy

Neuromuscular transmission:
Myaesthenia gravis

Muscular:
Muscular dystrophy
Duchenne, Becker
Myotonias
Dystrophia myotonica
Myotonia congenita
Metabolic myopathies
Congenital myopathies
Inflammatory myopathies e.g.
Dermatomyositis

Figure 14.8 Neuromuscular disorders

CLINICAL FEATURES

Neonatal presentation	Older children
In utero: • Polyhydramnios • Reduced fetal movements Arthogryphosis Hypotonia (floppy baby) Feeding difficulties Breathing difficulties (may need respiratory support)	Motor delay Gait abnormalities Muscle weakness Muscle fatiguability

SPECIFIC INVESTIGATIONS

(These are tailored depending on the clinical features)

EMG	Specific features may be seen, e.g. muscular dystrophy, myotonic dystrophy
Muscle imaging (USS, MRI)	Myopathies, muscular dystrophies
Muscle biopsy	SMA, Duchenne muscular dystrophy, myotonic dystrophy, congenital myopathies
Nerve stimulation test	Myaesthenia gravis
Nerve conduction studies	HMSN, SMA, Guillain–Barré disease
Sural nerve biopsy	HMSN
Creatinine phosphokinase	↑ In myotonic dystrophy and Duchenne muscular dystrophy
DNA analysis	Specific disorders, e.g. muscular dystrophy, myotonic dystrophy
Tensilon test	Myaesthenia gravis
Acetylcholine receptor antibodies	Myaesthenia gravis

THE FLOPPY BABY

The congenital neuromuscular disorders present as a neonatal hypotonia ('floppy baby'). There are many causes of floppy babies, which can be divided into **central** and **peripheral** (neuromuscular) causes. The latter are identified by the presence of **weakness** (limb movement absent or decreased) in addition, although in practice they can be difficult to differentiate:

Central causes (brain and spinal cord)	**Floppy only** (limb antigravity movement present)
Neuromuscular causes	**Floppy and weak** (no/reduced limb antigravity movement)

Causes (neonatal hypotonia)

Central causes	Neonatal sepsis Drugs, e.g. maternal pethidine during delivery Hypoxic–ischaemic encephalopathy Metabolic disease, e.g. hypothyroidism, peroxisomal disorders, MSUD Syndromic, e.g. Down syndrome, fetal alcohol syndrome, Prader–Willi syndrome
Neuromuscular causes	Anterior horn cell disorder, e.g. spinal muscular atrophy Neuromuscular junction disorder, e.g. transient neonatal myasthenia Skeletal muscle disorder, e.g. congenital myopathy, congenital myotonic dystrophy

---

Clinical features of floppy baby with neuromuscular disorder

- *In utero*: Polyhydramnios, reduced fetal movements
- Arthogryphosis
- Hypotonia   **Frog-like** position while resting
               Head lag (little or no head control)
               Neurological 'flip-over' examination demonstrates weakness in all positions
- Feeding difficulties
- Breathing difficulties

SPINAL MUSCULAR ATROPHY TYPE 1 (SMA, WERDNIG-HOFFMAN DISEASE)

Autosomal recessive, severe disease. Deletion in SMN1 gene 5q11–13. Incidence 4:100 000 approximately.

Due to **progressive degeneration of the anterior horn cells** as a result of failure of arrest of apoptosis.

Clinical features

- Severely affected – floppy and weak
- *In utero*: decreased fetal movements, arthrogryphosis
- Respiratory distress
- Tongue and other muscle **fasciculation**
- Extraocular muscles not affected
- Absent reflexes
- Progressive weakness

Death in infancy (from respiratory failure).

Investigations

Muscle biopsy   Characteristic perinatal denervation pattern
EMG   Few definitive changes
DNA testing   Possible to confirm diagnosis

NB: CK normal.

Management

Supportive only (physiotherapy, orthopaedic, occupational therapy).

POLIOMYELITIS

Due to infection with poliovirus type 1, 2 or 3. Transmission faecal–oral route.

Clinical features

Incubation 7–14 days. Subclinical infection (95%).

Abortive poliomyelitis (5%)   Fever, sore throat, myalgia
Non-paralytic poliomyelitis (2%)   Above plus meningeal irritation
Paralytic poliomyelitis (0.1%)   Initial fever, sore throat, myalgia, then meningeal irritation, muscle pain (neck
                                and lumbar region). Then asymmetrical paralysis:
                                • Spinal poliomyelitis – limbs, thorax, diaphragm, trunk
                                • Bulbar poliomyelitis (5–30%) motor cranial nerve paralysis
                                NB: No sensory involvement

Predisposing factors:
- Exercise early in illness
- Male
- Trauma, surgery, IM injection
- Tonsillitis (bulbar polio)

Investigations

- Clinical diagnosis
- Viral PCR and culture

Management

Supportive therapy, early bed rest.

Prevention

- Intramuscular inactivated polio vaccine

HEREDITARY MOTOR-SENSORY NEUROPATHIES (HMSN, CHARCOT–MARIE–TOOTH, CMT)

This is a group of many disorders in which there is progressive disease of the peripheral nerves involving demyelination and/or axonal degeneration. Treatment is supportive only.

HMSN Type 1 (CMT 1)

Autosomal dominant. Different genes found underlying different subtypes. Peripheral myelin protein 22 (PMP-22) gene mutations in CMT1A. Prevalence 15:100 000.

Clinical features

- Presentation in late childhood
- Progressive distal weakness: Weakness of dorsiflexion (foot drop), pes cavus
                                   Gait disturbance
                                   Inverted champagne bottle-shaped legs
- Absent tendon reflexes
- Milder involvement of hands
- Distal sensory loss – paraethesias, loss of proprioception and vibration

Investigations

DNA testing
Nerve conduction studies   Reduced motor and sensory velocities; differentiate demyelinating from axonal
Sural nerve biopsy   'Onion bulb' formations of Schwann cell cytoplasm (due to de- and re-myeliniation. Not necessary for diagnosis)

Management

Supportive only – foot splints, ankle fusion, pillows under legs at night.

GUILLAIN–BARRÉ DISEASE

This is a post-infectious demyelinating neuropathy, developing 1–3 weeks after an often trivial viral infection.

Clinical features

Trivial viral infection, then 1–3 weeks later:

- Distal limb weakness, ascending and symmetrical
- Areflexic
- Muscle pain and paraesthesia
- Respiratory muscle and facial weakness (20%)
- Urinary retention or incontinence
- Autonomic features rare (BP and heart rate lability)

Investigations

Clinical diagnosis.

Nerve conduction	Delay in motor and sensory conduction
LP	CSF Protein ↑ (×2 normal)
	Oligoclonal bands
	WCC normal, glucose normal
Respiratory function tests	Spirometry

Management

Supportive therapy with ventilation in severe cases. Spontaneous recovery usual in 2–3 weeks, though there may be some residual weakness.

Gamma-globulin (IV) reduces duration and severity. Plasmapheresis occasionally used.

Miller–Fischer syndrome

A rare, severe form involving:

- Ataxia
- Proximal muscle weakness
- External ophthalmoplegia

MYASTHENIA GRAVIS

A disease of immunological neuromuscular blockade in which there are **IgG antibodies to acetylcholine receptors (AchR)**.

Mostly acquired, may be hereditary. Incidence approximately 15:100 000. Female:male = 2:1. Average age of onset 30 years.

Associations	Drugs (D-penicillamine, lithium, propranolol)
	HLA-B8, DR3
	Hashimoto thyroiditis
	Collagen vascular disease

Clinical features

Eyes	External ocular muscle weakness, diplopia and ptosis
Bulbar	Dysphagia (bulbar muscle involvement)
Face	Sad facial expression (facial muscle weakness)
Limbs	Proximal weakness
	Reflexes fatiguable
Fatiguability	**Muscle fatiguability,** i.e. progressive weakness with *use* – a cardinal feature

Diagnosis

Tensilon test	An anticholinesterase, e.g. edrophonium, given IV, brings transient relief. NB: Cannot use edrophonium in neonates (causes arrhythmias)
Serum	AChR antibodies (90%)
Nerve stimulation	Fibrillation and decreased muscle response with repetition

Management

Anticholinesterase drugs	4–6 hourly, e.g. pyridostigmine, neostigmine
Antibody removal	Using thymectomy, steroids or plasmapharesis can be done

Care during anaesthetics.

Transient neonatal myaesthenia gravis

In a pregnant mother suffering from myaesthenia gravis, AChR antibodies will cross the placenta because they are IgG antibodies, and cause a transient neonatal disease, generally lasting 2–3 weeks.

Congenital myaesthenia gravis

This is a condition of *different* aetiology (due to congenital abnormality of AChR channels and not autoimmune disease) which has similar features to myasthenia gravis but is non-progressive.

MUSCULAR DYSTROPHIES

These are genetic myopathies involving progressive disease and death of muscle fibres.

	Inheritance	Features
Duchenne MD	XR (dystrophin absent)	See below
Becker MD	XR (dystrophin reduced) Dystrophin gene *abnormal*	Similar but less severe than Duchenne MD
Emery–Dreifuss MD	XR	Scapulohumeral weakness, contractures Cardiac involvement causes sudden death
Facioscapulohumeral MD	AD *Anticipation* occurs	A group of disorders Face and shoulder weakness Normal life expectancy
Limb girdle MD	AR, AD	A group of disorders Proximal limb weakness Calf hypertrophy may occur. Rate of progression varies but often wheelchair bound by 30 years

Duchenne muscular dystrophy

X-linked recessive, incidence 1:3600 live male infants. Due to absence of dystrophin (a muscle protein), caused by a mutation in the dystrophin gene on chromosome Xp21.3.

Clinical features

Normal early motor development	
Proximal limb weakness	Evident from 3 years of age
	Gower's sign evident at 3–6 years: A manoeuvre to stand from lying down involving rolling over, then using hands to 'climb up' the knees
	Waddling (Trendelenburg) gait
Calf muscle pseudohypertrophy	As a toddler
Progressive deterioration	Eventually wheelchair bound (usually by teenage years) with scoliosis
	Pharyngeal weakness and respiratory failure develop
Cardiac	Dilated cardiomyopathy, Q waves in left chest leads
Learning disability (33%)	

Investigations

Creatinine phosphokinase (CK)	Extremely elevated ($\uparrow$ 10 x normal)
Muscle biopsy	Fibre necrosis, fat infiltration, *no* dystrophin on staining
EMG	Myopathic pattern
Cardiac	ECG, CXR
Genetic testing	Dystrophin gene mutation looked for

Management

Supportive only at the present time, with physiotherapy, nutritional support, orthopaedic involvement and occupational therapy. The prognosis is poor with eventual death from respiratory complications.

Detection

- Female carriers – CK $\uparrow$ in 70%
- Antenatal detection is possible on CVS sampling using DNA probes

MYOTONIC DYSTROPHY

A progressive distal muscle weakness in which the cardinal feature is a **failure of muscle relaxation (myotonia)**.

Autosomal dominant. Chromosome 19q13 expansion with numerous trinucleotide CTG repeats. **Anticipation** occurs, i.e. more severe with each generation (see p. 16). Worse if inherited from the mother.

Clinical features

May present in the neonatal period or later.

Face	**Fish mouth** (inverted 'V' shaped upper lip)
	Facial muscle weakness, decreased muscle mass in temporal fossa, high-arched palate
Eyes	Ptosis, cataracts
Other muscles	Weakness of distal limbs and respiratory muscles
Cardiac	Cardiomyopathy, conduction defects
Mental	Learning disability (50%)
Hair	Frontal baldness in males
Endocrine	Hypogonadism, small pituitary fossa, glucose intolerance
Immunity	IgG $\downarrow$
Gastrointestinal	Constipation

Investigations

Diagnosis is clinical. Shake hands with the child (if old enough) and the parent and they *cannot* quickly let go.

Muscle biopsy	Prognostic value in neonates
EMG	Classic findings seen after infancy
Other	Endocrine, immunoglobulin and cardiac assessment is necessary

Management

- Phenytoin or carbamazepine may help with myotonia (increase depolarization threshold)
- Care must be taken during anaesthesia

MYOTONIA CONGENITA (THOMSEN DISEASE)

- Autosomal dominant (chromosome 7q35) or recessive
- Myotonia with generalized muscle hypertrophy – appearance of a body builder

CONGENITAL MYOPATHIES

The term congenital myopathies encompasses many unrelated congenital diseases of the muscles, which may be mild, causing little problem throughout life, or severe; they may also be either static or progressive.

Some are due to ultrastructural deformities of the muscles, and some to abnormalities within the mitochondrial DNA and involve metabolic defects and features in other organs. Muscle biopsy is usually involved in diagnosis.

General features

- Those of neuromuscular causes of floppy baby (see p. 363), i.e. neonatal hypotonia *with weakness*. They have a distinctive appearance with a thin muscle mass at birth and undescended testicles
- Features may be mild at birth but are often progressive

Myotubular myopathy

Usually X-linked recessive (also autosomal dominant and recessive forms).

Disorder of muscle ultrastructure, possibly due to developmental arrest.

Clinical features

In utero	Decreased fetal movements, polyhydramnios
Neonatal	Severe myopathy at birth. Ptosis prominent. Most die within few weeks of birth

Diagnosis

Muscle biopsy is diagnostic.

Congenital muscle fibre-type disproportion (CMFTD)

Sporadic, autosomal recessive. Features as in myotubular myopathy but less severe, with a high degree of clinical variability. Diagnosis on muscle biopsy.

Nemaline rod myopathy

Abnormal rod-shaped inclusions within muscle fibres (mostly α-actinin). Autosomal dominant or recessive. Variable penetrance of dominant form, with mildly affected individuals having poorly developed muscles only.

A severe neonatal form exists, with early death in most infants, and a milder form with motor delay, feeding difficulties and recurrent respiratory infections, dolicocephaly and high arched palate.

Diagnosis on muscle biopsy (nemaline rods are abnormal structures within the muscle fibres).

POTASSIUM-RELATED PERIODIC PARALYSES

Autosomal dominant. Involves periodic attacks of paralysis with transient alterations in serum potassium:

K ↓   Hypokalaemic periodic paralysis
K ↑   Hyperkalaemic periodic paralysis

Normal between attacks in childhood.

Episodes of paralysis, e.g. on awakening, lasting minutes or hours. Liquorice may precipitate attacks. Progressive disease with weakness in adulthood. Diaphragmatic muscles unaffected, ECG changes occur during attacks.

Care must be taken during anaesthesia.

HEREDITARY SENSORY NEUROPATHY, FAMILIAL DYSAUTONOMIA (RILEY–DAY SYNDROME)

Autosomal recessive. Gene at chromosome 9q31–33. Disease of peripheral nervous system involving reduced numbers of small nerve fibres (pain, temperature, taste, autonomic functions).

Associations   Eastern European Jews

Clinical features

Autonomic features	Excessive sweating, blotchy erythema, abnormal tearing
	'Crises' (labile BP, heart rate, vomiting, irritability, sweating, poor temperature control)
Peripheral neuropathy	Insensitivity to pain, feeding difficulties and aspirations, clumsy gait, scoliosis, corneal ulcers, slurred speech
CNS	Breath-holding seizures, mental retardation

Investigations

Diagnosis	Intradermal histamine produces no flare.
	Metacholine infusion causes exaggerated hypotensive response
	Metacholine eye drops produce miosis (no reaction normally)
Plasma	Dopamine-β-hydroxylase enzyme ↓
Urine	VMA ↓, HVA↑
Sural nerve biopsy	Decreased unmyelinated fibres
CXR	Chronic changes from aspirations
ECG	Prolonged QT

Management

- Eye drops, protection from injury
- Autonomic crises – anxiolytics, antiemetics, electrolyte control

Prognosis

Death in childhood from chronic pulmonary failure.

PSYCHIATRIC DISORDERS

ATTENTION DEFICIT HYPERACTIVITY DISORDER (ADHD)

Diagnostic criteria

- Inattention
- Hyperactivity
- Impulsivity

Lasting > 6 months and commencing < 7 years, and inconsistent with the child's developmental level. These features should be present in more than one setting, and cause significant social or school impairment.

Risk factors:

- Male > female 4:1
- Learning difficulties
- CNS disorder, e.g. epilepsy, cerebral palsy
- Specific developmental delay
- First-degree relative with ADHD
- Family member with depression, learning disability, antisocial personality or substance abuse

These children also have an increased risk of:

- Conduct disorder
- Anxiety disorder
- Aggression

A significant proportion of children with ADHD will become adults with antisocial personality and there is an increased incidence of criminal behaviour and substance abuse.

Management

Psychotherapy	Behavioural therapies
	Family therapy
Drugs	If behavioural therapy alone insufficient:
	Stimulants, e.g. methylphenidate (Ritalin), amphetamines (dexamphetamine)
	Side effects: insomnia, appetite suppression, headaches, abdominal pain, growth retardation (reversible on stopping drug)
Diet	Some children benefit noticeably from exclusion of certain foods from their diet, e.g. red food colouring, cow's milk
	This is not universal though, and any changes should be made with the assistance of a dietician

AUTISM (CLASSICAL OR REGRESSIVE)

Prevalence 5–6:10 000 (currently rising).

A developmental behavioural disorder of **social interaction and understanding**, which is the end-point of several organic aetiologies, e.g. prenatal insults, metabolic disorders, localized CNS lesions, postnatal infections (e.g. encephalitis). The specific organic cause is rarely found (< 10%). Features and severity very variable and thought to be part of a *spectrum*.

Genetic factors	Siblings have a 2–3% prevalence, i.e. 50–100 x greater than average incidence
	Monozygotic twin concordance 60%

Increased risk of epilepsy in teenage years.

Clinical features

- Diagnosis made at 2–3 years. Features noticeable from 1 year
- Severity varies greatly between individuals and over time in a single child
- Impairment of social interactions   Limited eye contact
  Child relates to *parts* of a person not the whole person
  Plays alone
- Narrow range of interests and repetitive behaviour   Repetitive play, fascination with movement
  Interest in detail
  Poor concentration span
  Early development of numbers
- Rigidity of thought and behaviour – difficulty in changing from one activity to the next or in stopping an activity
- Abnormal speech and language development – delay in speech, echolalia
- Developmental stasis or regression – seen in 25–30% at 15–18 months of age
- Most have low IQ

Management

1. *Assessment*   Detailed medical and developmental history (focusing on development and core behaviours)
   Medical examination and play observation
   Hearing and vision testing
   Other investigations if indicated, e.g. lead, FBC and iron studies, chromosomes and fragile X, Rett gene, thyroid function, PKU test
   Neuroimaging only if specific neurological signs. EEG if epilepsy
2. *Written report*   Produced for parents and all relevant professionals and an action plan is made for the family
3. *Interventions*   Behavioural therapies and educational programmes (several approaches may be used, none of which has been shown to be more effective than others)

ASPERGER SYNDROME

These children have a severe impairment in reciprocal social interaction, but are otherwise relatively normal.

- No delay in language, but have unusual language development, e.g. interpret literally, have one-sided conversations
- Variable fine and gross motor delay (clumsy, walk later than they speak)
- Difficulty in understanding non-verbal communication
- Generally high level of intelligence
- Develop all-absorbing special interests
- May be able to memorize large amounts of information, though not necessarily fully comprehend it

FURTHER READING

Aicardi J *Diseases of the Nervous System in Childhood*, 2nd edn. London: MacKeith Press with Blackwell Science Publications, 1998

15
Ophthalmology

- *Visual development*
- *Visual impairment*
- *Eye lid abnormalities*
- *Lacrimal system abnormalities*
- *Anterior segment, iris and lens malformations*
- *Optic nerve abnormalities*
- *Disc abnormalities*

- *Orbital abnormalities*
- *Refractive error and strabismus (squint)*
- *Infections and allergies*
- *Retinopathy of prematurity*
- *Non-accidental injury*
- *Phakomatoses*

VISUAL DEVELOPMENT

- Eye grows rapidly during the first 2 years of life
- Neonates have poor visual acuity (approx 6/200)
- By 6 months of age electrodiagnostic tests show that vision improves to 6/6
- Any untreated **obstruction or interference with focusing** on objects during the first 7 years of life prevents normal development of visual acuity (**amblyopia**)
- **Binocular vision** develops in the first 3–6 months of age
- **Depth perception** begins at 6–8 months, is accurate at 6–7 years and improves during adolescence

VISUAL ACUITY

- Top number is the **distance the subject is away from the chart** in metres
- Bottom number is the number written by the side of the letter on the chart. This number indicates the **maximum distance** (in metres) that a **normal sighted** person can see that letter
- In the UK normal vision is 6/6 since meters are used (20/20 in USA as feet are used)

Visual acuity testing

Age	Test
Birth	Face fixation, preference for patterned objects
6 weeks	Fixes and follows a face through 90° (not to the midline until 3 months old) 90 cm away
	Optokinetic nystagmus on looking at a moving striped target
3 months	Fixes and follows through 180° 90 cm away
6 months	Reaches for a toy
10 months	Picks up a raisin
1 year	Picks up hundreds and thousands
2 years	Identifies pictures of reducing size (Kays pictures)
3 years	Letter matching with single letter charts, e.g. Sheridan Gardiner, Stycar chart
5 years	Identifies letters on a Snellen chart by name or matching letters

VISUAL IMPAIRMENT

Causes

- Congenital – anophthalmos, optic nerve hypoplasia, cataracts
- Prematurity – retinopathy of prematurity
- Hypoxic–ischaemic encephalopathy
- Refractive error – amblyopia, myopia, hypermetropia
- Strabismus
- Optic atrophy
- Tumour, e.g. retinoblastoma
- Systemic condition, e.g. juvenile idiopathic arthritis (uveitis)
- Infection – orbital cellulitis, trachoma
- Delayed visual maturation (normal children with learning difficulties; they develop normal vision later)
- Cortical blindness, i.e. cortical defect, no eye abnormality

Clinical presentation

- Lack of eye contact
- Failure to smile by 6 weeks of age
- Visual inattention, failure to track objects or fix on face by 3 months
- Nystagmus
- Squint
- Photophobia
- White pupillary reflex (**leucocoria**) (see below)

Management

Initial assessment by a paediatrician, an ophthalmologist and a neurologist is necessary.

- Ophthalmological assessment: general eye examination and visual acuity
- Full neurological assessment

Investigations

These are led by the individual case history and examination, but may include:

Electrophysiological tests	**Electro-retinogram (ERG)** (abnormal in retinal defects)
	Visual evoked response (VER) (abnormal in both eye and cortical defects)
Bloods	Serology for congenital infection
	Pituitary function tests
	Inborn error of metabolism, e.g. galactosaemia
Brain CT/MRI	

Treatment

- Treat any treatable cause
- Specialized regular developmental assessment with help from teachers from the Royal National Institute for the Blind (RNIB)
- Maximize non-visual stimulation
- Education: Mainstream school or school for the blind
               Braille (if blind)
               Low vision aids (if impaired vision, e.g. high-power magnifiers, telescopic devices)
- Genetic counselling if appropriate

EYE LID ABNORMALITIES

Ptosis	Droopy lids, can cause amblyopia if obstructing the vision
Lid coloboma	Varying from a small notch to absence of lid (usually upper lid)
Epiblepharon	Horizontal fold of skin in upper or lower lid turning eye lashes in; usually resolves spontaneously by 2 years old
Dystichiasis	Extra row of eyelashes
	Autosomal dominant inheritance
	Associated with lymphoedema
Ectropion	Eversion of usually lower lid
Entropion	Inversion of usually the lower lid
Epicanthus	Vertical crescentic fold of skin between upper and lower lids
	May mimic strabismus
	Especially prominent in Asian children
Telecanthus	Wide interpupillary distance
Blepharophimosis	Shortening of palpebral fissures horizontally and vertically

LACRIMAL SYSTEM ABNORMALITIES

Nasolacrimal duct obstruction

- A persistent membrane across the lower end of the nasolacrimal duct is very common at birth, leading to a watery eye (about 5% of newborns)
- Normally disappears after the first year

- If the problem persists beyond 12 months the nasolacrimal ducts are probed under general anaesthetic. This usually gives immediate resolution and, if not, the procedure is repeated

Dacrocystocele

- Uncommon, cystic swelling of the nasolacrimal duct due to obstruction
- Can mimic a dermoid cyst, haemangioma or encephalocele
- Treatment is topical antibiotics and digital massage
- It may lead to dacrocystis if it becomes infected, and will need systemic antibiotics ± surgical decompression

ANTERIOR SEGMENT, IRIS AND LENS MALFORMATIONS

CORNEAL ABNORMALITIES

Keratoconus is thinning of central cornea leading to cone formation and astigmatism. Usually presents and progresses through adolescence.

Differential diagnosis of corneal opacities

- **Sclerocornea** – cornea indistinct from white scleral tissue with no apparent limbus. Rare
- **Forceps injury** causing a tear in Descemet's membrane in the cornea leading to corneal oedema
- **Mucopolysaccharidosis** and **mucolipidosis** (see p. 284)
- **Posterior corneal defects** – iris undifferentiated from cornea
- **Congenital hereditary endothelial dystrophy** – uncommon, hereditary dystrophy, onset at birth. Corneal oedema and clouding
- **Dermoid** – usually straddle the corneo-scleral limbus. Associated with Goldenhar syndrome
- **Infantile glaucoma** (see p. 377)
- **Congenital hereditary stromal dystrophy** – very rare, autosomal dominant corneal clouding
- **Other causes** – cystinosis, Wilson disease, congenital syphilis, Riley–Day syndrome

IRIS ABNORMALITIES

Aniridia	Iris hypoplasia. Sporadic or autosomal dominant
	Sporadic form: 1/3 develop Wilms tumours, therefore yearly abdominal USS and clinical evaluation for Wilms tumour needed
Iris coloboma	Notching of iris. May involve retina and optic nerve
	Associations: trisomy 13, triploidy, trisomy 18, Klinefelter, Turner syndrome, CHARGE, Walker–Warburg, Aicardi, Rubensten–Tayabi, Goldenhar syndrome
Brushfield's spots	Iris stromal hyperplasia surrounded by hypoplasia.
	Seen in 90% of Down syndrome
Heterochromia	Variation in colour between the two irises
	Occasionally associated with Wilms tumour
Hypochromic	Reduced iris pigmentation compared to other eye.
	E.g. congenital Horner, Fuchs heterocromia, Waardenburg-Klein syndrome, tumours
Hyperchromic	Increased iris pigmentation
	E.g. pigmented tumours, siderosis, ectropion uvea, oculodermal melanosis
Persistent pupillary membrane	Most common developmental abnormality of iris
	If especially prominent can lead to anterior polar cataracts

PUPIL ABNORMALITIES (ANISOCORIA)

Small pupil May be associated with other eye abnormalities, e.g. congenital rubella syndrome, Lowe oculocerebrorenal syndrome
Drugs, e.g. morphine

Large pupil Iris trauma
Drugs, e.g. ecstasy
Parasympathetic neurological disorder:
- Holmes–Adie pupil
- Unilateral VI nerve palsy (seen in ↑ ICP)

Causes of leucocoria (white pupil)

- Retinoblastoma
- Cataract
- Colobomas
- Infection – toxocaria, toxoplasma
- Retinopathy of prematurity
- Uveitis
- Coats disease
- Vitreous haemorrhage
- Retinal detachment
- Persistent hyperplastic primary vitreous

CAUSES OF CATARACT IN CHILDREN

Bilateral	Unilateral
Idiopathic	Idiopathic
Any congenital infection, e.g. CMV, toxoplasmosis, rubella, varicella, syphilis	Trauma
	Rubella
Hereditary: • AD (mostly), or AR or XLR • Down, Turner, Trisomy 13–15 and 18, Marfan, Alport, Fabry disease, Lowe syndrome, Conradi syndrome	Intraocular tumours
Anterior segment dysgenesis	
Drugs – corticosteroids	
Metabolic: • Hypoparathyroidism (hypocalcaemia) • Galactosaemia ('oil-drop' cataract) • Diabetic mother, diabetic child (uncommon, snowflake cataracts)	

CONGENITAL GLAUCOMA

- Primary congenital glaucoma incidence 1:10 000 births
- Mainly sporadic, may be autosomal recessive. Males > females
- Intraocular pressure rises due to maldevelopment of the drainage angle in the anterior chamber
- May present at birth or develop later (usually < 3 years old)

- May be secondary to Sturge–Weber syndrome, dysgenesis syndromes, Lowe syndrome, rubella, aniridia, neurofibromatosis, microcornea, ROP and retinoblastoma

Clinical features

- **Buphthalmos** (excessive corneal diameter [> 13 mm] due to stretching of the eye from the constant elevated intraocular pressure). Cornea becomes white and hazy due to corneal oedema
- Photophobia, lacrimation and eye rubbing
- Both eyes are usually affected but asymmetrically
- Eyes have a tendency to become myopic with disc cupping

Management

Involves topical antiglaucoma medication +/– drainage angle surgery, with regular follow-up and refraction.

OPTIC NERVE ABNORMALITIES

Morning glory disc	Very rare, usually unilateral, mostly sporadic inheritance
	Enlarged optic disc, with central area of white tissue
	Associated with high myopia and other developmental abnormalities, and poor visual development
Coloboma	Unilateral or bilateral, vision depends on area of retinal or optic nerve involvement
Myelinated nerve fibres	Bilateral in 20%. White flame-shaped area at disc, causing visual field defects
Tilted discs	Usually bilateral, associated with reduced vision and visual field defects
Persistent hyaloid membrane	Remnants of hyaloid artery which normally disappears before birth. Usually asymptomatic.
Optic nerve hypoplasia	Uni- or bi-lateral. Small, pale optic disc with crowded vessels at disc
	Causing visual field defects, nystagmus and amblyopia
	Associations: fetal alcohol syndrome, endocrine abnormalities, e.g. hypothalamic and pituitary dysfunction, CNS anomalies

DISC ABNORMALITIES

DISC SWELLING

Causes

Raised ICP	(Think of this first). **Papilloedema** is optic disc (papilla) swelling secondary to raised ICP
Optic (local)	Infiltration, e.g. leukaemia
	Retinal vein occlusion
	Ischaemic optic neuropathy
Disc drusen	(Whitish hyaline/calcific deposits at the disc, present in 0.3% of the normal population. Usually bilateral and may be present in other family members. Usually cause no ocular complications apart from very rarely a minor loss of visual field)
Hypermetropia	

Clinical features

Symptoms	Blurred vision
	Enlarged blind spot (later in disease)
Signs	**Disc**: blurring, erythema, heaping up of the disc margins, obliteration of the physiological cup, disc haemorrhages
	Retina: retinal vein dilatation and loss of venous pulsation, retinal haemorrhages

OPTIC ATROPHY

This is visible as disc pallor.

Causes

- Optic nerve compression, e.g. tumour, aneurysm
- Ischaemia, e.g. severe anaemia, arteritis
- Optic and retrobulbar neuritis, e.g. multiple sclerosis
- Deficiency, e.g. vitamin B_{12}
- DIDMOAD
- Hereditary optic neuropathy
- Infection, e.g. orbital cellulitis, syphilis
- Toxic neuropathy, e.g. methyl alcohol, quinine, tobacco
- Causes of papilloedema

ORBITAL ABNORMALITIES

Differential diagnosis of proptosis in children

Malignant	E.g. rhabdomyosarcoma, neuroblastoma
Benign	Inflammatory, e.g. orbital cellulitis, mucocele
	Traumatic, e.q. haematoma
	Metabolic, e.g. Graves disease
	Infiltrative, e.g. glioma
	Developmental, e.g. dermoid cyst

CRANIOFACIAL MALFORMATIONS AFFECTING OCULAR DEVELOPMENT

Craniosynostosis	Proptosis, corneal exposure, strabismus, papilloedema, optic atropy
Hypertelorism	Increased distance between the orbits. Associated with cleft lip and palate, and strabismus
Waardenburg syndrome	AD. Iris heterochromia, white hair, retinal hypopigmentation, confluent eyebrows ± deafness
Goldenhar syndrome	Facial asymmetry, small low set ears often with ear tags, wide mouth with jaw abnormalities, vertebral dysgenesis, strabismus, microphthalmos (small globe)
Treacher–Collins syndrome	Jaw and maxillary hypoplasia, ear abnormalities, lid defects
Pierre–Robin syndrome	Retinal detachment, cataracts, myopia, microphthalmia (see p. 125)
Fetal alcohol syndrome	Short horizontal palpebral apertures

REFRACTIVE ERROR AND STRABISMUS (SQUINT)

REFRACTIVE ERROR

Hypermetropia

- Long-sightedness
- Most common childhood refractive error
- Early correction (with glasses) necessary to prevent amblyopia

Myopia

- Short-sightedness
- Uncommon in childhood, often hereditary

Amblyopia

Amblyopia is **permanent impairment of visual acuity** in an eye that did not receive a clear image while vision was developing. Usually only one eye affected, known as a **'lazy eye.'**

Causes

It results from *any* interference with visual development:

- Refractive errors
- Squint
- Obstruction of vision, e.g. strawberry haemangioma occluding vision, ptosis

Treatment

- Patching the good eye for periods of time during the day to force the affected eye to work and therefore develop, and
- Treat underlying cause, e.g. correct any refractive error with glasses, treat squint
- Treatment while young is very important. After age 7 years, improvement is unlikely

SQUINT (STRABISMUS)

Squint is a common condition and is due to misalignment of the visual axes.

> Squints may be:
>
> - **Real** or **apparent**, e.g. unilateral epicanthic fold
> - **Convergent** (esotropia), **divergent** (exotropia) or **vertical**
> - **Constant** (manifest, i.e. -tropia), **intermittent** (latent, i.e. –phoria, only present during inattention, ocular alignment is maintained with effort) or **alternating**
> - **Comitant** (angle of deviation is constant) or **incomitant** (angle of deviation changes on direction of gaze)
> - **Non-paralytic** or **paralytic**

Convergent squint

The most common childhood squint. Usually related to accommodation and caused by an imbalance between accommodation and convergence. (Eyes **accommodate** and **converge** when looking at near objects. Accommodation is the process of altering the shape of the natural lens to focus the incoming light onto the retina).

Convergent squints are usually constant in childhood.

Accommodative convergent squint	**Refractive** (due to child being long-sighted/hypermetropic): Difficulty on focusing on near objects. The stimulation for convergence is increased by the eyes trying to accommodate to focus on a near object, causing a squint
	Non-refractive: No hypermetropia is present. The stimulation for convergence is disproportionately high for the stimulation of accommodation
Mixed accommodative convergent squint	Hypermetropia and an *abnormal* stimulation of accommodation and convergence is present. Squint is most noticeable when focusing on near objects

| *Essential infantile convergent squint* | Idiopathic squint which presents in the first 6 months. The child **alternates fixation** between the two eyes. Usually corrected surgically by the age 2 years |

Divergent squint

| *Intermittent divergent squint* | Usually presents around the age of 2 years as an intermittent squint
With tiredness or inattention this may become constant |
| *Constant divergent squint* | May be congenital, due to underlying visual impairment in older children or after surgical over-correction of a convergent squint |

Paralytic squints

Rare.

- Divergent, e.g. IIIrd nerve palsy
- Convergent, e.g. VIth nerve palsy
- Vertical, e.g. IVth nerve palsy (head tilt occurs)

NB: Young babies often have a squint at times (particularly on convergence looking at a close object) as they have not yet developed binocular vision. There should be no squint by age 4 months. Any squint present after **2–3 months of age** should be referred to the ophthalmologist as binocular vision should have developed by this time.

Tests for squint

Visual acuity must be assessed first.

1. Corneal light reflection test	Pen torch is shone to produce reflections in both corneas. If reflection is in different places in each cornea, a squint is present
2. Eye movements	Child is asked to look at an object/toy which is moved in a horizontal, vertical and diagonal direction at $1/3$ of a meter. Detects a paralytic squint
3. Cover test	Eyes covered individually with a card using a toy for visual fixation If the fixing eye is then covered, the squint eye moves to take up fixation On removal of the cover the eyes move again as the normal fixing eye takes up fixation (manifest squint) Used to detect a **latent squint** where the eye squints when covered An **alternating squint** is where each eye moves in turn when covered

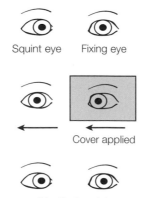

Figure 15.1 Cover test in a manifest squint of the right eye

Children should have fundoscopy and a refraction test for glasses if there is any history of squint. This should be repeated yearly as their refraction may change.

INFECTIONS AND ALLERGIES

CONJUNCTIVITIS

Clinical features

- Conjunctival injection
- Pus in the eye
- 'Gritty' or irritating eye
- Otitis media commonly associated with bacterial conjunctivitis, and should be examined for

Causes

Neonatal (ophthalmia neonatorum)	Child
(Notifiable disease in the UK)	
Staphylococcus aureus (usually presents early)	*Staphylococcus aureus*
Chlamydia trachomatis (florid pus on first day)	*Haemophilus influenzae*
Neisseria gonorrhoea (presents late [after 1ˢᵗ week])	*Streptococcus pneumoniae*
Escherichia coli ⎫	*Moxarella catarrhalis*
Haemophilus influenzae ⎬ Uncommon	Viral
Streptococcus pneumoniae ⎭	Allergic
Aseptic causes, i.e. chemical irritants	
Ophthalmia neonatorum is any purulent conjunctivitis occurring during the first 3 weeks of life.	

NB: Chlamydia, *Neisseria gonorrhoea*, streptococcus, chemical and herpes simplex can be acquired during delivery from the genital tract. *Neisseria gonorrhoea* is particularly dangerous as it can penetrate the cornea within 24 h.

Management

- Eye swab – microscopy (Gram stain) and culture. (Chlamydia and gonorrhoea require special media.) PCR for rapid detection
- Frequent eye and lid hygiene
- Neonate: Chloramphenicol or neomycin eye drops hourly or 2 hourly
  Chlamydia: oral erythromycin (2 weeks) plus tetracycline eye ointment
  Gonococcus: eye irrigation with crystalline penicillin hourly. IV penicillin 10 days
- Infant/child: Fusidic acid, chloramphenicol or neomycin eye drops
- Pseudomonas and *Haemophilus influenzae* type b – oral antibiotics needed

ORBITAL AND PRE-SEPTAL CELLULITIS

Preseptal cellulitis	Infection in the tissues anterior to the eyelid septum, with white conjunctiva, no diplopia, proptosis or loss of vision
Orbital (post-septal) cellulitis	Infection posterior to orbital septum, much more serious and can lead to loss of vision, cavernous sinus thrombosis, meningitis and septicaemia

Distinguishing clinical features

	Preseptal cellulitis	Orbital cellulitis
Conjunctiva/sclera	White	Inflamed oedematous
Ocular motility	Normal	Decreased/painful causing diplopia
Acuity	Normal	Impaired (if severe)
Colour vision	Normal	Impaired (if severe)
Pupillary reflex	Normal	Impaired (if severe)
Proptosis	None	Present
Fever and systemic upset	None (usually)	Present

NB: These features of orbital cellulitis are **danger signs** indicating possible need for surgery:

- An ophthalmologist should be contacted to help make the differentiation between pre- and post-septal cellulitis
- Orbital cellulitis may result from severe sinusitis, and therefore an ENT specialist should also be involved to assess the need for any urgent intervention
- Complications of orbital cellulitis include cavernous sinus thrombosis, meningitis, subdural and periosteal abscesses, and amblyopia/blindness if visual axis is interrupted.

Investigations

- Eye swab
- Blood cultures
- FBC
- Orbital and sinus CT scan (to show any involvement of the sinuses and intraorbital complications necessitating surgical drainage)

} If orbital cellulitis suspected

Treatment

Preseptal cellulitis   Oral antibiotics
Orbital cellultis   Broad spectrum IV antibiotics ± surgical intervention

ATOPIC CONJUNCTIVITIS

- Common, especially in boys aged 5–15
- Recurrent inflammation of the conjunctiva in spring and summer months, associated with severe itching and a milky white discharge
- Giant papillae form under the upper and lower lids which appear as large nodules
- Treatment involves topical antihistamines and occasionally low dose topical steroids

STEVENS–JOHNSON SYNDROME

A rare acute inflammatory reaction affecting the skin and mucous membranes, which is life threatening (see p. 298).

Ocular signs

- Conjunctivitis
- Scarring of the conjunctiva (corneal scarring may develop)
- Dry eye

Management of eye features

Lubricants and artificial tears.

RETINOPATHY OF PREMATURITY (ROP)

Thought to be due to proliferation of the retinal vasculature due to high oxygen saturation in the blood of premature babies. Normally retinal vasculature begins to develop from the optic disc in the 16th week *in utero*. The vessels reach the nasal peripheral edge of the retina by the 8th month of gestation. The temporal edge of the retina is vascularized by birth.

May result in:

- Decreased visual acuity
- Retinal detachment
- Blindness

Management

- Screening all premature infants at risk (< 1500 g at birth or < 32 weeks gestation) from 32 weeks by ophthalmologist
- Prevention by minimizing oxygen therapy to lowest necessary level
- Laser photocoagulation or cryotherapy if necessary

International classification of ROP

Location

Zone I   Circle around disc, with radius of twice the distance from the fovea to the disc

Zone II From edge of Zone I to nasal edge of peripheral retina

Zone III From edge of Zone I to temporal edge of retina

Extent

Expressed as clock hours around retina

Stage

Stage 1 Demarcation line in peripheral retina

Stage 2 Ridge of tissue in peripheral retina

Stage 3 Ridge with extraretinal fibrovascular proliferation

Stage 4 Sub-total retinal detachment

Stage 5 Total retinal detachment

Plus disease

The presence of dilated veins and tortuous arterioles with vitreous clouding and poor pupil dilatation

---

NON-ACCIDENTAL INJURY

Child abuse presents with eye signs in approximately 5% of total NAI presentations. A reliable clinical history is often difficult to obtain and often the **clinical signs do not match the timing or mechanism of the injury.**

Clinical features

- **Retinal haemorrhages** (most common), usually as a consequence of **shaking.** Usually < 1 year old
- Subconjunctival haemorrhage, hyphaema and periorbital bruising
- Cataract, lens dislocation and retinal detachment are signs of long-term abuse

A common feature of shaken baby syndrome is that there is often *no* external evidence of trauma around the eyes but there may be bruising on the child's limbs or trunk from where they have been held. **Intracranial haemorrhage** is often co-existent.

Other causes of retinal haemorrhages:

- Birth trauma (normally resolved by 1 month)
- Leukaemia
- Coagulation disorders
- Tussive injury, e.g. whooping cough

PHAKOMATOSES

Group of disorders with neurological abnormalities and congenital abnormalities of the skin, retina and other organs.

Neurofibromatosis   Autosomal dominant, cutaneous neurofibromas, café au lait spots, axillary freckling, tumours of the CNS, iris nodules, glaucoma, choroidal naevi, optic nerve and orbital tumours (see p. 352)

Von Hippel–Lindau   Autosomal dominant, haemangioblastoma, phaeochromocytoma, hypernephroma, retinal angioma, hypertensive retinopathy (see p. 353)

Tuberous sclerosis   Autosomal dominant, 50% sporadic mutations, mental handicap, epilepsy, adenoma sebaceum, shagreen patches, ash leaf patches, subungual fibromas, retinal tumours, iris hypopigmentation (see p. 352)

Sturge–Weber   Cutaneous angioma over trigeminal nerve 1st and 2nd divisions, leptomeningeal angiomas with epilepsy and/or seizures, glaucoma, choroidal haemangiomas (see p. 300)

16
Haematology

- *Physiology*

- *Anaemia*

- *Haemoglobinopathies*

- *Polycythaemia and thrombocythaemia*

- *Haemostasis*

- *The spleen*

PHYSIOLOGY

HAEMOGLOBIN

A red blood cell contains about 640 million molecules of haemoglobin (Hb). Haemoglobin is composed of four polypeptide chains (normal adult Hb has two α and two β chains, $\alpha_2\beta_2$), each with a haem group.

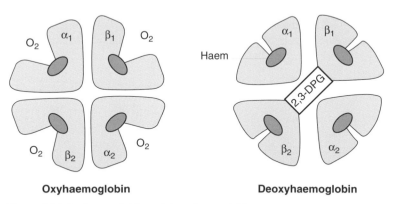

Figure 16.1 Oxyhaemoglobin and deoxyhaemoglobin

HAEMOGLOBIN FUNCTION

Haemoglobin carries oxygen from the lungs to the tissues. Each Hb molecule combines with four O_2 molecules to form oxyhaemoglobin. Deoxyhaemoglobin contains no oxygen molecules and has the metabolite 2,3-DPG in the centre, which acts to decrease its affinity to oxygen.

HAEM SYNTHESIS

This occurs in the mitochondria via a series of biochemical reactions:

Glycine + succinyl coenzyme A ⟶ Protoporphyrin
ALA (rate-limiting enzyme)   +   } → Haem
Vitamin B_6 (coenzyme)   Iron (Fe^{2+}, ferrous)

CONTROL OF ERYTHROPOIESIS

Substances necessary for erythropoeisis include:

- Hormones – erythropoietin, IL-3, stem cell factor, thyroxine and androgens
- Metals – iron, manganese, cobalt
- Vitamins – B_{12}, folate, C, E, B_6 (pyridoxine), thiamine, riboflavin, pantothenic acid
- Amino acids

ERYTHROPOIETIN

This is a hormone that regulates Hb synthesis. It is a glycosylated polypeptide made mostly in the peritubular complex of the kidney. A low O_2 tension in the kidneys stimulates erythropoietin synthesis.

Recombinant erythropoietin

This is given subcutaneously (or intravenously) three times per week. Indications include endstage renal failure, inherited haemoglobinopathies, e.g. thalassaemia, and anaemia of chronic disease. Side-effects include hypertension, high blood viscosity and, rarely, encephalopathy.

Shift to left ⟵
(increased affinity)
Acute alkalosis
Decreased temperature
pCO_2 ↓
2,3 DPG ↓
Carboxyhaemoglobin
Methaemoglobin
Abnormal haemoglobin (e.g. fetal
                                haemoglobin)
Cyanotic congenital heart disease

OXYHAEMOGLOBIN DISSOCIATION CURVE

The oxyhaemoglobin dissociation curve describes the relationship between the affinity of Hb for oxygen and the surrounding partial pressure of oxygen.

METHAEMOGLOBINAEMIA

This is a clinical state where Hb contains iron in the oxidized form (Fe^{3+}, ferric). This can be an inherited condition or result from a drug toxicity reaction oxidizing the iron (see p. 96).

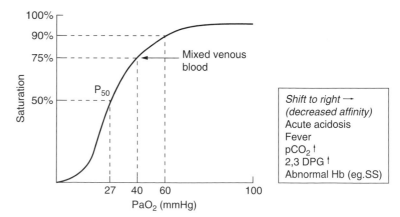

Shift to right ⟶
(decreased affinity)
Acute acidosis
Fever
pCO_2 ↑
2,3 DPG ↑
Abnormal Hb (eg.SS)

Figure 16.2 Oxyhaemoglobin dissociation curve

RED CELL METABOLISM

Red blood cells generate:

- Energy as ATP via the anaerobic Embden–Meyerhof pathway
- Reducing power as NADH via this pathway, or NADPH via the hexose–monophosphate pathway

Embden–Meyerhof (EM) pathway

Glucose
- ATP (helps RBC keep their shape)
- → Lactate
- NADH (reduces MetHb to Hb)

Hexose monophosphate (HM) pathway

Glucose-6-phosphate $\xrightarrow{\text{G6PD}}$ 6-Phosphogluconate ——→ Ribulose-5-phosphate

NADPH (maintains Fe in ferrous state)

Haemopoiesis sites			
Fetus	0–2 months	Yolk sac	
	2–7 months	Liver, spleen	
	5–9 months	Bone marrow	
Infant		Bone marrow (all bones)	
Adult		Bone marrow (vertebrae, ribs, pelvis, skull, sternum, proximal end femur)	
Extramedullary haemopoiesis is when Hb is synthesized in the liver and spleen outside fetal life.			

Haemoglobin types						
Fetal blood:	HbF	$\alpha_2\gamma_2$ (age dependent)	Adult blood:	HbA	$\alpha_2\beta_2$	(96–98%)
	HbA2	$\alpha_2\delta_2$ (age dependent)		HbA2	$\alpha_2\delta_2$	(1.5–3.2%)
				HbF	$\alpha_2\gamma_2$	(0.5–0.8%)
The switch from fetal haemoglobin (HbF) to adult haemoglobin occurs by 3–6 months of age.						

RED BLOOD CELLS

Cell	Condition
Target cells	Iron-deficiency anaemia Abnormal Hb, e.g. thalassaemia, HbSC disease ELCAT deficiency Lipid abnormalities, e.g. abetalipoproteinaemia, liver disease
Pencil cells	Iron-deficiency anaemia
Acanthocytes	Lipid abnormality, e.g. abetalipoproteinaemia, liver disease
Burr cells	Chronic renal failure
Heinz bodies*	G6PD deficiency
Basophilic tippling	Lead poisoning, thalassaemia, B_{12} deficiency
Ring sideroblasts (in bone marrow)	Sideroblastic anaemia
Howell–Jolly bodies	Post splenectomy, hyposplenism
Prickle cells	Pyruvate kinase (PK) deficiency
Red cell fragments	Microangiopathic anaemia
Bite cells	G6PD deficiency
Blister cells	G6PD deficiency
Dimorphic film	Post-transfusion B_{12}/folate + iron deficiency, e.g. coeliac disease Partially treated iron-deficiency anaemia Sideroblastic anaemia Chronic haemolysis with no folic acid

*Special stain needed.

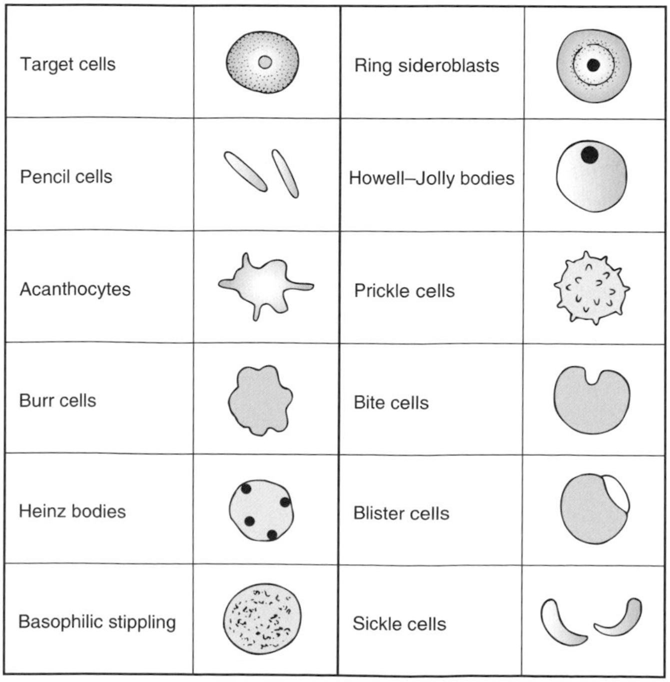

Figure 16.3 Red blood cells

ANAEMIA

Anaemia is an inadequate level of haemoglobin.

Normal ranges of Hb in childhood	
Age	Hb (g/dl)
Birth	14.9–23.7
2 weeks	13.4–19.8
2 months	9.4–13.0
6 months	11.1–14.1
1 year	11.3–14.1
2–6 years	11.5–13.5
6–18 years	11.5–16.0

Clinical features

Symptoms	Headaches, fatigue, fainting
	Breathlessness, palpitations
General signs	Pallor, faltering growth
	Tachycardia, tachpnoea, flow murmur, cardiac failure, retinal haemorrhages (if severe)
	Hydrops fetalis (*in utero*)
Specific signs	E.g. koilonychia (iron deficiency), jaundice (haemolysis) (see individual causes below)

Investigations

Full blood count	To assess degree of anaemia
Red cell indices	Size (**mean corpuscular volume [MCV]**) – normocytic, microcytic, macrocytic
	Haemoglobin content (**mean corpuscular haemoglobin [MCH]** and **mean corpuscular haemoglobin concentration [MCHC]**) – normochromic or hypochromic
Reticulocyte count	Rises within 2–3 days of a bleed. High in haemolysis
	Low count suggests marrow failure. Normal = 1.5–2%
Platelet and WCC	Low in pancytopenia
	Rise in haemolysis, haemorrhage or infection
Blood film	Red cell morphology
	Dimorphic blood film is when features of both microcytosis and macrocytosis are present
Haematinics	Iron studies, B_{12}, folate
Hb electrophoresis	If haemoglobinopathy suspected
Red cell enzymes	G6PD deficiency, pyruvate kinase deficiency
Coombs' test or DAT	Haemolytic anaemia
Membrane studies	Hereditary spherocytosis
Bone marrow	**Aspiration** – smear of bone marrow to view developing cells
	Trephine – core of bone and marrow, useful to view overall marrow architecture, cellularity and abnormal infiltrates

MICROCYTIC HYPOCHROMIC ANAEMIA

Causes

- Iron deficiency
- Thalassaemia
- Sideroblastic anaemia (congenital)
- Anaemia of chronic disease

Iron-deficiency anaemia

Iron-deficiency anaemia is very common among infants due to insufficient dietary iron. Infants have high iron requirements for their rapid growth and because they have small stores. Premature infants are particularly susceptible as they have lower iron stores and more to grow, and therefore oral iron supplements are recommended for these infants until the age of 2 years. Many formula milks contain added iron.

Iron metabolism

Iron absorption	(Maximum 3–4 mg/day) occurs in the duodenum and jejunum (as ferrous Fe^{2+}) mainly derived from cereals
	Absorbed iron is transported as transferrin (a β-globulin, with Fe^{2+}) in the plasma
Body iron	$2/3$ incorporated into Hb molecule
	$1/3$ in stores as ferritin $2/3$ or haemosiderin $1/3$ or other iron proteins. Stores are found in the RE cells of the liver, spleen and bone marrow, and in parenchymal liver cells
	Small fraction of ferritin circulates in the serum. The amount of serum ferritin is related to tissue iron stores.
Iron loss/use	Mainly in the stool (in iron-laden macrophages)
	Nail, hair and skin cell turnover
	Rapid growth periods and in pregnancy (high requirements)
	Menstruation accounts for significant losses in females

As iron can only be absorbed in the ferrous soluble form, much iron in the diet is unavailable and, as there is no physiological mechanism for excretion of iron, the control of iron balance is through absorption. Thus iron deficiency is the commonest cause of anaemia worldwide and iron overload may occur in certain situations. In iron overload, excess iron is transferred to parenchymal cells, e.g. those in the heart, pancreas, liver and endocrine organs.

Causes

- Inadequate intake – most common cause of anaemia in infants
- Malabsorption – coeliac disease
- Excess loss (bleeding) – gastrointestinal loss, e.g. hookworm, menstrual loss

Infants most at risk of inadequate iron intake:

- Premature infants (lower iron stores and more to grow)
- Inadequate solid food after 6 months of age (solid foods rich in iron provide more iron than milk), i.e. given too much milk. Seen especially in the developing world in predominantly breast-fed infants after 9–12 months of age
- Formula-fed infants (iron poorly absorbed)
- Those fed cow's milk under 1 year (iron from cow's milk is very poorly absorbed)

Factors which increase iron intake and absorption:

- Encourage breast feeding during first 6 months (iron absorbed better than from formula milk)
- If fed formula milk, use those fortified with iron

- Baby cereals contain extra iron
- Standard cow's milk not recommended below 1 year of age
- Fresh fruit and vegetables (vitamin C) enhance iron absorption by changing ferrous (predominant in vegetables) to the better absorbed ferric iron (predominant in meat)
- Food rich in iron (red meat, oily fish, dark green vegetables, beans and pulses, dried fruit and nuts)
- Avoid high-fibre foods and tannins (tea) as they decrease iron absorption

Clinical findings

- Usually asymptomatic. Discovered on incidental blood test
- General features of anaemia (see p. 390)
- Nails – brittle, ridged, spoon shaped (koilonychia)
- Mouth – angular stomatitis, painful smooth glossitis
- Gastrointestinal tract – pica (toddlers with iron deficiency), atrophic gastritis, if severe – oesophageal web
- Subtle neurological impairment in toddlers (low motor and cognitive scores and increased behavioural problems)

Specific investigations

RBC indices and film	Hypochromic, microcytic,
	Anisocytosis, target cells, pencil cells, moderately raised platelets
Serum iron	↓
Serum ferritin	↓
Total iron-binding capacity (TIBC)	↑
Free erythrocyte porphyrin (FEP)	↑
Bone marrow	No iron stores in macrophages, no siderotic granules in erythroblasts
	Small erythroblasts

Management

Investigate and treat underlying cause	Take full dietary and absorption history, do baseline investigations
	Coeliac screen if necessary
	Search for blood loss if necessary (endoscopy, colonoscopy, Meckel scan, check for hookworm, haematuria and menorrhagia)
Oral iron supplements	(Elixir or tablets):
	Ferrous sulphate (67 mg iron in 200 mg tablet)
	Ferrous gluconate (37 mg iron per 300 mg tablet)
	Dietary management if necessary
Parenteral iron	Rarely needed. It can be given IM or IV. Anaphylactic reactions can occur

Sideroblastic anaemia

This is an anaemia with hypochromic peripheral cells and increased marrow iron and **ring sideroblasts**. There is disordered haem synthesis.

Causes

Inherited	X-linked disease, mitochondrial (Pearson syndrome)
Acquired	**Primary –** myelodysplasia (RARS – refractory anaemia with ring sideroblasts)
	Secondary:
	• Malignant disease of marrow
	• Drugs, e.g. isoniazid, alcohol
	• Lead poisoning. NB: Basophilic stippling occurs
	• Other conditions, e.g. malabsorption, haemolytic anaemia

Investigations

1. Blood film. Microcytic, hypochromic, often dimorphic
2. Bone marrow. Erythroblasts with a ring of iron granules on staining with Perls' reaction

Management

- Withdraw cause
- Pyridoxine therapy (especially inherited disease) and folate therapy if deficient
- Repeated blood transfusions

Laboratory tests in hypochromic anaemias				
	Iron deficiency	**Chronic disease**	**Sideroblastic**	**Thalassaemia**
MCV, MCH,	↓	↓ or N	↓ (Congenital)	↓↓
MCHC			↑ (Acquired)	
Serum iron	↓	↓	↑	N
Serum ferritin	↓	N or ↑	↑	N or ↑
TIBC	↑	↓	N	N
Marrow iron stores	Absent	Present	↑ in nucleated RBCs (ring sideroblasts)	Present

MACROCYTIC ANAEMIA

This is divided into macrocytic and megaloblastic.

Causes

Megaloblastic anaemia	Macrocytosis
Vitamin B_{12} deficiency Folate deficiency	Newborn (fetal Hb) Reticulocytosis
DNA synthesis defects, e.g. orotic aciduria	Hypothyroidism Liver disease Pregnancy

Megaloblastic anaemia

In megaloblastic anaemia there are erythroblasts with delayed maturation of the nucleus present in the bone marrow due to defective DNA synthesis. There may also be platelet and WCC deficiencies. In children it is most commonly due to folate deficiency, and more rarely B_{12} deficiency.

Folate

Found in green vegetables, liver and kidney. Stores of 3–4 months present. Absorbed in the small intestine.

Causes of folate deficiency:

Inadequate intake	Special diets, coeliac disease, Crohn disease
Increased utilization	Physiological – prematurity, pregnancy
	Pathological:
	• Haemolysis
	• Malignant disease
	• Inflammatory disease
Increased urine loss	Acute liver disease
Antifolate drugs	Phenytoin, methotrexate, trimethoprim

Vitamin B_{12} metabolism

Found in animal produce only (liver, fish, dairy produce). Body stores of 2–3 years present.

Diet——→IF-B_{12} complex——→Absorbed in——→Plasma bound to——→Bone marrow
        (stomach)   terminal ileum   [TC I and TC II]   (TC II necessary)

IF = intrinsic factor (made by parietal cells); TC = transcobalamin (I and II).

Causes of B_{12} deficiency:

Low intake	Vegans
Impaired absorption	Ileal resection
	Bacterial overgrowth
	Crohn disease (impaired ileal mucosa), ileal TB
	Congenital intrinsic factor impairment (pernicious anaemia)
Abnormal metabolism	Nitrous oxide, transcobalamin II deficiency

Specific clinical features of megaloblastic anaemia

Mouth	Red, sore glossitis, angular stomatitis
Skin	Pale yellow (mild jaundice), purpura, melanin pigmentation (unknown mechanism)
Neuropathy	NB: This is in B_{12} deficiency only
	Polyneuropathy and subacute combined degeneration of the cord

Subacute combined degeneration of the cord:

- Progressive neuropathy of posterior and lateral columns (vibration, proprioception) of the spinal cord
- Difficulty walking, ataxia, tingling hands and feet
- Absent ankle jerks (peripheral), increased knee jerks (cord)
- Optic atrophy, retinal haemorrhage, dementia may also occur

Investigations

Blood film	Macrocytosis
	Neutrophils have hypersegmented nuclei (five or more lobes)
	WCC and platelets may be low
Bone marrow	Hypercellular marrow with megaloblastic changes
Chemistry	Unconjugated bilirubin $\uparrow$, hydroxybutyrate $\uparrow$, LDH $\uparrow$ (due to marrow cell breakdown from ineffective erythropoiesis)
Iron and ferritin	N or $\uparrow$

B_{12} and folate tests

Test	B_{12} deficiency	Folate deficiency
Serum B_{12}	↓	N
Serum folate	N, ↑	↓
Red cell folate	N, ↓	↓
Underlying cause: Dietary history, malabsorption tests and coeliac screen		

Schilling test

This is used to differentiate inadequate intake from malabsorption and pernicious anaemia. Oral radioactive-labelled cyanocobalamin is given. Absorption is measured by detecting the amount in a 24-h urine after 'flushing' it into the urine by giving a large unlabelled IM dose simultaneously, or by whole-body counting of labelled cyanocobalamin. The test is repeated with an IF preparation to see if this allows absorption to occur.

Management

- Treat underlying cause.
- Give supplements: Folate – oral supplements daily (1–5 mg)
                        B_{12} (hydroxycobalamin) regular intramuscular injections

HAEMOLYTIC ANAEMIAS

These result from an increased rate of red cell destruction. Clinical features due to the anaemia, increased requirements and increased red cell breakdown products (causing jaundice). Intravascular haemolysis causes specific features (see below). Normal RBC lifespan is 120 days.

Causes

Hereditary   Membrane – spherocytosis, elliptocytosis
              Metabolism – G6PD deficiency,* PK deficiency
              Haemoglobin – HbS, HbC, thalassaemias
Acquired   Immune:
              - Autoimmune:* Warm Ab, e.g. SLE, dermatomyositis
                            Cold Ab, e.g. CMV, mycoplasma

              - Alloimmune: Transfusion reactions*
                               Haemolytic disease of the newborn
                               Transplant, e.g. BMT, cardiac transplant
              - Drug-induced antibodies,* e.g. quinine
              Red cell fragmentation syndromes:*
              - ECMO
              - Prostheses, e.g. cardiac valves
              - Microangiopathic: HUS, TTP, DIC
                                  Meningococcal septicaemia
                                  Kassabach–Merritt syndrome
              Systemic disease, e.g. renal, liver
              Infections,* e.g. malaria
              Toxins, e.g. burns, drugs (diapsone, sulphasalazine)
              Membrane defect, e.g. paroxysmal nocturnal haemoglobinuria (PNH)*

*Denotes that intravascular haemolysis may occur.

Clinical features

- Features of anaemia (pallor, breathlessness, etc.)
- Fluctuating mild jaundice (acholuric, urobilinogen in the urine)
- Folate deficiency (due to rapid Hb turnover)
- Splenomegaly
- Pigment gallstones
- Aplastic crises precipitated by parvovirus, e.g. SS disease

Investigations

Increased RBC production	Reticulocytosis
	Erythroid hyperplasia of bone marrow
Increased RBC breakdown	Unconjugated hyperbilirubinaemia (albumin bound)
	Urine urobilinogen ↑
	Faecal stercobilinogen ↑
	No serum haptoglobins (become saturated with Hb and removed)
Damaged RBCs	Microspherocytes, elliptocytes, fragments
	Osmotic fragility ↑
	Autohaemolysis
	Shortened RBC survival (using chromium labelling)
Autoimmune tests	Coombs' test, other Abs
Red cell enzymes	G6PD deficiency, PK deficiency
Membrane studies	Hereditary spherocytosis and elliptocytosis

Intravascular haemolysis

This is destruction of the RBC within the circulation. The particular features are:

- Haemoglobinaemia, haemoglobinuria
- Haemosiderinuria (from breakdown of Hb in renal tubules)
- Methaemoglobinaemia
- Red cell fragments

Hereditary spherocytosis (HS)

Autosomal dominant, variable expression. Spherical RBCs, i.e. not biconcave discs, due to a defect in a membrane protein (spectrin, ankyrin or band 3). Their shape results in the cells being unable to pass through the splenic micro-circulation, so they die prematurely.

Associations   Northern Europeans (incidence 1:3000)

Clinical manifestations (very variable even within families)

- Neonatal jaundice
- Symptoms of mild haemolytic anaemia as above, particularly: Splenomegaly
  Pigment gallstones, leg ulcers
  Aplastic or anaemic crises especially with parvovirus
- May be asymptomatic

Investigations

Blood	Anaemia (may be mild)
Film	Reticulocyte counts of 5–20%
	Microspherocytes

Membrane studies	Defect in membrane protein
Others	Autohaemolysis ↑

Management

Splenectomy after childhood if severe anaemia requiring transfusion or impaired growth. Folic acid supplements. No treatment if mild.

Hereditary elliptocytosis

Autosomal dominant.

Similar to spherocytosis. Cells are elliptical and the clinical features milder.

Glucose-6-phosphate dehydrogenase deficiency (G6PD deficiency)

X-linked recessive. Females may be mildly affected. NB: Carrier state protects against *Falciparum malariae*. Millions affected worldwide.

G6PD is an enzyme involved in the hexose–monophosphate pathway (see p. 388), and is the only source of NADPH for a red blood cell, which prevents oxidant damage to the cell. Defective activity of the enzyme results in a susceptibility of the RBC to acute haemolysis with oxidant stress.

There are several types, the commonest being:

- Type A, African type – milder, young RBCs have normal enzyme activity
- Type B, Mediterranean type – severe, all RBCs affected

Clinical features

- Neonatal jaundice
- Haemolytic crises (rapidly developing intravascular haemolysis) induced by oxidant stress, including:
  Sepsis
  Drugs, e.g. antimalarials (primaquine, chloroquine, fansidar, maloprim), sulphonamides (co-trimoxazole), chloramphenicol, naphthalene (moth balls)
  Fava beans (type B only).

Investigations

Diagnosis	G6PD levels in RBC. NB: These may be normal during a crisis
During a crisis	Intravascular haemolysis, bite cells, blister cells, Heinz bodies, reticulocytes
	NB: *No* spherocytes
	(Hb normal between attacks)

Management of a crisis

- Treat the cause (sepsis, stop suspected drug)
- High fluid input (IV)
- Transfusions as required

Pyruvate kinase deficiency (PKD)

Autosomal recessive. Prevalence: thousands worldwide

Pyruvate kinase is an enzyme involved in the Embden–Meyerhof pathway. Deficiency results in a reduction in ATP formation and rigid RBCs.

Clinical features

- Anaemia (Hb 4–10 g/dl) with relatively mild symptoms due to compensatory increased 2,3-DPG levels
- Splenomegaly, jaundice, gallstones, frontal bossing

Investigations

Diagnosis	Direct assay of PK levels
Blood film	Prickle cells, poikilocytes, reticulocytes
Blood	Features of autohaemolysis

Management

- Repeated transfusions
- Splenectomy if necessary

Autoimmune haemolytic anaemias (AIHA)

These occur as a result of autoantibody production. They are divided into 'warm' and 'cold' types, depending on the temperature at which the antibody reacts better with the red cells. They all have a positive direct antiglobulin test (DAT, Coombs' test).

	Cold AIHA	Warm AIHA
Type of Ab IgG	IgM	IgG
Best temperature for attachment of Ab to RBC	4°C	37°C
Causes	Idiopathic Infections: EBV, CMV Mycoplasma Lymphomas Paroxysmal cold haemoglobinuria (NB: IgG Ab)	Idiopathic Autoimmune: SLE, RhA Lymphomas CLL Methyldopa
Clinical features	Haemolytic anaemia Splenomegaly Acrocyanosis (blue peripheries)	Haemolytic anaemia Splenomegaly **Evans syndrome =** warm AIHA and ITP ± neutropenia
Investigations	Those of haemolytic anaemia Less spherocytosis Positive Coombs' test	Those of haemolytic anaemia Spherocytosis in peripheral blood Positive Coombs' test
Management options	Remove cause Keep warm Alkylating agents may help	Remove cause Steroids (high dose initially) Splenectomy (if poor response to steroids) Immunosuppression, e.g. azathioprine, cyclophosphamide Folic acid and blood transfusions as necessary High-dose immunoglobulin

Red cell fragmentation syndromes

These result from physical damage to red cells from:

- Abnormal surfaces, e.g. artificial heart valves or grafts
- Microangiopathic anaemia when red cells pass through:
  Fibrin strands in small vessels during DIC
  Damaged vessels in HUS, TTP or meningococcal sepsis

Investigations as listed above (for intravascular haemolysis).

Paroxysmal nocturnal haemoglobinaemia (PNH)

Acquired defect of red cells making them susceptible to destruction by complement. Platelets and WBCs may also be affected.

Clinical features

- Haemolysis
- Dark urine (haemosiderinuria, haemoglobinuria)
- Thrombosis

Specific investigations

Ham's test – red cell lysis occurs at low pH (due to complement activation at low pH).

Management

- Supportive only
- Consider anticoagulation
- Development into leukaemia or aplastic anaemia may occur

APLASTIC ANAEMIAS

Aplastic anaemia is due to bone marrow aplasia, causing a pancytopenia (anaemia, leucopenia and thrombocytopenia).

Causes

Primary	Congenital:	Fanconi anaemia
		Dyskeratosis congenita
	Idiopathic (most cases)	
Secondary	Drugs:	Regular effect, e.g. cytotoxics
		Sporadic effect, e.g. chloramphenicol, azathioprine, penicillamine
	Infection – viral hepatitis, measles, EBV, parvovirus,TB	
	Radiation	
	Pregnancy	

Clinical features

Those of bone marrow suppression.

Investigations

Blood film	Anaemia (normocytic, normochromic or macrocytic, low reticulocytes)
	Leucopenia (particularly neutrophils)
	Thrombocytopenia
Bone marrow	Trephine biopsy (hypoplasia with replacement with fat cells)

Management

- Remove any cause
- Initial supportive therapy (blood and platelet transfusions, antibiotics for infections)
- Specific therapy options: Stem cell transplant can offer a cure
                                Drugs, e.g. haemopoietic growth factors, methylprednisolone, immunosuppressants
                                (e.g. antilymphocyte globulin and cyclosporin)

Fanconi anaemia

Autosomal recessive. Presentation at 5–10 years.

Clinical features

- Aplastic anaemia (developing during childhood)
- Growth retardation
- Absent radii or thumbs, microcephaly
- Pelvic or horseshoe kidney
- Mental retardation (25%)
- Café-au-lait patches, hypopigmented macules
- Increased chromosomal breakages, with AML often developing

Management

Stem cell transplant is the only chance of cure (androgen therapy delays progression of disease).

Prognosis

Without SCT, most die from bone marrow failure or AML at < 30 years.

RED CELL APLASIA

This is an isolated anaemia due to reduced or absent erythroblasts in the bone marrow. It may be an acute, transient disease lasting 2–3 months, or a chronic problem.

Causes

Chronic disease

Congenital	Diamond–Blackfan syndrome
Acquired	Idiopathic
	Thymoma, SLE, leukaemia

Acute disease

Infections	Parvovirus infection in patients with shortened red cell survival, e.g. SS, spherocytosis
	Infants following viral infection (transient erythroblastopenia of infancy)
Drugs	E.g. azathioprine, co-trimoxazole

Management

- Supportive therapy with regular transfusions and iron chelation
- Specific treatments include steroid therapy and growth factors
- BMT rarely needed

Diamond–Blackfan syndrome

- A pure red cell aplasia, presenting with profound anaemia by 2–6 months of age. Other congenital anomalies, e.g. dysmorphic facies, triphalangeal thumbs, in 30%. Autosomal recessive
- Blood film shows a macrocytic anaemia, young red cell population and reduced reticulocytes. Thrombocytosis and neutropenia may be present initially. Bone marrow shows reduced erythrocyte precursors
- Treatment is with steroids and transfusions as necessary. If steroid unresponsive, immunosuppression, androgens and stem cell transplant may be tried

HAEMOGLOBINOPATHIES

SICKLE CELL HAEMOGLOBINOPATHIES

These involve synthesis of an abnormal haemoglobin. Sickle haemoglobin (HbS) = Hb $\alpha_2\beta^S_2$ (in the β chain, valine is substituted for glutamic acid on codon 6).

HbS is insoluble at low O_2 tensions and polymerizes as long fibres, resulting in the red cells becoming sickle shaped. The sickle cells block areas of the microcirculation and result in microinfarcts. HbS also releases O_2 in the tissues more readily than HbA, i.e. the oxyhaemoglobin dissociation curve shifted to the right.

Sickle cell anaemia	HbSS (homozygous disease) 85–95% HbS, 5–15% HhF, no HbA
Sickle cell trait	HbSA (heterozygous disease) 40% HbS, 60% HbA

Sickle cell anaemia

HbSS disease, seen in Africans, Mediterraneans and Indians.

Clinical features

Clinical features vary depending on any co-existing haemoglobinopathies, e.g. HbSS + β-thalassaemia is mild.

The clinical features are due to:

- Anaemia – severe haemolytic, and
- Intermittent crises

Sickle crises

Painful (vascular-occlusive) crises	Vascular-occlusive episodes precipitated by cold, hypoxia, infection or dehydration. They occur in: • Bone (commonest) • Chest (**sickle chest syndrome**) • Dactylitis (hand–foot syndrome) (digital infarcts, usually in small children, resulting in fingers and toes of differing lengths) • Cerebral (strokes) • Spleen (results in autosplenectomy usually by age 5 years) • Also kidney, liver, heart
Haemolytic crises	Haemolysis, usually accompanying a painful crisis
Acute sequestration	Sickling within organs with blood pooling Occur in the spleen, chest and liver
Aplastic crises	Sudden fall in Hb and reticulocytes Occur with parvovirus B19 infection

Infection

Increased risk of infection with encapsulated bacteria, especially *Streptococcus pneumoniae*, *Haemophilus influenzae* B, meningococcus and salmonella. At risk of overwhelming infection (meningitis, pneumonia, septicaemia), particularly < 3 years of age.

Long-term problems

- Faltering growth (due to chronic disease)
- Pigment gallstones (due to haemolysis)
- Salmonella osteomyelitis
- Asceptic necrosis of the hip
- Priapism (pooling of blood within the corpora cavernosa)
- Renal failure
- Congestive heart failure
- Proliferative retinopathy
- Leg ulcers
- Splenomegaly in infancy with autosplenectomy (due to splenic crises) later

Investigations

Blood film	Hb 6–8 g/dl
	Sickle cells, target cells, Howell–Jolly bodies
Sickledex test	HbS blood sickles when deoxygenated with dithionate and Na_2HPO_4
Hb electrophoresis	To detect relative quantities of HbS, HbF and HbA

Management

General	Folic acid 5 mg daily
	Oral penicillin daily (because of autosplenectomy)
	Triple vaccination (pneumococcal, Hib and meningovax) essential (splenic protection)
	Regular influenzae vaccination
	Avoid crisis precipitants
Crises	Admit to hospital
	Check FBC, film, reticulocytes, group and save, U&Es, LFTs
	CXR if respiratory symptoms/signs, ECG if chest pain
	MSU and blood cultures if infection suspected
	Analgesia (strong, usually IV opiates)
	Fluids (IV, 50% above usual formula)
	Bed rest and keep warm
	Monitor closely (saturations, pulse, BP, respiratory rate, pain and nausea)
	IV antibiotics if infection present or suspected
	Transfusion if necessary (multiple may be needed)
	Exchange transfusion if indicated (severe painful crises, neurological damage, sequestration, sickle chest syndrome, priapism)
Surgery	Transfusions are performed preoperatively for major surgery to reduce HbS fraction to < 30%
	Anaesthetic care is taken to keep patient warm, well oxygenated and hydrated, and avoid acidosis, and pain free
New therapies	Stem cell transplant (if unaffected HLA-identical sibling and severe disease)
	Hydroxyurea (may increase HbF and decrease frequency of crises)

Sickle trait

Heterozygous expression of the sickle Hb gene (HbSA). HbS makes up 30–40% of the haemoglobin. This blood type appears to protect against *Falciparum malariae*, and is thus genetically selected for.

Clinical course is usually benign with no anaemia. In severe hypoxia, sickling can occur, with resulting ischaemic consequences. Haematuria is the commonest symptom. Care is needed with general anaesthetics and pregnancy.

Diagnosis by Sickledex test and Hb electrophoresis.

HAEMOGLOBIN C

In HbC, lysine replaces glutamic acid on codon 6 on the β chain.

Heterozygous state (HbAC)	No anaemia, target cells
Homozygous state (HbCC)	Haemolytic anaemia, splenomegaly, target cells
HbSC disease (HbS and HbC genes)	Hb 9–10 g/dl, target cells
	Less severe than HbSS
	Thrombosis, pulmonary embolism and retinal vascular changes
	Large spleen

THALASSAEMIAS

These are a heterogeneous group of disorders in which there is a partial or complete deletion of globin chain genes, resulting in a *reduced rate* of synthesis of normal α- or β-chains and *precipitation* of the other excess chains in the red cells which causes **haemolysis**. Other Hb types, e.g. HbA2, are also made with increased frequency.

Thalassaemia comes from the Greek '*thalassa*' meaning 'sea', as the disease was found in people on the shores of the Mediterranean. It is found in tropical and subtropical areas (Asia, N. Africa and the Mediterranean).

β-thalassaemia   Due to reduced or absent β-globin chains (excess α-chains precipitate)

α-thalassaemia   Due to reduced or absent α-globin chains (excess β-chains precipitate)

Chromosome 16 codes for α-globin. Chromosome 11 codes for β, δ and γ-globins.

In α-thalassaemias whole α-globin genes are deleted, whereas in β-thalassaemia mainly point mutations within the β-globin genes occur (> 100 mutations have been identified)

Diagnosis

Suspicion of thalassaemia may be made clinically and is confirmed by the blood film. Specific identification of the type of thalassaemia is made from Hb electrophoresis and DNA analysis:

- α-Thalassaemias
- β-Thalassaemia major
- Thalassaemia intermedia
- Thalassaemia minor

Haemoglobin types seen in thalassaemias	
HbA	$\alpha_2 \beta_2$
HbA2	$\alpha_2 \delta_2$
HbF	$\alpha_2 \gamma_2$
HbH	β_4
HbBarts	γ_4 (no oxygen carrying ability)

β-Thalassaemia major

Homozygous disease. Affected children have either no (β°) or very small amounts (β⁺) of β-chains.

Haemoglobin electrophoresis	HbF 70–90%
	HbA2 2%
	± HbA 0–20%

Clinical features

The clinical features are a result of:

- **Haemolytic anaemia**
- Attempt by the body to make more Hb (**medullary and extramedullary haemopoesis**) and the effects of multiple transfusions (**iron overload**, **infections**)

Severe anaemia from 3–6 months	When switch from γ to β-chain production normally occurs
Hepatosplenomegaly	Due to haemolysis and haemopoiesis
Extramedullary and	Thalassaemic facies (frontal bossing, maxillary hyperplasia)
medullary haemopoiesis	'Hair on end' skull X-ray appearance
	Cortical thinning with fractures
Iron overload	See below. Due to multiple transfusions
Infections	Hepatitis B and C (multiple blood transfusions)
	Yersinia enterocolytica (seen with desferrioxamine therapy)
	Encapsulated organisms (autosplenectomy)
Faltering growth	

Investigations

Blood film	Microcytic hypochromic anaemia
	Target cells, basophilic stippling, nucleated red cells
Hb electrophoresis	As above
DNA analysis	May be used to identify the mutation

Management

Transfusions	4–6 weekly (transfuse when Hb ≤ 10 g/dl; this is 'hypertransfusion')
Folic acid	5 mg daily
Iron chelation	Subcutaneous desferrioxamine for 8–12 h, overnight, 5 days per week. Chelated iron is excreted in the urine and stools
	NB: Auditory and ophthalmological assessments needed while on desferrioxamine
Vitamin C	200 mg/day. Increases iron excretion
Splenectomy	May be needed to decrease blood requirements (usually done only if > 6 years old)
Endocrine therapy	As necessary (insulin, thyroid, parathyroid and pituitary hormones)
Stem cell transplant	Recommended in childhood if unaffected HLA-identical sibling is present

Effects of iron overload	
Liver	Cirrhosis, hepatoma
Heart	Cardiomyopathy (arrhythmias, cardiac failure)
Endocrine	IDDM, growth failure, delayed puberty, hypothyroidism, hypoparathyroidism, osteoporosis
Skin	'Slate-grey' appearance

β-Thalassaemia minor (trait)

Heterozygous disease with reduced β-chains.

Clinical features	Asymptomatic, picked up as incidental finding
Blood film	Mild or no anaemia (Hb 10–15 g/dl)
	Microcytic, hypochromic picture, target cells
Hb electrophoresis	HbA
	HbA2 > 3.5%
	HbF 1–3%

NB: It is important to check iron status to exclude **iron deficiency**.

Thalassaemia intermedia

This is a clinical syndrome, resulting from several different gene defects:

- Homozygous β-thalassaemia with persisting HbF
- Homozygous β-thalassaemia with coexisting α-thalassaemia
- Heterozygous β-thalassaemia (trait) with coexisting extra α-chains

Clinical features

Variable.

- Symptomatic anaemia (Hb 7–10 mg/dl)
- Splenomegaly, hepatomegaly, extramedullary haemopoiesis, infections, leg ulcers, gallstones

Management

- Transfusions may be required
- Hydroxyurea
- Splenectomy if necessary

α-Thalassaemias

These all involve decreased synthesis of α-chains. There are *four* genes for α-globin because the gene is duplicated on chromosome 16. Deletion of one α-globin gene results in a silent carrier with only a mild microcytosis (α-thalassaemia trait).

Disease	α-Globin genes deleted	Hb electrophoresis	Blood film
α-thalassaemia trait	1 or 2 α-/αα α-/α- αα/--	Normal ± HbH	Hypochromic, microcytic cells ± mild anaemia
HbH disease	3 --/α-	HbH, HbA, Hb Barts	Hypochromic, microcytic anaemia Golf ball cells
Hydrops fetalis (Hb Barts)	4 --/--	Hb Barts only	

α-Thalassaemia trait

One or two α-globin genes are deleted. Asymptomatic.

Hb electrophoresis   Normal ± HbH

Blood film	No/mild anaemia, hypochromic, microcytic cells
Globin chain synthesis studies	α:β-chain synthesis ratio is reduced
DNA studies	

HbH disease

Three α-globin genes are deleted.

Hb electrophoresis	HbH, HbA, Hb Barts (in fetus)
Blood film	Microcytic, hypochromic anaemia (Hb 7–10 g/dl)
	'Golf ball' cells (aggregates of β-globin chains)
Splenomegaly	Thalassaemia intermedia syndrome

No treatment required.

Hydrops fetalis (Hb Barts)

No α-chains (four genes deleted).

Hb electrophoresis	Hb Barts (γ4)
	No HbF

Death occurs *in utero* due to lack of HbF, unless there is early prenatal diagnosis and intrauterine transfusions.

ANTENATAL AND NEONATAL DIAGNOSIS OF SICKLE CELL AND THALASSAEMIA

Antenatal diagnosis	Chorionic villous sampling (first trimester) (8–10 weeks) ⎫ Fetal DNA analysis
	Amniotic fluid (second trimester) ⎭
	Fetal blood sampling – umbilical cord blood in second trimester (18–20 weeks) to check normal chain manufacture (electrophoresis)
Neonatal diagnosis	Hb electrophoresis can be done at birth but the switch from γ-chains (HbF) to β-chains occurs at 3–6 months, making testing at 6 months accurate. DNA analysis can be used to identify the defect on each allele

POLYCYTHAEMIA AND THROMBOCYTHAEMIA

POLYCYTHAEMIA

Polycythaemia is an increased **Hb level** to above the upper limit of normal and increased **haematocrit**. It may be 'relative', due to decreased circulating volume.

Causes

Secondary	Appropriate:	Cyanotic heart disease
		Lung disease
		Central hypoventilation
		High altitude
	Inappropriate:	Renal disease, e.g. hydronephrosis, cysts, tumour
		Adrenal disease, e.g. CAH, Cushing syndrome
		Tumour, e.g. cerebellar haemangioblastoma
		Neonatal, e.g. infant of diabetic mother, IUGR, twin–twin transfusion
Relative	Dehydration, e.g. gastrointestinal losses, burns	
	Stress polycythaemia	
Primary	Polycythaemia rubra vera (PV) (very rare in children)	

Clinical features

- Haemorrhage or thrombosis
- Headaches

Management

- Treat cause
- Venesection if necessary

THROMBOCYTHAEMIA

Thrombocythaemia is increased **platelet levels** to above upper limit of normal.

Causes

Reactive	Haemorrhage
	Postoperative
	Kawasaki disease
	Acute infection, e.g. URTI
	Chronic infections, e.g. TB
	Postsplenectomy
	Iron-deficiency and haemolytic anaemia
	Connective tissue disease
	Chronic renal disease
	Drugs, e.g. steroids
	Malignancies
Endogenous	CML (very rare in childhood)

Clinical features

Usually asymptomatic; risk of thrombosis is low.

Management

Often no treatment is required. To reduce the risk of thrombosis, platelet pheresis, low-dose aspirin or anagrelide (antiplatelet drug) may be used.

HAEMOSTASIS

Haemostasis involves:

- Normal vasculature
- Platelets
- Coagulation factors

PLATELETS

Produced from megakaryocytes in the bone marrow, lifespan 7–10 days.

Functions

Mechanical plug formation in vascular trauma. This involves adhesion (vWF involved), secretion of granule contents (including arachidonic acid), aggregation and procoagulant activity (involving PF3 and coagulation factors).

BLOOD COAGULATION CASCADE

This involves activation of the blood coagulation factors, resulting in production of thrombin and a fibrin clot. Fibrin stabilizes the initial platelet plug.

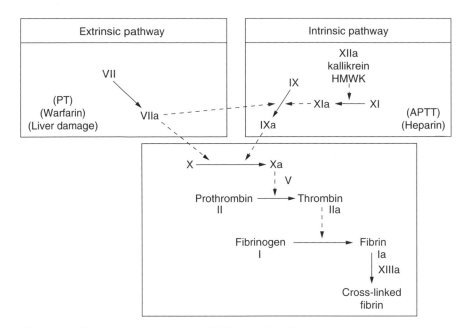

Figure 16.4 Blood coagulation cascade: HMWK = High molecular weight kininogen

INVESTIGATIONS OF CLOTTING DISORDERS

Blood count and film	Platelets (morphology and count). Abnormalities of other blood cells
Bleeding time	Measures platelet plug formation *in vivo* Prolonged in thrombocytopenia and platelet function disorders and von Willebrand disease
Prothrombin time (PT)	Measures factors VII, X, V, prothrombin and fibrinogen (extrinsic and common pathways). Tissue thromboplastin and calcium added to sample Normal = 10–14 s (INR = 1) May be expressed as international normalized ratio (INR) Prolonged in liver disease, vitamin K-dependent clotting factors Used to monitor warfarin therapy
Activated partial thromboplastin time (APTT)	Measures factors V, VIII, IX, X, XI, XII, prothrombin and fibrinogen (intrinsic and common pathways) Surface activator, phospholipid and calcium added Normal = 30–40 s Used to monitor heparin therapy

Thrombin clotting time (TT)	Abnormal in fibrinogen deficiency or thrombin inhibition Thrombin added to sample. Normal = 14–16 s

NB: Prolonged PT or APTT due to factor deficiency are corrected when normal plasma is added.
If correction is incomplete with normal plasma, then an **inhibitor of coagulation** may be present,
e.g. lupus anticoagulant.

Coagulation factors	Specific assays of individual clotting factors
Fibrinolysis tests	Detection of fibrinogen or fibrin degradation products (FDPs). Plasminogen ($\downarrow$ in enhanced fibrinolysis) and plasminogen activator ($\uparrow$)

DISORDERS OF THE VASCULATURE

These involve abnormalities in the vessels or the perivascular connective tissues.

Causes

Inherited	Connective tissue disorders, e.g. Ehlers–Danlos syndrome Hereditary haemorrhagic telangiectasia
Acquired	Easy bruising syndrome Henoch–Schönlein purpura (HSP) Infections, e.g. meningitis Scurvy Drugs, e.g. steroids

Clinical features

Features generally mild. Skin and mucous membrane bleeding (easy bruising, petechiae, ecchymoses).

Investigations

Screening tests all normal (including the bleeding time).

Hereditary haemorrhagic telangiectasia

Autosomal dominant. Telangiectasia in the skin, mucous membranes and internal organs, becoming more numerous throughout life. Recurrent GI bleeding occurs.

PLATELET DISORDERS

These include **thrombocytopenia** and **platelet function disorders**.

Thrombocytopenia

Causes

Decreased production	Isolated megakaryocyte depression:	Infections Drugs Thrombocytopenia and absent radii (TAR) syndrome
	Abnormal megakaryocytes – Wiskott–Aldrich syndrome	
	Bone marrow failure – aplastic anaemias	

Increased consumption	Immune disease:	ITP
		Drug induced, e.g. trimethoprim, quinine, heparin
		Post-infectious, e.g. malaria
		Neonatal isoimmune ITP (maternal antiplatelet antibodies)
		Post-transfusional (Pl^{A1} antibodies)
		SLE
		DIC
		HUS, TTP
Abnormal distribution	Splenomegaly	

Immune thrombocytopenia (ITP, idiopathic thrombocytopenic purpura)

Common in children. Thought to be due to immune complex platelet destruction.

Clinical features

1–4 weeks post-infection, e.g. chicken pox, measles, EBV, or vaccination: bleeding, bruising, petechiae, mucosal bleeding (if platelets < 20 x10^9/L). Intracranial bleeds (very rare).

Investigations

Blood film	Platelets ↓ (< 10–20 × 10^9/L)
	Hb and WCC normal
Bone marrow	Megakaryocytes ↑ or N
Antibodies	Antiplatelet IgG, antiplatelet IgM

Management options

- Monitoring only (clinically and platelet count)
- Oral steroids for 2–3 weeks
- Intravenous immunoglobulin (IVIG)
- Platelet transfusions (in emergency, as they are quickly destroyed)
- Immunosuppression and/or splenectomy only if no response to above treatments and chronic disease
- Avoid aspirin and contact sports.

Prognosis

| *Spontaneous remission* | Most cases |
| *Chronic disease* | 5–10% in childhood (commoner in adults) |

Thrombotic thrombocytopenic purpura (TTP)

This is a serious disease involving thrombocytopenia with arteriolar thrombi. Features are similar to HUS, with more widespread involvement.

Clinical features

A classic pentad of:

1. Fevers
2. Haemolytic anaemia
3. Thrombocytopenia – purpura
4. CNS – fluctuating neurological signs
5. Renal – ischaemic damage

Investigations

Blood film   Platelets ↓
                  Microangiopathic anaemia
Serum   LDH ↑

Management options

- Plasmapheresis, FFP
- Steroids, cytotoxics, antiplatelet drugs

Thrombocytopenia absent radius (TAR) syndrome

This involves:

- Thrombocytopenia, megakaryocytes ↓, anaemia, eosinophilia
- Bilateral absent radii and thumbs, abnormal humerus and ulnar
- Leg involvement (50%) – CDH, patella and knee dislocations, small feet, tibial torsion
- Other associations – CHD, renal abnormalities, mental retardation, spina bifida, 100% have cow's milk protein intolerance

Platelet function disorders

Causes

Hereditary   Bernard–Soulier syndrome
             Glanzmann disease
             Grey platelet syndrome
             Hermansky–Pudlak syndrome (platelet function albinism)

Acquired   Drugs: aspirin (cyclo-oxygenase inhibition), heparin (inhibits segregation and secretion)
             Myeloproliferative disorders
             Uraemia

Investigations

Blood film   Normal platelet count
Bleeding time Prolonged
Specific tests   Platelet aggregation studies with ADP, adrenaline, collagen, ristocetin
             Other tests, e.g. adhesion studies, nucleotide pool measurement
             von Willebrand factor assay
             Factor VIII assay

Bernard–Soulier syndrome

- Autosomal recessive, deficiency of membrane glycoprotein Ib
- Platelet adhesion defects (no aggregation with ristocetin)
- Large platelets with some thrombocytopenia

Glanzmann disease

Autosomal recessive, failure of platelet aggregation due to deficiency of membrane glycoproteins IIb and IIIa.

CLOTTING FACTOR DISORDERS

Haemophilia A

- Incidence 30–100:1 000 000
- X-linked recessive, 30% spontaneous mutation rate
- Gene located at Xq2.8
- Disease due to absent or low factor VIII

Clinical features

Spontaneous bleeding	Joints (haemarthroses), painful and swollen, resulting in deformity (arthritis) unless rapidly treated
	Muscle haematomas
	'Pseudotumours' in bones (due to subperiosteal bleeds)
	Haematuria
	Intracerebral bleeds (rare)
Excessive traumatic bleeding	Surgery, e.g. post-circumcision, dental extractions
Infection (transfusion related)	Hepatitis B and C (subclinical liver disease), HIV (now all screened for)

Severity varies dependent on the level of factor VIII (% of normal) present:

< 1% of normal	Severe disease. Frequent spontaneous bleeds
1–5% of normal	Moderate disease. Severe bleeds with injury, occasional spontaneous bleeds
> 5% of normal	Mild disease. Bleed a lot after surgery

Investigations

- Factor VIIIc activity ($\downarrow$ or absent)
- APTT $\uparrow$

Management

- Prophylactic recombinant factor VIII infusions – aim to keep > 2% of normal, usually given 2–3 times per week
- Recombinant factor VIII infusions after injury or prior to surgery:

Injury	Factor VIII levels aimed for (% of normal)
Minor bleed	> 30%
Severe bleed	> 50%
Pre major surgery	100%

- Desmopressin (DDAVP) infusion – used in mild disease. Causes a rise in the patient's own factor VIII levels
- Fibrinolytic inhibitor, e.g. tranexamic acid. May be given with DDAVP
- Advice – avoid contact sports, maintain good oral hygiene

Factor VIII antibodies

These develop in 10% of haemophiliacs as a result of frequent factor VIII transfusions. They inhibit future factor VIII treatment. Management options include:

- Give very large doses of factor VIII
- Immunosuppression
- Give factor IX concentrate, which bypasses the factor VIII, recombinant factor VIII or porcine factor VIII

Carrier female detection	Analyse plasma factor VIII activity (usually half normal in carrier female)
	DNA analysis (more accurate)
Antenatal screening	Chorionic villous sampling (8–10 weeks)
	Fetal blood sampling for factor VIII activity (18–20 weeks)

Haemophilia B (Christmas disease)

- Incidence 1:30 000 males
- X-linked recessive, gene at Xq2.6
- Due to deficiency of factor IX
- Clinical features identical to haemophilia A
- Management is with infusions of factor IX concentrate

von Willebrand disease

Incidence 3–10:100 000. Autosomal dominant, variable expression, worse in females.

Disorder of:

- Low vWF (causing low factor VIII activity)
- Platelet adhesion abnormalities

von Willebrand factor (vWF) is the carrier protein for factor VIII and promotes platelet adhesion.

Clinical features

These are variable.

Excessive traumatic bleeding	From cuts, operative, mucous membranes (epistaxis, gums, menorrhagia)
Spontaneous bleeds	Haemarthroses and muscle bleeds (both rare except in homozygotes)

Investigations

Bleeding time	Prolonged
Factor VIIIc activity	↓
vWF levels	↓
Platelet aggregation with ristocetin	↓

Management

Acute bleeds treated with factor VIII concentrate containing vWF in severe disease, and DDAVP or fibrinolytic inhibitors in milder disease.

Vitamin K deficiency

Vitamin K is a fat-soluble vitamin, present in green vegetables and synthesized in the gut. Deficiency affects the vitamin K-dependent clotting factors **II**, **VII**, **IX** and **X**.

Causes of vitamin K-dependent clotting factor deficiency

Low vitamin K stores	Haemorrhagic disease of the newborn (see p. 455)
	Inadequate diet
Malabsorption of fat-soluble vitamins	Cystic fibrosis
	Small bowel disease, e.g. coeliac disease
	Hepatic obstruction
Vitamin K antagonists	Phenytoin, rifampicin, warfarin

Investigations

PT   ↑↑
APTT   ↑ or N

Management

Vitamin K	IV (takes 6 h to work)
	IM or oral (as prophylaxis)
Fresh frozen plasma (FFP)	Immediate effect
Prothrombin concentrates	Immediate effect

Disseminated intravascular coagulation (DIC)

This is a state of consumption of platelets and clotting factors with widespread intravascular fibrin deposition due to uncontrolled activation of the clotting cascade. It may be acute or more rarely chronic.

Causes

Sepsis	Meningococcal, Gram-negative, viral (purpura fulminans)
Widespread tissue damage	Trauma, burns, surgery
Hypersensitivity reactions	Anaphylaxis
Malignancy	Acute promyelocytic leukaemia
Other	Hypoxia, hypothermia, snake venom, Kasabach–Merritt syndrome

Clinical features

Severely unwell patient with generalized bleeding (acute disease).

Investigations

Blood count and film	Platelets (↓), microangiopathic anaemia
TT	↑
APTT	↑
PT	↑
FDPs	↑, fibrinogen ↓
Factors	V and VIII (↓)

NB: Chronic disease may have normal screening results, due to production of new factors.

Management

1. Treat the underlying cause
2. Supportive therapy (blood, FFP, fibrinogen, platelets)

Haemostasis tests								
	BT	Plts	PT	APTT	TT	FVIIIc	FIX	vWFAg
Haemophilia A	N	N	N	↑	N	↓	N	N
Haemophilia B	N	N	N	↑	N	N	↓	N
vW disease	↑	N	N	↑ or N	N	↓	N	↓
Liver disease	N, ↑	↓	↑	↑	N, ↑	N	↓	N
DIC	N, ↑	↓	↑	↑	↑↑	↓	↓	↓
APTT, activated partial thromboplastin time; BT, bleeding time; Plts, platelets; PT, prothrombin time; TT, thromboplastin time								

THROMBOSIS

Pathogenesis of thrombosis is related to Virchow's triad of:

1. Hypercoagulability
2. Intravascular stasis
3. Vessel wall damage: Arterial thrombosis occurs mainly as a result of vessel wall damage, e.g. arteriosclerosis
   Venous thrombosis occurs mainly as a result of hypercoagulability and venous stasis

Causes of venous thrombosis

Hypercoagulability	Congenital:	Antithrombin III deficiency (involved in inhibition of thrombin and factor X)
		Protein C deficiency (protein C inactivates factors V and VIII and stimulates fibrinolysis)
		Protein S deficiency (a co-factor for protein C)
		Factor V Leiden (abnormal factor V protein)
		Increased fibrinogen or factor VIII levels
		Abnormal plasminogen or fibrinogen
	Acquired:	Thrombocytosis
		Trauma
		Lupus anticoagulant
		Pregnancy and OCP
		Malignancy
Intravascular stasis	Dehydration	
	Immobilization	
	Venous obstruction	
	Pump failure	

Investigations

These may include:

Blood count and film	Platelets ($\uparrow$), haematocrit ($\uparrow$), malignancy
PT, APTT	May be shortened. NB: If prolonged and does not correct with normal plasma, suggests lupus anticoagulant
TT, reptilase time	Prolonged if fibrinogen abnormal
Fibrinogen assay	
Protein S and C assay	
Antithrombin III assay	
Factor V Leiden (PCR)	

THE SPLEEN

SPLENECTOMY

This may occur naturally (autosplenectomy, e.g. sickle cell anaemia) or as a result of therapeutic surgical therapy, e.g. ITP, or secondary to trauma.

The consequences are:

| *Immediate* | Marked thrombocytosis (platelets > 1000 x 10^9/L), usually for 2–3 weeks, then moderate increase |
| *Long-term* | Susceptibility to encapsulated organisms, e.g. pneumococcus, and malaria infection. Young infants at particular risk of infection with *Streptococcus pneumoniae*, *Haemophilus influenzae* and *Niesseria meningitides* |

Blood count and film findings in hyposplenism

- Platelets may be high
- Monocytosis, lymphocytosis
- Howell–Jolly bodies, Pappenheimer granules, target cells, irregular contracted red cells

Management

- Try to avoid splenectomy in children < 6 years (increased susceptibility to infections)
- Prophylactic penicillin for life
- Triple vaccination > 2 weeks prior to splenectomy (pneumococcal, *Haemophilus influenzae* and meningococcal C)
- Malaria prophylaxis when travelling to endemic areas

SPLENOMEGALY

This can result in abdominal discomfort and a pancytopenia (hypersplenism), as the spleen sequesters and destroys cells.

Causes

Infections	Acute: EBV, SBE, septicaemia
	Chronic: TB, brucellosis, schistosomiasis
Extra-medullary haemopoeisis	Haemolytic anaemias, haemoglobinopathies, osteopetrosis
Neoplasm	Leukaemia, lymphoma, haemangioma
Storage diseases	Gaucher disease, Niemann–Pick, Langerhans' cell histiocytosis, mucopolysaccharoidoses
Portal hypertension	
Systemic disease	JIA, SLE, amyloidosis
Massive splenomegaly	Malaria, Kalar–Azar, CML, myelofibrosis

FURTHER READING

Hann IM, Lake BD, Lilleyman J, Pritchard J, Weatherall DJ *Colour Atlas of Paediatric Haematology*. Oxford: Oxford University Press, 1996

Lilleyman JS, Hann IM, Blanchette VS *Paediatric Haematology,* 2nd edn. Edinburgh: Churchill Livingstone, 1999

Nathan DG, Orkin SH, Look T, Ginsburg D (eds) *Nathan & Oski's Hematology of Infancy and Childhood*, 6th edn, Vol 1 and 2. Philadephia: WB Saunders, 2003

17
Oncology

- *Mechanisms of carcinogenesis*
- *Incidence of childhood cancer*
- *Cancer treatment*
- *Neuroblastoma*
- *Nephroblastoma (Wilms tumour)*
- *Soft tissue sarcomas*
- *Bone tumours*

- *Retinoblastoma*
- *Gonadal and germ cell tumours*
- *Liver tumours*
- *Brain tumours*
- *Leukaemias*
- *Lymphoma*
- *Childhood histiocytosis syndromes*

MECHANISMS OF CARCINOGENESIS

- Cancer develops when there is genetic alteration of the normal **cell regulatory system** (growth and development) via mutation(s)
- Cancer-causing genes fall into three types (see below)
- Mutations activating the cancer genes can be **germline** (familial/inherited), **somatic** (most) or both
- The environment can increase the *frequency* of genetic mutations (see below)

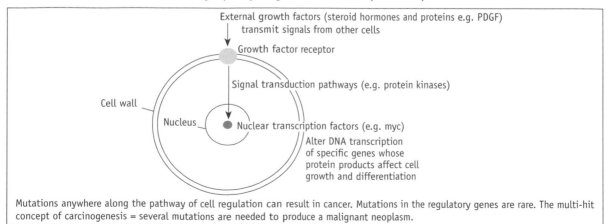

Figure 17.1 Normal cell regulation of growth and differentiation

CANCER GENES

Types

There are three major categories of cancer genes:

Tumour suppressor genes	Involved in restricting cell proliferation
	Inactivation can result in tumours
	E.g. RB1 gene (ch 13q14) – retinoblastoma, osteosarcoma
	WT1 gene (ch 11p13) – Wilms tumour
Oncogenes	Genes whose product can lead to unregulated cell growth
	Most arise from mutations in **proto-oncogenes**
	E.g. *Bcr-abl* gene – ALL, CLL
	MYCN amplification – neuroblastoma
DNA repair genes	DNA repair and replication continually occur throughout life
	Some inherited disorders involve defective DNA repair mechanisms, and thus the chances of cancers developing secondary to somatic mutations is increased, e.g. ataxia telangiectasia, xeroderma pigmentosum

Mechanism of activation

The above genes may be altered by:

- Single gene germline mutations – sporadic or inherited, e.g. retinoblastoma, or
- Somatic mutations, or
- Both

Two-hit theory of carcinogenesis is that a tumour will develop only when both copies of a gene are damaged. In many inherited cancers, the first allele is a germline mutation and the second a somatic mutation. This would explain why not all children who inherit the retinoblastoma mutation develop the tumour, and that they develop it at different ages.

Environmental factors

Environmental factors can increase the risk of mutations. **Carcinogens** are environmental cancer causing agents, i.e. increase the frequency of genetic cancer-causing events:

- Ionizing radiation, e.g. leukaemia, thyroid carcinoma, breast cancer
- Ultraviolet radiation, e.g. skin cancers
- Viruses, e.g. EB virus (Hodgkin disease, Burkitt lymphoma and nasopharyngeal carcinoma)
- Drugs, e.g. immunosuppressive drugs (non-Hodgkin lymphoma), diethylstilboestrol in pregnancy – vaginal adeno-carcinoma in the daughter

Tumour types	
Carcinoma	Epithelial
Sarcoma	Connective tissue
Lymphoma	Lymphatic tissue
Glioma	CNS glial cells
Leukaemia	Haematopoietic cells

INCIDENCE OF CHILDHOOD CANCER

1:650 children develop cancer by age 16 years.

Relative frequencies of type of cancer:		Relative frequency of cause of death	
Leukaemia	31%	ALL	20%
AML	10%		
Brain tumours	24%	Brain	24%
Lymphomas	10%	Hodgkin disease	0.2%
Neuroblastoma	6%	End (neuroblastoma)	11%
Wilms tumour	6%	Renal tract	3%
Bone tumours	5%	Bone & cartilage	5%
Rhabdomyosarcoma	4%	Soft tissue	6%
Retinoblastoma	3%	Other	20%
		(From: Cancer deaths in England and Wales 1995–99 ages 0–15 years)	

CANCER TREATMENT

Cancer management is multifactorial involving many specialists and therapists, and includes:

- Chemotherapy
- Radiotherapy
- Surgery
- Stem cell transplantation (which acts by either high-dose therapy or immunological means)
- Immunotherapy

CHEMOTHERAPY

Many different drugs and regimens are used, and new developments are continually being made in this area, so that many children are treated as part of continually evolving drug trials. These drugs preferentially target rapidly dividing cells, e.g. cancer cells, but also affect normal cells that rapidly divide, e.g. bone marrow progenitors, gut epithelium.

Chemotherapeutic agents

Drug group	Examples	Action	Toxicity
Antimetabolites	Methotrexate	Folic acid antagonist Inhibits dihydrofolate reductase	Severe enteritis Liver damage, dermatitis, stomatitis Myelosuppression Renal impairment
	6-Mercaptopurine (6-MP)	Purine analogue Inhibits purine synthesis	Myelosuppression Hepatic necrosis

Drug group	Examples	Action	Toxicity
Alkylating agents	Cyclophosphamide	Inhibits DNA synthesis	Myelosuppression Haemorrhagic cystitis (give Mesna) Secondary malignancy Sterility Lung fibrosis SIADH
Vinca alkaloids	Vincristine	Inhibits microtubule formation	Peripheral neuropathy Ptosis Constipation Extravasation injury Minimal myelosuppression Jaw pain Seizures, SIADH
	Vinblastine	Inhibits microtubule formation	Cellulitis Myelosuppression Peripheral neuropathy (not as severe as vincristine)
Antibiotics	Doxorubicin and daunorubicin	Bind to DNA	Myelosuppression Necrosis on extravasation Cardiotoxicity
	Bleomycin	Bind to DNA	Myelosuppression Dermatitis, stomatitis Lung fibrosis
Enzymes	L-asparaginase	L-asparagine depletion	Pancreatitis, hyperglycaemia Allergies Coagulopathy Encephalopathy
Others	Cisplatin	Inhibits DNA synthesis	Nephrotoxic Neurotoxic, ototoxic Myelosuppression
	Etoposide	Topoisomerase inhibitor	Myelosuppression Secondary AML

Side-effects common to most agents

- Bone marrow suppression: Anaemia
  Thrombocytopenia
  Immunosuppression (neutropenia, most marked 10 days after chemotherapy commenced. Infections treated with broad-spectrum antibiotics)
- Nausea and vomiting
- Mouth ulcers
- Tumour lysis syndrome
- Hair loss
- Secondary malignancy – many agents, especially alkylating agents

Tumour lysis syndrome

The high rate of cellular breakdown in fast-growing tumours (especially with high WCC ALL and bulky NHL) after chemotherapy can cause this potentially life-threatening syndrome of:

1. Rise in urate
2. Then $PO_4 \uparrow$ with simultaneous Ca $\downarrow$ (within 1–2 days)
3. Then rapid development of hyperkalaemia

Prevention

Prevention with hyperhydration and the use of allopurinol and rasburicase are essential. If the syndrome develops, then treatment with dialysis may be necessary. Haemofiltration removes less solute than dialysis and is reserved for milder cases.

- Intravenous fluids (with no added K) and some units feel that alkalinization prior to chemotherapy is beneficial
- Regular monitoring of biochemistry
- Allopurinol/rasburicase
- Dialysis or haemofiltration (used prophylactically in bulky tumours)

Nausea and vomiting

These are common side-effects of chemotherapy.

Centres involved:

- Visceral afferents
- Chemoreceptor trigger zone (CTZ)
- Vomiting centre (in the medulla)
- Higher centres (emotional)
- Vestibular apparatus

Common antiemetics

Drug	Action	Adverse effects
Ondansetron	5-HT3 antagonist	Elevated transaminases
Metoclopramide	CTZ + peripheral gut	Acute dystonic reactions (oculogyrate crises, spasms)
Cyclizine	Antihistamine	Those of antihistamines (drowsiness, dry mouth, blurred vision)

RADIOTHERAPY

This is often used as an adjunct to chemotherapy, e.g. cranial irradiation in ALL. Side-effects include:

Early Nausea and fatigue, inflammation of skin, gut and bladder
Late Organ damage dependent on location of treatment:
- Brain – cognitive impairment
- Skin – radiation damage, skin malignancies
- Gonads – infertility
- Other organs – secondary malignancy

SURGERY

Direct initial surgical excision may be done, or the tumour may be 'pre-shrunk' using chemo- or radio-therapy, and then excised. Regional lymph nodes are generally also excised if affected or for staging of the disease.

SMALL MOLECULE INHIBITORS

A new class of drugs called small molecule inhibitors, e.g. Glivec, that target signal transduction pathways are being used in CML.

IMMUNOTHERAPY

Immunotherapy is being developed with both non-specific mediators of immune defence, e.g. interferon-α, and cancer-targeted therapies using monoclonal antibodies and T-cell based tumour vaccines.

STEM CELL TRANSPLANTATION (SCT)

Haemopoietic stem cells replace the diseased marrow with normal marrow cells. The child's diseased marrow is ablated with high-dose chemotherapy + radiotherapy and then the child is rescued with the SCT. Used for therapy after relapse of leukaemia and also in initial consolidation therapy.

Autologous SCT

The child acts as their own donor. Their own marrow is harvested before ablation, purged of malignant cells, cryopreserved and then re-infused into the child after marrow ablation. Alternatively, *peripheral* blood stem cells may be harvested with granulocyte colony-stimulating factor (G-CSF).

Complications

- Residual cancer cells may cause relapse
- Conditioning toxicity (including infertility and secondary malignancy)
- Infections in cytopaenic phase (2 weeks for peripheral blood stem cell transplant, 4 weeks for BMT)

Allogeneic SCT

Marrow from a matched donor (HLA screened, preferably an HLA-identical sibling) is used. The conditioning with chemotherapy and radiotherapy here is also used to destroy the patient's immune system to prevent rejection.

Complications

- Marrow rejection
- GvHD (acute or chronic)
- Infections
- Acute regimen-related toxicity (initial ablative therapy causes veno-occlusive disease, pneumonitis, haemorrhagic cystitis)

Graft-versus-host disease (GvHD)

This is due to the **donor T cells** mounting an immune response to the host major histocompatibility complex (MHC) antigens. It may be acute or chronic, though the former can transform into the latter:

Acute GvHD	< 100 days of SCT (usually 10–14 days post SCT)
	Fever
	Rash – fine pruritic maculopapular may progress to bullae or exfoliation of ears, palms, soles, then trunk
	Enteritis – bloody diarrhoea, protein-losing enteropathy
	Cholestatic hepatitis
	Predisposing factors: HLA differences between donor and host, sex mismatch, active malignancy at time of BMT

	Prevention: T-cell depletion of donor marrow
Chronic GvHD	> 100 days post-SCT
	Rash – hyperpigmented nodules, lichenoid, erythema, hypopigmented, then scleroderma-like
	Arthritis
	Malabsorption
	Obstructive jaundice
	Autoimmune features – SLE, scleroderma, Sjögren syndrome, primary biliary cirrhosis
	Predisposing factors: acute GvHD, increasing age, buffy coat transfusions

A beneficial graft-versus-leukaemia effect occurs in the process and helps eliminate any remaining cancer cells.

Management

Further immunosuppression, e.g. cyclosporin A, steroids.

NEUROBLASTOMA

A tumour arising from **neural crest cells** of the **sympathetic nervous system** developing in:

- Adrenal medulla – 50%
- Sympathetic chain – 50% (anywhere from the posterior cranial fossa to the coccyx)

Tumours of neural crest cells may be benign ganglioneuromas, ganglioneuroblastomas or malignant neuroblastomas, and may spontaneously regress in infants.

Clinical features

Usually < 5 years	
Abdominal mass	
Metastatic disease (70%)	Bone pain, limp
	Proptosis, periorbital bruising
	Massive hepatosplenomegaly
	Skin nodules, lymphadenopathy
	Weight loss, pallor, malaise
	Cord compression (paraplegia) – usually direct extension not metastasis
	Horner syndrome – again direct pressure from thoracic primary

Diagnostic investigations

Urine catecholamine metabolites	↑ Homovanillic acid (HVA) and vanillylmandelic acid (VMA)
CT or MRI scan	
Meta-iodobenzylguanidine (MIBG) scan	(A catecholamine precursor; will also outline metastases)
Tissue biopsy or positive bone marrow	Necessary to confirm diagnosis and define molecular features that determine prognosis and therapy

Staging is complex. Stage 4S refers to neonates with small adrenal tumour and metastases in skin, liver or bone marrow only (can undergo spontaneous remission).

Cytogenetic abnormalities

A poor prognosis if these are present.

- Chromosome 1p partial deletion
- Chromosome 17q gain
- Amplification of N-myc (MYCN) oncogene

Management

Treatment is dependent on the child's age, tumour stage and biology (presence or absence of the *MYCN* oncogene).

Low-risk disease	Surgical resection ± chemotherapy
	Subtype (stage 4S) resolves with no therapy
High-risk disease	More aggressive chemotherapy, surgery, high dose chemotherapy with stem cell rescue, local radiotherapy and differentiation treatment
Differentiation therapy	Use of retinoic acid derivatives to force cells to differentiate past a point of development so that they lose the capacity to grow quickly and spread

New therapies using targeted radiation therapy with ^{131}I-MIBG monoclonal antibodies are being trialed. (High-dose therapy with stem cell rescue is standard treatment.)

Prognosis

Low-risk tumours	> 90% cure rate
High-risk tumours	10–40% cure rate

NEPHROBLASTOMA (WILMS TUMOUR)

Nephroblastoma is tumour of **embryonic renal precursor cells**. Incidence 7.8:million.

Associations	Genitourinary anomalies
	Overgrowth disorders (hemihypertrophy, Beckwith–Wiedemann syndrome)
	Aniridia
	Chromosome 11 short arm deletions involving one of two Wilms genes, e.g. *WIT* gene (11p13)

Clinical features

- Mean age 3 years
- Abdominal mass (the most common presentation)
- Abdominal pain and vomiting
- Hypertension
- Haematuria

5% have bilateral disease at presentation.

Investigations

Imaging	Abdominal USS, CT or MRI scan abdomen and CXR (lung metastases)
Urine	Haematuria (micro- or macro-scopic)

Staging (determined after tumour resection)

I	Completely resected disease of kidney only
II	Disease beyond the kidney but completely resected
III	Residual disease post-surgery or nodal involvement
IV	Metastatic disease (bilateral used to be called stage V but now just called bilateral)

Management

Dependent on the stage.

- Initial chemotherapy then nephrectomy is now standard in the UK and rest of Europe
- Primary nephrectomy then chemotherapy is still used in the USA

• Radiotherapy is used as part of a combined strategy for local residual disease post-surgery and for pulmonary metastatic disease

Prognosis

This is related to both histology and disease stage, tumour size and child's age.

Favourable histology	89–98% 2-year survival
Poor histology	17–70% 4-year survival (variation due predominantly to precise histology of tumour)

SOFT TISSUE SARCOMAS

Incidence 1.4:million per year.

These comprise:

• Rhabdomyosarcoma (50%)
• Non-rhabdomyosarcoma soft tissue tumours (NRSTs), e.g. liposarcoma, angiosarcoma, leiomyosarcoma, neuro-fibrosarcoma and fibrosarcoma

RHABDOMYOSARCOMA

Rhabdomysarcoma is a tumour of **primitive mesenchymal tissue** (which striated skeletal muscle arises from).

Associations	Neurofibromatosis type 1
	Beckwith-Wiedemann syndrome

These tumours may occur anywhere, but the most common sites are:

• Head and neck
• Genitourinary tract
• Extremities

Clinical features

Head and neck tumour	Proptosis
	Facial swelling
	Nasal obstruction, blood-stained nasal discharge
	Cranial nerve palsies
GU tract tumour	Urinary tract obstruction
	Dysuria
	Blood-stained vaginal discharge

Investigations

Imaging of relevant area	CT, USS, MRI scan
Metastases search	Bone scan, CXR and CT, bone marrow
Tumour tissue	Histology

Staging

I	Completely resected
II	Microscopic residual tumour
III	Macroscopic residual tumour
IV	Metastatic disease

Management

This depends on the resectability, stage, location, histology and presence of metastases.

- Initial surgical resection then chemotherapy
- If unresectable initially, chemotherapy, second-look surgery ± radiotherapy

Prognosis

Localized standard-risk histology disease has a 70% 5-year survival.

BONE TUMOURS

The two most common bone tumours are **osteosarcoma** (the most common) and **Ewing sarcoma**. Rarer tumours include chondrosarcoma and fibrosarcoma.

Incidence 5.6:million (whites > blacks). Commonly present in adolescence. Male > female.

	Osteosarcoma	Ewing sarcoma
Associations	Most common Retinoblastoma Osteogenesis imperfecta	11:22 translocation and variants
Site	Metaphysis (proximal end) of long bones Knee, proximal humerus	Diaphysis of long bones Flat bones, e.g. ribs, pelvis
Presentation	Bone pain and mass	Bone pain and mass, and soft tissue component
X-ray findings	Sclerotic with 'skip lesions'	Lytic lesions 'Onion skinning' periosteal reaction
Tumour cells	Spindle cells	Small round cells*
Metastases	Lung and bones	Lung and bones
Management	Surgery and chemotherapy	Surgery or radiotherapy to primary then chemotherapy
Prognosis	50% survival if non-metastatic < 20% survival if metastatic	65–70% survival if non-metastatic 25–30% survival if metastatic

*Similar small round cell undifferentiated neoplasms include primitive neuroectodermal tumours (PNET).

RETINOBLASTOMA

Retinoblastoma is a tumour arising in the retina. Usually develops in the posterior portion of the retina. Incidence approximately 4:million children.

Both hereditary and sporadic forms exist.

Hereditary tumour (40%)	All the bilateral tumours May be unilateral (75%)
Sporadic tumour (60%)	Unilateral tumours

Hereditary tumours

- Retinoblastoma (RB1) gene on chromosome 13q (tumour suppressor gene)
- Autosomal dominant, incomplete penetrance
- Increased incidence of secondary malignancies (osteosarcoma, soft tissue sarcoma and melanoma)

Clinical features

- Leucocoria (white pupillary reflex)
- Squint (any *new* squint in a child should be investigated, though retinoblastoma will be an unusual finding in these children. Ophthalmological problems and brain tumours will be more common pathologies)
- Decreased vision
- If advanced disease – proptosis, raised ICP, orbital pain

Investigations

- Fundoscopy
- Orbital imaging – CT or MRI of orbits, USS orbits

Management

- Local therapy (radiotherapy, photocoagulation or cryotherapy)
- Enucleation of the eye if unavoidable
- Chemotherapy to reduce tumour volume prior to local therapy or if residual or metastatic disease

Treatment that minimizes radiotherapy to improve visual sparing and reduce the incidence of future secondary tumours is being optimized.

Prognosis

- Overall survival > 90%
- Poor survival if extensive or metastatic disease

GONADAL AND GERM CELL TUMOURS

These are tumours arising from **primitive pluripotent germ cells**, which migrate from the fetal yolk sac to form the gonads. Extragonadal tumours occur due to abherrant germ cell migration. They are mostly benign.

Associations   Cryptorchidism, gonadal dysgenesis

Classification is based on the differentiation pathway:

Embryonic differentiation	Teratoma (usually benign), e.g. sacrococcygeal teratoma	
	Embryonal carcinoma	
Extraembryonic differentiation	Choriocarcinoma	Highly malignant
		Gonadal or extragonadal
		β-hCG ↑
	Yolk sac carcinoma	AFP ↑
Suppressed differentiation	Germinoma	
	Seminoma	
	Dysgerminoma (ovarian tumours)	

SACROCOCCYGEAL TERATOMA

Most common neonatal tumour. Rectum and urinary tract may be involved and 90% have an external component.

10% are malignant at birth, but if benign teratomas are left unresected malignant transformation can occur. Malignancy is defined by a tumour that secretes AFP or β-hCG or has particular histological appearance (yolk sac tumour).

Investigations

Imaging	CT or MRI scan of affected area, bone scan, chest CT
Biological markers	AFP ↑ and β-hCG
Histology of lesion	(Biopsy or resected specimen)

Management

This involves surgical resection wherever possible for benign tumours. Malignant tumours should be treated with chemotherapy before surgery to minimize morbidity.

Prognosis

Excellent if benign, and 60–90% 5-year survival if malignant.

TESTICULAR GERM CELL TUMOURS

Present as	Testicular swelling (painless or painful)
	Gynaecomastia (if secretes hCG)
	Metastases (retroperitoneal, LN, lung)
Seminoma ($^1/_3$)	Dysgerminoma is the ovarian counterpart
Teratoma ($^2/_3$)	

OVARIAN GERM CELL TUMOURS

Present as	Abdominal pain (acute or chronic) and swelling
	Abdominal mass

LIVER TUMOURS

Liver tumours may be:

Primary	Benign (50%)	Haemangioma, liver cell adenoma
		Haemangioendothelioma
		Hamartoma, focal nodular hyperplasia
	Malignant (50%)	Hepatoblastoma (65%)
		Hepatocellular carcinoma (35%)
Metastatic	Neuroblastoma, Wilms tumour	

	Hepatoblastoma	Hepatocellular carcinoma (HCC)
Age	<3 years	12–15 years
Associations	Hemihypertrophy	Pre-existing cirrhosis (33%)
	Beckwith–Wiedemann syndrome	
	Meckel diverticulum	
	Renal anomalies	
Clinical features	Abdominal mass	Abdominal mass
	Systemic features uncommon	Systemic features more common
Tumour cells	Immature hepatic epithelium	Abnormal hepatocytes
Markers	AFP ↑ in 60% of patients	AFP ↑ in 50% of patients
Metastases	Lung, lymph nodes	Lung, lymph nodes
Prognosis	3-year survival:	Very poor survival figures
	75% if resectable	Recurrence common
	(but only if successful liver	
	transplant fully removes tumour)	
	65% if unresectable	
	10–20% if metastatic	

Investigations

Include CT or MRI scans to search for extent of tumour and metastases. It can be difficult to differentiate between the two tumours.

Management

- Hepatoblastoma is chemosensitive and primary chemotherapy followed by surgery should be used
- Primary surgical excision (possible in 50% of hepatoblastomas and 33% of HCC)
- Chemotherapy (preoperatively if initially unresectable or for metastases)
- Liver transplantation is indicated in a minority

BRAIN TUMOURS

Brain tumours are almost always primary in children. They can be divided into

- Supratentorial
- Infratentorial (posterior fossa)

<2 years	Equal frequencies of posterior fossa and supratentorial tumours
2–12 years	²/₃ are infratentorial (posterior fossa)

Clinical features

Signs of raised ICP	Morning headache, drowsiness, vomiting
	Diplopia, strabismus, papilloedema (a late sign in young children)
	Nystagmus: Horizontal in unilateral cerebellar tumours, worse on looking to the side of the lesion
	All directions in cerebellar vermis or fourth ventricle tumours
	Horizontal, vertical and rotatory in brainstem tumours

	Head tilting and nuchal rigidity
	Bulging fontanelle with loss of pulsation, macrocephaly
	Cranial nerve palsies (IV and VI)
Focal neurological signs	Long-tract signs: hemiparesis
	Seizures: complex partial seizures
	Ataxia: Truncal (cerebellar vermis)
	Ipsilateral (cerebellar hemisphere)
Other features	Endocrinopathies, e.g. diabetes insipidus
	Behavioural change

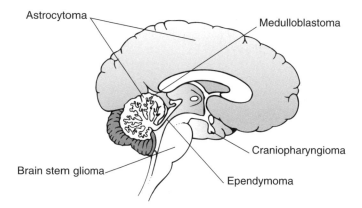

Figure 17.2 Location of brain tumours

INFRATENTORIAL TUMOURS

Medulloblastoma (20%)

- Usually midline
- Present with truncal ataxia and ICP ↑
- 20% have spinal metastases at diagnosis
- Treatment is surgical resection followed by chemotherapy and radiotherapy
- Standard risk tumours have 80% long-term disease control; poor risk have 20% long-term disease control
- Neurocognitive sequelae problematic secondary to tumour, raised ICP, radiotherapy and probably chemotherapy

Brainstem glioma (10%)

- May be: 1. Diffusely infiltrating the pons (most cases; very poor outlook)
          2. Low-grade focal midbrain or cervicomedullary tumours (good outlook if resectable)
- Present with ataxia, cranial nerve palsies and long-tract signs
- Treatment is mostly radiotherapy, unless low-grade focal tumour is resectable

Astrocytoma (20%)

- Usually cystic, slow growing
- May be in a cerebellar hemisphere or midline
- Present with ICP ↑ by blocking the fourth ventricle or aqueduct of Sylvius
- Treatment is surgical resection ± chemotherapy and radiotherapy
- 5-year survival 90–95%

Ependymoma (10%)

- Locally invasive
- Presents with ICP ↑ and cranial nerve signs
- Treatment is surgery and radiotherapy, though chemotherapy has a role in younger children
- 5-year survival 50%

SUPRATENTORIAL TUMOURS

Craniopharyngioma (see p. 235)

- Develops from a squamous remnant of Rathke's pouch in the sella turcica
- Solid and cystic areas; 90% show calcification on skull X-ray
- Presents with endocrine abnormalities, ICP ↑, bitemporal hemianopia
- Treatment is surgical resection ± radiotherapy

Optic nerve glioma

- $1/3$ associated with neurofibromatosis
- Presents with: Decreased acuity and disc pallor
  Diencephalic syndrome – anorexia, or increased appetite, emaciation, hyperalert, euphoric (occurs if hypothalamus invaded)
- Treatment is dependent on site, age and presence of neurofibromatosis. In isolated optic nerve tumours in a blind eye, surgical resection may be indicated. In other tumours, chemotherapy or radiotherapy are the major modalities. No treatment until progression is observed as the natural history is variable with spontaneous stabilization or even regression of tumour occurring in patients with NF1

Astrocytoma

Prognosis is dependent on age, site and histology of the tumour. Supratentorial low-grade astrocytomas amenable to surgical resection do well, whereas high-grade tumours of the thalamus do badly.

Choroid plexus papilloma

- Predominantly tumours of very young children
- Secrete CSF and cause slowly progressive hydrocephalus
- Prognosis is excellent after resection
- Choroid plexus carcinoma carries a much worse prognosis

Pineal tumours

- Variety of tumour types can occur in the pineal gland in children
- Therapy and prognosis are dependent on the histology and the age of the patient

LEUKAEMIAS

The leukaemias are the most common form of childhood cancer. They include:

- Acute lymphoblastic leukaemia (ALL) (75%) – peak incidence 4 years
- Acute myeloid leukaemia (AML) (20%) – stable incidence < 10 years, higher incidence during adolescence and older
- Chronic myeloid leukaemia (CML) (3%)
- Juvenile CML and the myelodysplastic syndromes (2–3%)

The leukaemias are classified according to morphology and cytochemistry, immunophenotyping, chromosome analysis and gene rearrangements.

ACUTE LYMPHOBLASTIC LEUKAEMIA (ALL)

The most common form of childhood cancer. Arises from early cells in the lymphoid series.

Genetic associations   Down syndrome
Hyperdiploidy (good prognosis)
Hypodiploidy (poor prognosis)
Translocations, e.g. t (9:22) Philadelphia chromosome } Poor risk leukaemias,
t (4:11) infant ALL } SCT indicated in first remission

Classification

Immunophenotypes classification
Precursor B-ALL (75%) (includes C-ALL [common], null-ALL and pre-B-ALL)
T-ALL (20%) M > F
B-ALL (5%) Mediastinal mass, 'Burkitt', t (8:14), t (2:8) and t (22:8)

French–American–British (FAB) system (morphological)	
L1	Small lymphoblasts, little cytoplasm (good prognosis)
L2	Larger and pleomorphic lymphoblasts, more cytoplasm
L3	Cytoplasmic vacuoles, finely stippled nuclear chromatin

Clinical features

Bone marrow failure   Hb ($\downarrow$)   Pallor, lethargy
WCC ($\downarrow$ or N)   Infections, fever
Platelets ($\downarrow$)   Bruising, bleeding gums, menorrhagia
Infiltration   Hepatosplenomegaly
Lymphadenopathy
Testicular swelling
Limp (bone pain)
Acute renal failure
Meningeal syndrome (ICP $\uparrow$, papilloedema, retinal haemorrhage)
Anterior mediastinal mass (on CT scan, in T-ALL)

Investigations

Peripheral FBC and film   Anaemia (normochromic, normocytic)
Blasts present
WCC $\downarrow$, N or $\uparrow$
Platelets $\downarrow$
Bone marrow (aspirate or biopsy) $\geqslant$ 30% leukaemic blast cells
CXR   Mediastinal mass (in T-ALL)
CSF   Blasts seen in cytospin if CNS involvement
Renal function + uric acid   Impaired renal function with $\uparrow$ uric acid if renal infiltration or tumour lysis syndrome
Special classification tests   Chromosomal analysis, immunocytochemistry, immunophenotyping, Immunoglobulin and T-cell receptor (TCR) gene rearrangement studies

Treatment

1. *Induction of remission* Multiagent chemotherapy: vincristine, daunorubicin, asparagine, steroid
2. *Consolidation of remission* Intensive multiagent chemotherapy: ara-c, cyclophosphamide, etoposide
   CNS prophylaxis (treatment that crosses the blood–brain barrier), e.g. high dose IV methotrexate, intrathecal chemotherapy, CNS radiotherapy
3. *Intensification* 2–3 blocks of intensive, multiagent chemotherapy
   Aim to clear submicroscopic or minimal residual disease
4. *Maintenance chemotherapy* 2 years chemotherapy. An outpatient treatment usually with oral 6-MP, vincristine and prednisolone or dexamethasone

Consider allogeneic SCT if very poor features such as initial WCC > 100, Philadelphia positive or t (4:11).

Relapse

- Common sites are the bone marrow, CNS and testes
- Treated with intensive chemotherapy (and cranial irradiation in CNS relapse)
- Stem cell transplant may offer the best chance of cure

Prognosis

- Dependent on type and other factors (see below)
- Overall 5-year survival is 70–80%

Prognostic indicators

Good	Bad
Low initial WCC	High initial WCC (> 50)
Female	Male
2–10 years	< 2 years or $\geq$ 10 years
$\leq$ 4 weeks to remission	> 4 weeks to remission
t (12:21)	t (9:22), t (4:11)
Hyperdiploidy	Hypoploidy
C-ALL or L1	CNS involvement

ACUTE MYELOID LEUKAEMIA (AML)

The predominant form of congenital leukaemia that probably arises from a pluripotent cell or myeloid progenitor committed to erythroid, granulocytic–monocytic or megakaryocytic lines.

Associations Down syndrome
Aplastic anaemia
Fanconi anaemia
Bloom syndrome
Previous chemotherapy (secondary AML)

Classification

French–American–British (FAB) system		
M0	Undifferentiated	No Auer rods
M1	Myeloblastic, no maturation	Few Auer rods
M2	Myeloblastic, some maturation	t (8:21), good prognosis, chloroma common, Auer rods common
M3	Acute promyelocytic	t (15:17), DIC common, many Auer rods. Retinoic acid as initial therapy, good prognosis
M4	Myelomonocytic	Chromosome 16 material inversion, eosinophilia, good prognosis
M5	Monocytic	Renal damage common, meningeal involvement, gum hypertrophy
M6	Erythroleukaemia	Poor prognosis
M7	Megakaryoblastic	Marrow fibrosis

Clinical features

Bone marrow failure   As in ALL (WCC may be ↓, N or ↑)
Other   Gum hypertrophy (M4 and M5 especially)
    DIC (M3)
    Chloroma (a localized mass of leukaemoid cells; common sites are retro-orbital, skin and epidural)
    Bone pain less common than in ALL

Investigations

As for ALL. Bone marrow must contain at least 30% blast cells (blasts may contain Auer rods).

Management

1. *Induction of remission*   Chemotherapy, e.g. daunorubicin, cytosine arabinoside, thioguanine or etoposide
    > 80% achieve remission (if not achieved SCT is necessary)
2. *Consolidation*   E.g. daunorubicin, cytosine arabinoside, thioguanine or etoposide
    Intrathecal chemotherapy (± cranial irradiation) if CNS leukaemia at diagnosis or CNS relapse
3. *Further consolidation*   Total of 4–5 courses of multiagent chemotherapy, e.g. etoposide, ara-c, m-amascrine
    SCT is usually only considered after relapse of AML in children
Other treatments   All-*trans*-retinoic acid (ATRA) given in M3

Prognosis

Overall cure rate 60–70%. Cure rates depend on type (highest for M3 AML), and decreases with increasing age.

MYELODYSPLASTIC SYNDROMES

Juvenile myelomonocytic leukaemia (JMML)

This is unlike adult CML, generally occurring at a young age and having features of AML. Philadelphia chromosome is *not* present.

Predominant findings	Abnormal monocytes on the blood film
	HbF elevated
	Platelets ↓
	Leucocytosis
	Hepatosplenomegaly, lymphadenopathy, bleeding tendency, eczema
	Chronic desquamative maculopapular rash

Due to resistance to treatment, allogeneic SCT is recommended.

Myelodysplasia (including monosomy 7)

Children initially develop only anaemia, thrombocytopenia or leucopenia. The bone marrow has characteristic dysplastic features and blast cells.

Associated chromosomal changes	Trisomy 8
	Complete or partial deletion of chromosome 5 or 7
	Monosomy 7 (the most common abnormality in infants with myelodysplasia and AML)

The condition usually evolves into AML and so patients are treated as for AML. BMT is considered more often as this condition is more resistant to chemotherapy.

CHRONIC MYELOGENOUS LEUKAEMIA (CML, ADULT TYPE)

This is a malignancy of a haematopoietic stem cell capable of entering both myeloid and lymphoid lineages and containing the Philadelphia (Ph) chromosome. The Ph chromosome has the translocation: t (9:22). This produces a fusion gene (*bcr–abl*) which encodes the bcr-abl protein, i.e. activates the *abl* oncogene.

Phases in CML

Chronic phase	3–4 years. Cell counts easily controlled with chemotherapy
Accelerated phase	More difficult to control
Blast crisis	ALL or AML

Clinical features

- Hypermetabolism – fever, weight loss, anorexia, night sweats
- Massive splenomegaly
- Anaemia, bleeding, bruising
- Leucostasis – visual disturbance, priapism
- Renal failure and gout

Investigations

Peripheral blood film	Hb N or ↓, platelets ↑, N or ↓,WCC ↑↑,immature myeloid cells but few blasts on film
Bone marrow	Hypercellular, myeloid hyperplasia
Others	Neutrophil alkaline phosphatase score ↓, uric acid ↑, B_{12} ↑
Cytogenetic studies	Philadelphia chromosome (⩾ 95%)

Management

Chemotherapy	E.g. busulphan, hydroxyurea,
	α-Interferon (suppresses the Ph chromosome); signal transduction inhibitors (STI) are in trial with encouraging results
SCT in chronic phase	Only known cure

Prognosis

- If BMT during chronic phase, survival is 80% (matched sibling), 50–60% (partially matched or unrelated)
- If BMT during accelerated phase, survival is 20–30%
- If BMT during blast crisis, survival is 0–10%

LYMPHOMA

These malignancies of lymphoid tissue are classified into:

- Hodgkin disease
- Non-Hodgkin lymphoma

Incidence 13:million children per year.

HODGKIN DISEASE

A malignancy of lymphoid tissue with Reed–Sternberg (RS) cells and Hodgkin cells seen on histology. It is a B-cell malignancy, but the exact origin of the malignant cells is unclear.

Bimodal age distribution: peak in mid-20s and > 50 years. Male > female, 2:1.

Histological classification

Nodular sclerosing (50%)	Good prognosis. Females > males, mediastinal mass common
Mixed cellularity (40%)	Present with more advanced disease
Lymphocyte predominant (10%)	Best prognosis
Lymphocyte depleted (v. rare)	Present with disseminated disease, poor prognosis

Clinical features

Lymphadenopathy	Painless, firm lymph nodes
	Cervical, supraclavicular, axillary, inguinal
	Mediastinal (cough, airway compression)
	Retroperitoneal
'B' symptoms	Fever (*Pel–Epstein*)
	Night sweats
	Weight loss
Other constitutional symptoms	Fatigue, pruritis, anorexia
Extranodal involvement	Hepatosplenomegaly, bone pain, skin deposits, SVC obstruction, bone marrow failure (rare)

Investigations

Careful clinical examination essential.

Bloods	FBC: Normocytic normochromic anaemia
	Neutrophils ↑, eosinophils ↑
	Platelets (initially high, low in advanced disease)
	ESR ↑ (used to monitor disease progress)
	LDH ↑ (poor prognosis)
	LFTs ↑ (poor prognosis)

Lymph node biopsy	For diagnosis and histological classification
CT chest/abdomen/pelvis	For staging
Other (if necessary)	Bone marrow aspirate
	Bone scan
	Liver biopsy
	MRI scan
	Laparotomy

Stages

I	Single lymph node region (LNR)
II	$\geq$ 2 LNR same side diaphragm
III	LNR both sides diaphragm
	$\pm$ spleen
IV	Disseminated involvement of extralymphatic organs, e.g. bone marrow, liver

The stage is also **A** absence of 'B' symptoms
       or **B** presence of 'B' symptoms

Management

Stages IA and IIA	Radiotherapy only or chemotherapy (ABVD)
Advanced disease	Chemotherapy, e.g. adriamycin (doxorubicin), bleomycin, vinblastine, dacarbazine (ABVD)
	$\pm$ Radiotherapy
Relapse	Alternative combination chemotherapy, e.g. MOPP, and autologous stem cell transplant

Prognosis

Stage I and II	>90% 5-year survival
Stage IIIA	>80% 5-year survival
Stage IIIB, IV	>70% 5-year survival

NON-HODGKIN LYMPHOMA

Arises from abnormal T or B lymphocytes.

Associations	Autoimmune disorders
	Congenital immunodeficiency disorders, HIV

Children have high-grade, diffuse disease.

Classification

There are several classifications.

National Cancer Institute histological classification of high-grade non-Hodgkin lymphomas	
Small non-cleaved cell (SNCC) (Burkitt)	B-cell tumours (like B-ALL)
	All have chromosomal translocations, either: t (8:14), t (2:8) or t (8:22), which contain the *c-myc* oncogene and an immunoglobulin gene (μ, κ or λ)
Lymphoblastic	T cell tumours (like T-ALL)
Large cell	T cell, B cell or non-B non-T cell phenotypes (anaplastic)

Clinical features

These are dependent on the site of the primary.

Systemic symptoms	Fever, night sweats, weight loss
Abdomen (31%)	Abdominal distension, nausea, vomiting, acute abdomen, hepatosplenomegaly
Mediastinum (26%)	Dyspnoea, pleural effusions, SVC obstruction
Oropharyngeal	Sore throat, stridor
Lymph nodes	Painless hard lymph nodes. Cervical LN most commonly affected
Bone marrow	Bone marrow failure symptoms and signs
CNS	Headache, raised ICP, cranial nerve palsies
Other organ	Skin deposits, testes mass

Investigations

Excision biopsy or fine-needle aspirate	Of lymph node or other mass
Bloods	FBC (anaemia, neutropenia, lymphoma cells platelets $\downarrow$)
	Urea and creatinine $\uparrow$, uric acid $\uparrow$, bone profile
	LDH $\uparrow$ (prognostic marker)
Bone marrow aspirate or trephine	(Involvement in around 20%)
CSF	CNS involvement
Imaging	CT scan chest/abdomen/pelvis and bone scan
Special tests	Chromosome analysis, immunological markers

Staging

This is as for Hodgkin disease, though it is less clearly related to prognosis than is the histological type.

Management

This depends on the grade of malignancy. High-grade malignancy in children is usually treated with multiagent chemotherapy, like ALL protocols.

Relapses are treated with intensive chemotherapy, radiotherapy and SCT.

Prognosis

Limited-stage disease	> 90% cure
Stage III and IV	70% cure

Burkitt lymphoma

An unusual B-cell lymphoma, related to EBV infection. Endemic in Africa (jaw involvement seen). Sporadic in developed countries (abdominal involvement seen).

Clinical features

- Massive jaw lesions
- Abdominal extranodal involvement
- Ovarian involvement

Specific investigations

Lymph node biopsy	'Starry sky' appearance (a few histiocytes amongst masses of lymphocytes)

Cell culture	For EBV
Chromosome analysis	t (8:14) usually present

Management

Intensive sequential chemotherapy (four cycles), with SCT in relapse. Recently very good results have been obtained (70% cure).

CHILDHOOD HISTIOCYTOSIS SYNDROMES

The histiocytoses are a group of disorders involving proliferation of histiocytic cells in the bone marrow of the **dendritic cell** or **monocyte–macrophage** systems. Many are benign proliferations, though some are malignant. They are classified on the basis of histology.

CLASS I HISTIOCYTOSES: DENDRITIC CELL DISORDERS

Langerhans' cell histiocytosis (LCH)

Langerhans' cells are skin histiocytes with antigen-presenting function (part of the antigen-specific immune response). They are CD1a positive. Identified on EM with the cytoplasmic organelles **Birbeck granules**, which look like tennis rackets.

The cause of LCH is unknown.

2–5 cases:million children annually, peak incidence age 1–3 years, males > females.

Clinical features

Features are a result of **infiltration** with Langerhans' cells and the subsequent immunological reaction to these cells. Presentation and extent of involvement vary widely: it may be single system or disseminated.

Bone pain and swelling	Due to isolated or multiple lytic lesions: • Punched-out skull lesions, mastoid necrosis with middle ear involvement • Jaw (floating teeth), orbit (proptosis), vertebral fractures, long bone lesions Bone marrow infiltration seen Skeletal survey should be performed at diagnosis
Skin rash	Pink or brown papules becoming eczematous, scaly and pruritic Involving face, scalp, behind ears, axillary and inguinal folds, back and nappy area
Ear discharge *Lymphadenopathy* *Hepatosplenomegaly*	
Other	*Lung* – infiltration causing cough, tachypnoea, chest pain (CXR: diffuse micronodules, later reticulonodular pattern) *Endocrine* – e.g. hypothalamic–pituitary infiltration causing endocrine abnormalities, especially diabetes insipidus *GIT* – infiltration causing abdominal pain, vomiting, diarrhoea, protein-losing enteropathy *CNS* – involvement, e.g. ataxia, pyramidal signs, tremor, encephalopathy (all rare)

Treatment

Single system disease	Observation alone Topical treatment (rash), analgesia, steroids and chemotherapy if necessary
Multisystem disease	Chemotherapy then SCT if necessary, i.e. non-responders with bone marrow disease

Prognosis

May regress spontaneously or progress to life-threatening disease. The prognosis is worse if multisystem, < 1 year old and with active disease.

CLASS II HISTIOCYTOSES: MACROPHAGE DISORDERS

These are proliferations involving macrophages and the many different types are divided into systemic and cutaneous forms.

Systemic

Haemophagocytic lymphohistiocytosis (HLH)

This may be:

- **Primary** (familial or sporadic). Mutations in the perforin gene found (10q21–22) in some cases (with absent perforin granules in cytotoxic lymphocytes), or
- **Secondary** (to infections, immunosuppression, metabolic disorders, fat infusions or malignancy)

It is a disorder involving **immune dysregulation**. Cytotoxic lymphocyte defects have been found:

- CD8 and CD56 T cells in perforin gene defects
- NK cells in EB virus associated disease

Diagnostic criteria are:

- Fevers
- Splenomegaly
- Pancytopenia
- High triglyceride or low fibrinogen
- Typical histology (with haemophagocytosis)

Other features include lymphadenopathy, skin rash, LFT $\uparrow$, ferritin $\uparrow$.

Treatment is:

Primary disease	Chemotherapy then BMT if needed (persistent or familial disease)
Secondary disease	May resolve with treatment of the precipitating factor

Primary HLH is generally fatal without BMT.

Future pregnancy risk is 1:4 for familial disease and there are no predictive tests currently available.

Rosai-Dorfman disease (sinus histiocytosis with massive lymphadenopathy)

This is usually a benign disorder with spontaneous regression involving massive cervical lymphadenopathy, fever, weight loss and skin papules, nodules or plaques.

Cutaneous

Juvenile xanthogranuloma (JXG)

- Single or multiple yellow–orange papules
- Lipid-laden macrophages seen on histology
- Usually regresses over a few years
- Systemic involvement (most commonly ocular) is rare

CLASS III HISTIOCYTOSES

These are the malignant histiocytoses of monocytic/myeloid origin.

Examples   Acute monocytic leukaemia (M5)
               Acute myelomonocytic leukaemia (M4)

Treatment is with chemotherapy or SCT.

FURTHER READING

Pizzo PA, Poplack DG *Principles and Practice of Pediatric Oncology,* 5th edn. New York, Lippincott Raven, 2005

18
Neonatology

- *Neonatal definitions and statistics*
- *Antenatal screening and diagnosis*
- *Pregnancy food and drug advice*
- *Fetal medicine*
- *Congenital infections*
- *Delivery*
- *Normal newborn*
- *Infant feeding*
- *Birth injuries*
- *Intrapartum and postnatal infections*
- *Neonatal intensive care*

- *Intrauterine growth retardation*
- *Large for gestational age*
- *Prematurity*
- *Respiratory disorders*
- *Cardiac disorders*
- *Neurological disorders*
- *Neonatal convulsions and jitteriness*
- *Gastrointestinal disorders*
- *Osteopenia of prematurity*
- *Haematological disorders*
- *Hypoglycaemia*

NEONATAL DEFINITIONS AND STATISTICS

Definitions

Embryo	< 9 weeks' gestation
Fetus	9 weeks' gestation–delivery
Stillbirth	Fetal death and expulsion from the uterus > 24 weeks' gestation
Miscarriage/abortion	Fetal death and expulsion from the uterus < 24 weeks' gestation
Term	37–42 weeks
Neonate	Infant < 28 days old

Low birthweight (LBW)	Infant ≤ 2500 g at birth
Very low birthweight (VLBW)	Infant ≤ 1500 g at birth
Extremely low birthweight (ELBW)	Infant ≤ 1000 g at birth
Small for gestational age (SGA)	Birthweight < 10th centile
Large for gestational age (LGA)	Birthweight > 90th centile
Appropriate for gestational age (AGA)	Birthweight between the 10th–90th centiles

Mortality rates

Stillbirth rate	Number of stillbirths per 1000 deliveries
Perinatal mortality rate	Number of stillbirths + deaths within the first 7 days per 1000 deliveries
Neonatal mortality rate	Number of deaths of liveborn infants within 28 days of birth per 1000 live births
Post-neonatal mortality rate	Number of deaths between 28 days and 1 year per 1000 live births
Infant mortality rate	Number of deaths between birth and 1 year per 1000 live births

Birth statistics

Total UK births	650 000/year
Perinatal mortality rate (PNM)	6–10/1000

Predicted survival percentage for infants admitted for neonatal care (adapted from Draper E et al Tables for predicting survival for preterm births are updated. BMJ 2003;**327**:872)

By gestation

Gestation (weeks)	22	23	24	25	26	27	28	29	30
European male	18	27	39	53	67	79	88	93	97
European female	21	31	45	59	73	83	90	94	97
Asian	9	19	35	54	73	85	93	96	98

By birthweight

Birthweight (g)	250–500	500–750	750–1000	1000–1250	1250–1500	1500–1750	1750–2000
European male	7	37	75	91	96	98	99
European female	12	51	84	95	98	99	99
Asian	13	54	85	95	98	98	99

ANTENATAL SCREENING AND DIAGNOSIS

Test	Timing	Details
General maternal	< 12 weeks	Blood group and antibodies (Rhesus and other red cell antigens)
Blood tests		FBC
		Rubella, syphilis and hepatitis B serology
		HIV status (with maternal consent)
		Haemoglobinopathy screening (sickle and thalassaemia)
	28, 34 weeks	Rhesus Abs if Rh negative (at same time as IM anti-D)
	26 weeks	Oral glucose tolerance test or random blood sugar (some centres)
	34 weeks	FBC
Maternal urine	Regularly	Dipstick for glucose, leucocytes, nitrites and protein
Ultrasound scans		
Dating scan	8–12 weeks	(crown–rump length)
Nuchal scan	11–14 weeks	Nuchal fold thickness measured – ↑ in Down syndrome: <ul><li>77% sensitive for 5% false-positive rate</li><li>Improved to 92% by combining results of serum PAPP-A and inhibin levels sampled at similar gestation (**combined test**), and up to 97% if presence/absence of nasal bone is included</li><li>Gives an individual risk for Down, trisomy 13 and 18, and aids prediction of other genetic syndromes</li><li>Congenital cardiac anomalies and early onset twin–twin transfusion syndrome in monochorionic twins</li><li>Also acts as a dating scan, early anomaly scan and allows early diagnosis of twins and assessment of the uteroplacental circulation and cervical integrity (length)</li></ul>
Anomaly scan	20–24 weeks	Detailed scan to look for fetal growth and biometry consistent with gestational dates, major congenital malformations and soft markers for aneuploidy. Neural tube defect > 98% accuracy
Growth scans	> 20 weeks	Done only if concern about fetal growth or wellbeing
		Biparietal diameter (BPD), head circumference (HC), femur length (FL) and abdominal circumference (AC)

Disorders diagnosable by ultrasound at 20 week anomaly scan

Anencephaly	Gastroschisis	Diaphragmatic hernia
Encephalocoele	Exomphalos	Limb defects
Holoprosencephaly	Renal agenesis	Hydronephrosis (not a disorder as such)
Hydrocephalus	Cleft lip	
Polycystic kidneys	Congenital heart disease	
Hydrops fetalis	Skeletal abnormalities	

NB: If nuchal scanning is not available, at **14–22 weeks** maternal serum screening for Down and other trisomies is done (the **triple test**):

Maternal serum Free β-hCG ↑
Unconjugated oestradiol (uE3) ↓ } in Down's
α-Fetoprotein (AFP) ↓

Provides data to calculate an individual risk in a woman with known gestational dates with a 62% sensitivity for identifying as high risk of Down fetus for a 5% false-positive rate.

INVASIVE TESTS

Chorionic villous sampling (CVS)	11–14 weeks	1% procedure-related risk (overall 3–4%) of miscarriage. Chorionic villous cells sampled. Earlier than amniocentesis
		• *Chromosome analysis* (PCR – 24 h result informing on major trisomies and sex chromosome aneuploidies. Full karyotype reporting in 10–14 days of cell culture)
		• *Enzyme analysis* (inborn errors of metabolism)
		• *Congenital infection* (viral particle DNA using PCR)
Amniocentesis	16 weeks onwards	1% procedure-related risk (overall 1.5–2%) of miscarriage
		• Tests as for CVS using fetal cells in amniotic fluid
Fetal blood sampling	> 20 weeks	Used to confirm suspicions of severe fetal anaemia or thrombocytopenia due to alloimmunization requiring intrauterine transfusion of RBCs or platelets as part of the same procedure

Future screening methods

Non-invasive techniques are being developed. These include:

- Diagnostic techniques using fetal DNA obtained from fetal cells in the maternal circulation or free fetal DNA in maternal plasma
- 3D USS
- Fetal MRI scanning } Looking for structural anomalies

PREGNANCY FOOD AND DRUG ADVICE

Things to take

Supplements Folic acid:
- Pre-conceptually *and* for the first trimester
- Reduces incidence of neural tube defects
- (Low dose all women [400 μg daily], high dose [5 mg daily] if previous neural tube defect)

Foods Oily fish:
- Important for neonatal brain development.
- Omega-3 oils reduce incidence of preterm labour
- (Avoid excess salmon or tuna due to high mercury content)

Things to avoid

Foods	Non-pasteurized products, soft cheeses	
	Pâté, chicken, raw vegetables	
	Over the counter warm pre-cooked meats	*Listeria monocytogenes* (see p. 452)
	Blue vein cheeses	
	Uncooked and smoked meats (lamb or pork)	
	Raw eggs, e.g. mayonnaise	Toxoplasmosis
	Unwashed fruits and vegetables	
	Liver – keep to minimum as the high levels of vitamin A it contains are potentially teratogenic	
Drugs	Avoid all drugs if possible due to possible teratogenic effects (see below)	
	No routine iron	
	Drug abuse – teratogenic effects (not opiates), fetal ischaemia with cocaine, IUGR, placental abruption, prematurity, neonatal addiction	
	Alcohol (limit quantity) – fetal alcohol syndrome if excessive alcohol (> 6 units/day)	
Smoking	Avoid – IUGR, increased risk of miscarriage, stillbirth and SIDS (including passive smoking from partner/work/social)	
Cats and cat litter	Avoid – toxoplasmosis risk from cat faeces	

FETAL MEDICINE

Fetal medicine is concerned with **antenatal detection, pregnancy management and treatment** (where applicable) of fetal disorders. This includes:

- **Antenatal screening** (see above) and additional diagnostic tests where indicated, including interventional tests, e.g. CVS, and counselling of options should they be abnormal
- Genetic counselling
- **Treatment during pregnancy** (see below) and termination of pregnancy where appropriate

---

FETAL THERAPY

Multiple fetal pregnancy reduction	Triplets and other higher multiples
Selective termination	Abnormality in multiple pregnancy
Laser ablation/multiple amniocentesis/selective fetocide	Severe twin–twin transfusion syndrome
Shunting for megacystis	Posterior urethral valves, pleural effusion
Fetal blood sampling	Intravascular transfusion (alloimmune red cell and platelet disorders)
	Diagnosis of fetal karyotype, infection, genetic, metabolic, biochemical abnormality
	Rarely for intrauterine therapy, e.g. antiarrhythmic drugs in persistent fetal tachycardia
Amniodrainage	Polyhydramnios (prevents preterm labour and unstable lie)
Amnioinfusion	Diagnostic – confirms ruptured membranes, better visualization of certain defects, e.g. renal agenesis
Needle aspiration of cysts	Megacystis, ovarian, lung, bowel
Laser ablation of tumours	Sacrococcygeal teratomas, cardiac rhabdomyomas

HIGH-RISK PREGNANCIES

Pregnancies are classified as high-risk due to:

Pre-existing maternal disease	**Chronic disease**, e.g. diabetes mellitus, heart disease, renal disease, asthma
	Nutritional disorders resulting in excessively low or high BMI and deficient dietary intake
	Maternal alloimmune disease (see below)
Antenatally detected fetal disorder	**Identified genetic abnormality**, e.g. Down syndrome, cystic fibrosis
	Fetal structural abnormality diagnosed via antenatal USS, e.g. spina bifida, renal abnormality
	Fetal arrhythmia
Pregnancy complication/indication	Multiple pregnancy
	Oligo- or poly-hydramnios
	Antepartum haemorrhage
	Pregnancy induced hypertension and pre-eclampsia (toxaemia of pregnancy)

MULTIPLE PREGNANCY

- Twin, triplet and higher multiple pregnancies are associated with specific increased risks to both the mother and the fetuses
- Establishing chorionicity (indirect aids zygosity testing) in the first trimester gives best results
- Growth discordance affects all twins after 32 weeks (monochorionic more so). Triplets > 30 weeks
- Regular scanning in pregnancy required – dichorionic: 4 weekly; monochorionic: 2 weekly

Monozygotic (identical)

- Single fertilized egg, incidence 3.5:1000 pregnancies
- These may be: Single chorion and amnion
  - Mixed (separate amnion, but monochorionic), or
  - Separate chorion and amnion
- Risk: twin–twin transfusion syndrome. A monoamniotic pregnancy may also lead to fatal cord entanglement and locked twins at delivery

Dizygotic (non-identical)

- Familial, variable rate. 1:66 spontaneous rate
- Two separately fertilized eggs
- Dichorionic placenta

Risks associated with multiple pregnancy

- Prematurity
- IUGR, discordant growth
- Asphyxia

- Second twin at particularly increased risk of asphyxia, trauma and respiratory distress syndrome
- Monozygotic twins: Increased congenital anomalies

  If single chorion and amnion: twin–twin transfusion syndrome, cord entanglement, discordant growth
- Increased fetal and maternal mortality

Twin–twin transfusion syndrome

This can occur *in utero* between monochorionic twins, i.e. share the same placenta, and is defined as a difference in Hb of > 5 g between the twins. If untreated, death of both twins occurs in > 90%; if treated, both twins survive in 66%. Essentially one twin has the majority of the placental blood flow (and nutrients), and hence grows larger and is plethoric, while the other twin is anaemic and smaller. It is the large plethoric twin who is at higher risk because diminished blood flow through smaller vessels (secondary to high haematocrit) can cause multiorgan damage.

Anaemic twin	Plethoric twin
IUGR	May have IUGR
Preterm delivery	Preterm delivery
Severe anaemia	*Cardiac*: cardiac failure and pulmonary hypertension
Hydrops fetalis	*CNS*: apnoeas and seizures
	Gastro: NEC
	Renal: renal vein thrombosis
	Other: hypoglycaemia, hypocalcaemia, jaundice

Antenatal treatments include amnioreduction (repeated removal of amniotic fluid) and laser septostomy, or selective fetal reduction.

MATERNAL DISEASES ASSOCIATED WITH MALFORMATIONS AND NEONATAL DISORDERS

- Maternal illness has a *general impact* on fetal growth and wellbeing, e.g. pre-eclampsia, chronic renal disease
- They can cause **fetal malformations**, e.g. diabetes, **fetal damage**, **premature delivery** or result in **temporary neonatal disease** due to a maternal transfer of IgG antibodies (IgG will cross the placenta), e.g. autoimmune thrombocytopenia. Sometimes, a transient transfer of antibodies can result in permanent consequences for the infant, e.g. congenital heart block in maternal lupus

Examples

Maternal illness	Malformation/disorder
Diabetes mellitus	Macrosomia (difficult labour), transient neonatal hypoglycaemia (from fetal hyperinsulinism) RDS, polycythaemia x 2 risk of any congenital anomaly Caudal regression syndrome (sacral agenesis) Renal vein thrombosis CHD, e.g. VSD, coarctation, TGA, hypertrophic subaortic Stenosis, hypertrophic obstructive cardiomyopathy
Phenylketonuria	CHD, microcephaly, mental retardation (only if high maternal phenylalanine levels during pregnancy) (see p. 00)
Placental antibody transfer	
Rhesus disease	Fetal anaemia
Lupus erythematosis	Neonatal lupus, congenital heart block (see p. 106)
Hyperthyroidism	Transient neonatal thyrotoxicosis (see p. 245)
Autoimmune thrombocytopenia	Transient neonatal thrombocytopenia
Myasthenia gravis	Transient neonatal disease and arthrogryphosis (see p. 367)

CONGENITAL INFECTIONS

Cytomegalovirus (2000/year in the UK)	Herpes simplex virus (HSV)
Rubella (6 cases in last 5 years in the UK)	Neisseria gonorrhoea
Toxoplasmosis	Listeria monocytogenes
Varicella	Group B streptococcus
HIV	*Escherichia coli*
Chlamydia trachomatis	Hepatitis A, B and C
Malaria	Parvovirus B19
Syphilis	

Vertical transmission may be:

- Transplacental
- Intrapartum (cervical secretions, haematogenous) or
- Postnatal (breast milk, saliva, urine)

Features that would arouse suspicion of a congenital infection:

- IUGR
- Petechial rash
- Hepatosplenomegaly
- Brain – fits, microcephaly, developmental delay, calcification
- Eye – cataracts, chorioretinitis, microphthalmia
- Deafness

- Cardiac defects
- Pneumonitis

Congenital infection may also result in miscarriage or stillbirth.

CYTOMEGALOVIRUS (CMV)

- Most common congenital infection. Approximate incidence: 2000/year in the UK live births
- 50% fetal infections are asymptomatic, around 5% will have clinical infection at birth, others presenting later. Up to 10% develop neurological sequelae (mainly deafness)
- Primary maternal CMV infection during pregnancy is associated with a worse prognosis than reactivation. It can be postnatally acquired

Clinical features

Brain **Cerebral periventricular calcifications**
  Sensorineural deafness (can be progressive)
  Developmental delay (mild or severe)
  Microcephaly, encephalitis
IUGR
Skin **Petechial rash**
Liver **Hepatosplenomegaly, jaundice**
Lungs **Pneumonitis** (usually with postnatally acquired)
Eyes Chorioretinitis, optic atrophy
Teeth Dental defects

Diagnosis

Urine PCR, blood PCR.

TOXOPLASMOSIS

Intracellular parasite, acquired from raw meat, unwashed vegetables and fruit, and cat faeces (kittens with primary infection can be high excretors).

Incidence of primary maternal infection during pregnancy is 1:1000. The risk of infant infection is inversely related to gestational age at the time of primary maternal infection:

First trimester maternal infection 15% risk
Second trimester infection 45% risk
Third trimester infection 65% risk

The severity of disease in the infant is dependent on the gestation. Highest risk at 24–30 weeks. Overall 10% have clinical features.

The recent BPSU study, however, found 12 cases per year in the UK, highlighting an inconsistency between the above figures.

Clinical features

Infection particularly affects the developing brain. Most have *no* apparent symptoms, but intracranial calcification is often present with neurological consequences.

Brain **Cerebral calcifications diffusely scattered dense, round lesions, basal ganglia curvilinear streaks**
  Seizures, hydrocephalus, microcephaly, encephalitis, developmental delay (mild or severe)

Eyes   **Chorioretinitis, cataract**
Liver   **Hepatosplenomegaly, jaundice**
Blood   **Anaemia**
Lungs   Pneumonitis

CONGENITAL RUBELLA

This is now very rare (only 6 cases reported in the UK in the last 5 years).

Risk and severity are dependent on gestation at maternal infection:

Very high risk   < 8 weeks gestation
High risk   < 18 weeks
Low risk   > 18 weeks

Clinical features

Eyes   **Cataracts, corneal opacities, glaucoma, microphthalmia**
Brain   **Sensorineural deafness**, psychomotor delay (mild to severe), behavioural problems, autism, progressive degenerative brain disorder
Liver   **Hepatosplenomegaly**, hepatitis
Skin/haem   **Petechial rash, thrombocytopenia**
Cardiac   **PDA, pulmonary artery stenosis, aortic stenosis, VSDs**
Lung   Pneumonitis
Bone   **Radiolucent bone lesions**
IUGR
Endocrine   Juvenile diabetes, thyroid disorders, precocious puberty

Diagnosis

Urine and blood rubella-specific IgM ↑.

VARICELLA

Congenital varicella infection

Primary maternal infection during pregnancy may rarely (< 2% of cases of maternal infection) produce **congenital varicella syndrome**:

Skin   Cicatrix (zigzag scarring), skin loss
Limbs   Malformation and shortening, paresis
Eyes   Cataracts, chorioretinitis, microphthalmia
CNS   Microcephaly, hydrocephaly, brain aplasia

It is thought to result from viral reactivation *in utero* rather than the initial fetal infection.

Maternal chicken pox around delivery (< 5 days pre–2 days after)

May cause *severe* chicken pox illness in the infant (high titres of virus, with no maternal antibodies yet made to protect the infant). These infants are given:

- Anti-varicella zoster IgG (VZIG) IM (post-exposure prophylaxis)
- If any vesicles develop, commence IV aciclovir

Indications to give VZIG to baby

- Maternal infection < 5 days pre–2 days after delivery
- < 28 weeks' gestation or < 1000 g, regardless of maternal history (little antibody crosses placenta < third trimester)
- Other babies on the ward who may have been exposed if < 28 weeks' gestation or mother non-immune

LISTERIA MONOCYTOGENES

This may be acquired transplacentally or by ascending infection and may present in different ways.

Source   Unpasturized cheeses and milk products, soft cheeses, chicken, raw vegetables
Uncooked meats, over-the-counter reheated foods

Clinical features

- Premature delivery, abortion or stillbirth, maternal flu-like illness
- Meconium passed *in utero* (in premature delivery)
- Pneumonia, meningitis, septicaemia
- Disseminated infection (fits, rash and hepatosplenomegaly)
- Hydrocephalus is a common sequelae

Treatment

Ampicillin IV and gentamicin IV.

CONGENITAL SYPHILIS

High transmission rate, 40% mortality untreated.

Clinical features

Infancy   Snuffles, congenital nephrotic syndrome, glaucoma, chorioretinitis
Hepatosplenomegaly, lymphadenopathy, osteochondritis, periostitis
Rash (desquamation hands and feet, maculopapular, bullous, condylomata)
Childhood   **Hutchinson teeth** (peg-shaped incisors with central notch)
(>2 years) **Sabre tibia**, saddle nose deformity, frontal bossing
Meningovascular involvement
Optic atrophy, corneal calcification (blindness), photophobia
Vertigo and deafness (VIII nerve involvement)
Paroxysmal nocturnal haemoglobinuria

OTHER CONGENITAL INFECTIONS

- Hepatitis B (see p. 192)
- HIV (see p. 36)
- Parvovirus B19 (see p. 53)

DELIVERY

RESUSCITATION

A minority of infants do not establish respiration rapidly after birth (they are 'flat'), and they need immediate assessment and intervention. Apgar scores are performed on all babies directly after birth (at 1, 5 and 10 min after birth, and longer if necessary) in order to assess their condition. These are a poorly predictive indicator of later adverse outcome. Five parameters are assessed, each scoring 0–2, and the total (out of 10) give the **Apgar** at that time.

Apgar scores

	Score		
Physical sign	**0**	**1**	**2**
Appearance	Pale	Blue extremities	Pink
Pulse	Absent	< 100 bpm	> 100 bpm
Grimace on suction	None	Grimace	Cry, cough
Activity	Flaccid	Some limb flexion	Active
Respiratory effort	Absent	Irregular	Regular

Basic resuscitation	Start the clock
	Dry and stimulate baby, and keep it warm
	Bag and mask ventilation
	External cardiac massage
Advanced resuscitation	Endotracheal intubation and ventilation
	Drug therapy
	Blood/fluid therapy via umbilical venous catheter
	Transfer to NICU

NB: Infants of 3 kg lose 1°C per min in ambient theatre temperature.

Drug therapy

Adrenaline IV or ETT	0.1–0.3 ml/kg of 1:10 000 (10 µg/kg) repeated as needed every 3–5 min
	0.1 ml/kg of 1:1000 (100 µg/kg) if required after two doses as above
Glucose 10% IV	2 ml/kg
Blood/4.5% albumin	10–20 ml/kg
Sodium bicarbonate (4.2% soln) IV	1 mmol/kg

ETT sizes and lengths		
Weight	**ETT size**	**ETT length (tip-to-lip)**
1 kg	2.5	7 cm
2 kg	3.0	8 cm
3 kg	3.5	9 cm
4 kg	3.5/4.0	$\geqslant$ 9 cm

HIGH-RISK DELIVERIES

Fetal/delivery	Maternal conditions
Acute fetal hypoxia (fetal distress)	Pyrexia
Meconium-stained liquor	Diabetes hyperthyroidism
Preterm delivery/big baby/small baby	Severe pre-eclampsia/toxaemia
Difficult airway, e.g. face presentation, hypertonus, laryngomalacia, tumour)	Any severe chronic illness, e.g. cardiac or renal disease
Instrumental delivery (hypoxia, intracranial bleed, fractures, cervical and brachial plexus injury, shoulder dystocia)	Autoimmune disorder with placental antibody transfer, e.g. Rhesus disease, AITP, myasthenia gravis
Caesarian (dependent on indication) (direct fetal laceration/trauma. Head may be stuck in second stage with breech)	
Multiple pregnancy	
Abnormal baby	
Breech vaginal delivery	

NORMAL NEWBORN

NEONATAL EXAMINATION

All infants should be given a general examination within 24 h of birth.

Measurements Gestational age, weight (length), head circumference
General Appearance (dysmorphic), posture, movements
Skin Colour (cyanosis, jaundice, anaemic, plethoric), birthmarks
Head Fontanelles (normal size, pressure, fused sutures), head shape
Face Features of dysmorphism
Ears Size, formation, position
Mouth Size, other abnormality (cleft lip/palate), neonatal teeth
Palate Inspect and palpate (cleft palate), sucking reflex checked
Eyes Red reflex, discharge, colobomas, size
Neck Any swellings (cystic hygroma, sternomastoid 'tumour')
Respiratory Respiratory movements, rate, auscultation
Cardiovascular Auscultation, femoral pulses
Abdominal Palpation (masses)
Genitalia Inspection (malformations, ambiguous genitalia), testes (both fully descended)
Anus Patent. NB: Meconium normally passes within 48 h of birth (and within 24 h in 95%). Most units ask surgeons to review if no meconium by 24 h
Back Check spine (midline defects)
Muscle tone Observation and holding baby prone
Reflexes Moro reflex
Hips Check for CDH (see below). Enquire if breech or family history in which case a hip USS is arranged

NEONATAL HIP EXAMINATION

The baby should be relaxed while this is carried out.

The pelvis is **stabilized** with one hand and the middle finger of the other hand is placed over the greater trochanter and the thumb around the femur. The hip is **flexed**. Then:

Barlow manoeuvre	To check if the hip is dislocatable
	The femoral head is gently pushed downwards. If dislocatable, the femoral head will be pushed out of the acetabulum with a clunk
Ortolani manoeuvre	To see if the hip is dislocated and can be relocated into the acetabulum
	The hip is abducted and upward pressure applied by the finger on the greater trochanter. If the hip was dislocated, it will clunk back into position

NB: Insignificant mild **clicks** due to ligaments may be heard.

VITAMIN K

- Prophylactic vitamin K is recommended for all newborns to prevent haemorrhagic disease of the newborn
- Vitamin K is given intramuscularly, or orally shortly after birth if bottle feeding
- Oral vitamin K given after birth, at 1 week and at 6 weeks if breast feeding

Haemorrhagic disease of the newborn

- Due to low vitamin K-dependent clotting factors at birth (immature liver, low gut bacteria) and a further fall in breast-fed babies (breast milk is a poor source of vitamin K)
- Presents as bleeding on day 2–6, usually mild but may be catastrophic
- Late presentation (rarely) may occur up to 6 weeks
- If bleeding occurs, give IV vitamin K, FFP, blood and plasma as needed and check for hepatic dysfunction, e.g. α_1-antitrypsin deficiency

Now rare (< 10 cases per year in the UK).

GUTHRIE TEST

This is a biochemical screen to detect some metabolic defects and is performed on all infants at the end of the first week of life via a blood test (usually a heel prick sample). The screen can detect:

Disease	Compound detected
Phenylketonuria	Phenylalanine
Hypothyroidism	TSH level
Not universal:	
Cystic fibrosis	IRT
Galactosaemia	Galactose
Maple syrup urine disease	Leucine
Homocystinuria	Methionine
Histidinaemia	Histidine
Sickle, haemoglobinopathy screen	

(It is often also used anonymously to determine prevalence of HIV within a population.)

Tandom mass spectroscopy is used to detect the rare metabolic conditions.

INFANT FEEDING

Infant requirements

Infant feeding	Purely milk feeding for the first 4-6 months	
	Then solid food is gradually introduced (**weaning**)	
Energy requirements	Term	100
(kcal/kg/day)	Premature	120
	SGA	140
Vitamin supplementation	Vitamin A (iu)	500–1500
(recommended daily dosage)	Vitamin D (iu)	400
	Vitamin E (iu)	5
	Vitamin C (mg)	35
	Folate (µg)	50

Breast milk

- For the first few days it is composed of **colostrum** (thick bright yellow–orange) with high protein, phospholipid, cholesterol and immunoglobulin content
- Major differences to formula milk:
  Casein:whey ratio (high whey in breast milk)
  Fat (higher in breast milk)
  Na, Ca, phosphorus
  Vitamin K } Lower in breast milk
  Iron
- Cow's milk is vastly different, and therefore should not be used as a substitute

Breast feeding

Establishment	In the first few days after birth is critical. It is important that time and energy is used to help the mother at this critical time
	Cup feeds of formula milk should be used if additional feeding is necessary whilst tying to establish breast feeding (to avoid nipple confusion)
Continuation	Proven to benefit the baby for the first 6 months and recommended by the WHO
	Many women commence well, but then stop after only a few weeks
	69% of women initiated breast feeding in 2000. At 6 weeks, 42% were still breast feeding and 21% at 6 months
	Higher social classes have higher rates of breast feeding
	Help is available from breast-feeding councillors and health visitors in particular

Advantages

- **Nutrition optimum**, e.g. fatty acids, arachidonic acid and docosohexaenoic acid needed for infant brain development
- Immunological protection transferred (IgA especially). In the developing world it gives very significant protection against respiratory and gastrointestinal diseases
- Uterine involution (oxytocin release) and maternal weight loss expediated
- Contraceptive (lactation amenorrhoea) – as effective as the combined oral contraceptive pill during first 6 months

- Convenient and cheap
- Decreases the risk of breast cancer (x 4.3 % per year of breast feeding)
- Reduces incidence of atopic disease throughout childhood and adolescence
- Helps to establish maternal–infant bonding

Problems

Social	It is finally becoming socially acceptable
Fatigue	The mother need not do all the feeding, as expressed breast milk can be given by other carers
Financial	The mother cannot go back to work while fully breast feeding (though some milk may be expressed at work, depending on the type of employment). It may be financially necessary for the mother to return to work prior to 6 months after delivery, though the current direction of employment legislation is toward providing prolonged maternity pay (up to 2 years in some countries)

Twins and higher multiples can be breast fed, though often supplemental formula feeds are necessary.

Reasons for not breast feeding

Maternal	Infant
Maternal drugs, e.g. cytotoxics } Contraindications Maternal HIV (in UK)	Acute illness
Unable to establish feeding	Cleft lip/palate (may manage breast feeding)
Maternal dislike	Metabolic disease, e.g. galactosaemia
Breast abscess (can use other breast)	
Maternal acute illness	
NB: Inverted nipples is not a contraindication	

Special infant formulae

Milk substitute	Composition
Nutramigen	Casein hydrolysate (protein hydrolysed to peptides of 15 amino acids or less)
Pregestamil	Casein hydrolysate
Peptijunior	Partial whey hydrolysate (contains some peptides of > 15 amino acids)
Neocate	Amino acids
These formulae are used for cow's milk protein allergy and lactose deficiency. Soya-based milks are not recommended as there is cross-reactivity with cow's milk protein intolerance of approximately 40%.	

Weaning

This is the introduction of solid food and is done gradually from around 6 months (or 4 months). Different puréed foods are introduced every few days initially. Babies generally like sweet things (as breast milk is very sweet), but it is important to introduce a wide variety of flavours early. Cow's milk should not be introduced before 1 year.

BIRTH INJURIES

HEAD INJURIES

Caput succedaneum	Very common. Bruising and oedema of the presenting part of the head
Chignon	Bruising from a Ventouse suction cap.
Cephalhaematoma	A bleed beneath the periosteum due to torn veins (therefore limited to one skull bone)
	Resolves spontaneously over a few weeks

Complications: Neonatal jaundice
Underlying skull fracture (present in 20% but rarely needs treatment)
Associated intracranial haemorrhage
Eventual calcification (leaving permanent bump on head)

Subaponeurotic haemorrhage	An uncommon bleed beneath the occipitofrontalis aponeurosis
	This may spread over the scalp to become large and result in shock. High mortality if not diagnosed

NERVE INJURIES

Erb palsy	Common injury (1:2000 deliveries) to the upper nerve roots of the brachial plexus (C5, 6 $\pm$ 7)
	Often follows shoulder dystocia
	Arm held in adduction, elbow extended, internally rotated, forearm pronated and wrist flexed (**'waiter's tip'** position)
	A few also have phrenic nerve involvement (causing ipsilateral diaphragmatic paralysis, a pneumothorax and/or Horner syndrome)
Facial nerve palsy	Mostly LMN due to forceps injury, prolonged pressure on maternal sacral promontory
	A few are UMN secondary to brain injury or nuclear agenesis (Moebius syndrome)
	The lesions are difficult to distinguish clinically and result in an asymmetrical face when crying and inability to close the eye on the affected side
Klumpke palsy	Injury to the lower (C7 + 8 + T1) nerve roots of the brachial plexus
	A wrist drop and paralysis of the small muscles of the hand result in 'claw hand'
	Around 30% also have a Horner syndrome

Management

Physiotherapy is given to prevent contractures. If there is no improvement at 2–3 months, refer to specialist unit. For facial nerve injury, eye patching and artificial tears are needed if eye closure incomplete.

MUSCLE INJURY

Sternomastoid tumour	Injury to the sternocleidomastoid muscle. May be from traumatic delivery or secondary to position *in utero*
	Manifest as a firm **swelling** within the sternomastoid muscle and a **torticollis**
	Swift and regular physiotherapy (taught to parents) results in resolution of the swelling over a few weeks.
	The preferential turning of the head to one side only can result in plagiocephaly and permanent postural deformity

BONE INJURIES

Clavicle fracture	Most common delivery injury, often not detected.
	Heals on its own but may need analgesia
	Seen in large babies with impacted shoulders, e.g. infant of diabetic mother
Humerus fracture	Usually upper third fractured. Radial nerve injury may occur
	Heals on its own but may need analgesia and immobilization

INTRAPARTUM AND POSTNATAL INFECTIONS

Infections which may be acquired during delivery

Sepsis (Group B β-haemolytic streptococcus, *Escherichia coli, Staphylococcus epidermidis*)

Conjunctivitis (see p. 382)

Herpes simplex

Umbilical infection (*E. coli, Staph. aureus*)

HIV infection

Chlamydia trachomatis

Gonococcal infection

GROUP B β-HAEMOLYTIC STREPTOCOCCUS (GBS)

Colonization of the vagina with Group B *β-haemolytic streptococcus* occurs in approximately 30% of women. At least 10% of babies will become colonized during delivery. 1% of colonized babies develop Group B strep sepsis, with about a 10% mortality (= 70 deaths in the UK/year).

Risk factors for sepsis are maternal pyrexia, premature rupture of membranes or the infant is preterm and inadequate labour prophylaxis was given (the infant should be treated).

Group B streptococcal neonatal infection causes *serious* disease with:

- **Early** lethargy, poor feeding, temperature instability, irritability, apnoeas, jaundice. Then features of sepsis and shock, meningitis and pneumonia
- **Late-onset** from 48 h

Investigations

- FBC, CRP and septic screen (blood culture in particular)
- CXR (diffuse or lobular changes)
- Check maternal high vaginal swab result

Treatment

Intravenous antibiotics, e.g. gentamicin and penicillin.

There is now increasing pressure to establish a mother's Group B streptococcus status before delivery and to give intrapartum prophylaxis with penicillin or clindamycin to colonized mothers.

NB: Any neonate in whom serious infection is suspected should be covered for Group B β-haemolytic streptococcus.

Causes of neonatal sepsis and meningitis

- Group B β-haemolytic streptococcus
- *Escherichia coli*
- *Staphylococcus epidermidis*

NEONATAL HERPES SIMPLEX INFECTION

Rare. In the UK the incidence is approximately 2:100 000 live births.

Acquired from the birth canal during delivery (in most cases the mother is asymptomatic). Primary maternal infection (with the greatest risk to the infant) during pregnancy is rare.

- Primary maternal infection – up to 50% infants infected
- Recurrent maternal infection – 3% infants infected
- Increased risk of neonatal infection with IUGR, prematurity, prolonged rupture of membranes (> 6 h) and fetal scalp monitoring (direct viral skin inoculation)

Infection may be localized skin vesicles only or widespread vesicles develop within the first week of life and rapid CNS involvement develops (meningoencephalitis). Infection in neonates may be severe (mortality 80% untreated).

Treatment is intravenous aciclovir.

CHLAMYDIA TRACHOMATIS

Chlamydia is found in the vagina in 4% of pregnant women and 70% of infected babies are asymptomatic.

Clinical features

- Conjuctivitis (purulent, like gonococcal) presenting in the 2nd week; cf. gonococcal presenting on days 1–2
- Pneumonia (may be present at 1–3 months of age), middle ear infection

Diagnosis

Organism identified on Giemsa staining and culture on special medium and immunofluorescence.

Treatment

- Oral erythromycin
- Tetracycline eye drops

UMBILICAL INFECTION

Omphalitis is umbilical stump infection. **Funisitis** is umbilical cord infection.

Usually due to *Staph. aureus* or *E. coli*. May lead to portal vein infection with subsequent portal hypertension.

Management

- Swab umbilicus (M, C & S)
- Gentle cleansing
- IV antibiotics if signs of spread (cellulitis around umbilicus)

NEONATAL INTENSIVE CARE

The neonatal intensive care unit (NICU) is a specialist unit to provide care to premature and sick neonates.

THERMAL STABILITY

Incubators provide a stable warm environment designed to be **thermoneutral**, i.e. neither too hot requiring the neonate to expend energy to keep cool, nor too cool requiring the neonate to expend energy to keep warm.

MONITORING

Heart rate	
Respiratory rate	
Temperature	
(ambient and that of infant)	
BP	Via umbilical artery or peripheral arterial line
	Or BP cuff (less accurate)
Oxygenation	Pulse oximetry (O_2 saturation)
	Transcutaneous (O_2 tension)
CO_2 levels	Transcutaneous (CO_2 tension)
Blood gases	Transcutaneous, via arterial line or capillary analysis from heel prick samples
Bloods	Regular samples (heel prick, venous or via arterial line) to monitor gases and blood glucose

Blood gas acid–base monitoring

The following **disturbances** may exist:

Acidosis	**Respiratory acidosis** (high CO_2), e.g. underventilated
	Metabolic acidosis (low bicarbonate), e.g. sick infant
Alkalosis	**Respiratory alkalosis** (low CO_2), e.g. overventilated
	Metabolic alkalosis (high bicarbonate)

These will be **compensated** for (but never enough to bring the pH to normal) by:

- Metabolic means by altering the bicarbonate level
- Respiratory means by altering the CO_2 level

To calculate the disturbance present:

1. Look at the pH to decide if acidosis or alkalosis
2. Look at the CO_2 and bicarbonate to see which one has caused this primary defect
3. Look at the other agent (CO_2 or bicarbonate) to confirm that it is trying to compensate (if not, a mixed picture exists)

VENTILATION

Ambient oxygen (room air) or oxygen via head box/in incubator may be sufficient.

Continuous positive airway pressure (CPAP)

Continuous flow of oxygen via nasal cannulae, face mask, or endotracheal tube. This keeps the terminal bronchials open in respiration and prevents them from collapsing.

Intermittent positive pressure ventilation (IPPV)

There are different types of IPPV:

Continuous mandatory ventilation (CMV)	Full ventilation
Intermittent mandatory ventilation (IMV)	Only occasional breaths given by the ventilator
	Used to wean a baby who is making some respiratory effort off the ventilator
Patient triggered ventilation (PTV)	Ventilator assists breath after triggered by baby
	Used to wean babies off the ventilator

Paralysis and sedation may be required for ventilation if a baby is struggling and 'fighting' the ventilator.

Ventilators

Ventilators are pressure and time cycled. Adjustments may be made to:

FiO$_2$	As low as able to avoid retinopathy of prematurity	
Rate	A fast rate will reduce CO$_2$	
Pressure	**PIP**	Peak inspiratory pressure
	PEEP	Positive end expiratory pressure. Used while ventilating, acts as CPAP does
	High pressures needed for stiff lungs (low compliance) but risk of pneumothorax	
Time	Inspiratory and expiratory times and their relative ratio may be altered	

High frequency oscillatory ventilation (HFOV)

Very high frequency rate (10 Hz or 600/min) ventilation via ETT. Useful in infants with severe lung disease, e.g. meconium aspiration syndrome.

Extracorporeal membrane oxygenation (ECMO)

Used only if other ventilatory methods fail in severe cases, and particularly useful for meconium aspiration syndrome in which the lungs are very stiff, and for ventilation perfusion (V:Q) mismatch. The extracorporeal circuit oxygenates the blood outside of the body. It can only be used on infants > 2.5 kg, and is only available in a few UK centres.

Complications and contraindications include intracranial haemorrhage (heparinization is necessary for ECMO).

Nitric oxide

A specific vasodilator acting particularly on the pulmonary artery smooth muscle. Produced by vascular endothelium and macrophages. It also acts as a vasodilator via increasing cGMP levels. Therefore used in persistent pulmonary hypertension of the newborn (PPHN) to decrease pulmonary hypertension (see p. 470).

Side-effects	Methaemoglobinaemia
	Platelet function affected

CIRCULATORY SUPPORT

Intravenous fluids given as 10% dextrose with added electrolytes (sodium 2–3 mmol/kg/day, potassium 2 mmol/kg/day and calcium 1 mmol/kg/day). The daily amount of fluid (ml/kg/day) increases over the first few days of life, and then stabilizes. Inotropes, e.g. dopamine and dobutamine, given if needed (if the mean arterial pressure is low). TPN can be given from day 1 if a long stay is anticipated.

FEEDING

Enteral feeds	Breast or formula milk.
	Given by breast or bottle (usually able if > 34 weeks' gestation) or bolus nasogastric feeds if unable to feed
	NB: Special formulae exist for premature infants who require a very high calorie intake
Total parenteral nutrition (TPN)	Used if enteral feeds are not tolerated or contraindicated, e.g. extreme prematurity, NEC
	Given via umbilical venous catheter (UVC) or a peripheral long line
	High calorie feed individually prepared to provide each infant's nutritional requirements (fat, carbohydrate, protein, elements, iron, calcium and trace metals)

Complications: Sepsis
TPN cholestasis
Microemboli

Supplements

Children's vitamin drops	Started when enteral feeds commenced until age 5 years
Iron	Commence oral supplements (if bodyweight < 2.5 kg or < 36 weeks' gestation) when 4 weeks old until on solid feeds

INTRAUTERINE GROWTH RETARDATION (IUGR)

Growth may be restricted *in utero* for many reasons. This is sometimes defined as growth < 3rd centile and sometimes < 10th centile.

The term IUGR (also known as small for gestational age [SGA]) should be reserved for those infants who have not reached their genetic potential.

These babies may be:

Asymmetrical	Weight on lower centile than head circumference due to relative sparing of the brain
	Due to placental failure late in pregnancy
	Have rapid weight gain after birth

Causes: Pre-eclampsia
Multiple gestation
Maternal cardiac or renal disease
Uterine malformation

Symmetrical	Head and body equally small
	Results from prolonged intrauterine growth failure
	Fetus is usually normal, though may be abnormal
	Postnatal growth is also poor

Causes: Smoking, malnutrition, chronic illness
Chromosomal disorder
Congenital infection

Associated problems

- Hypoglycaemia (small fat and glycogen stores). Need frequent feeds
- Hypothermia (large surface area:weight ratio and not much fat insulation)
- Infection
- Hypoxic–ischaemic encephalopathy (HIE)
- Hypocalcaemia
- Polycythaemia

LARGE FOR GESTATIONAL AGE (LGA)

Large for gestational age (LGA) is newborn weight > 90th percentile.

Causes

- Diabetic mother
- Familial, i.e. large parents
- Beckwith–Wiedemann syndrome

Associated problems

- Hypoglycaemia (hyperinsulinism)
- Birth trauma (difficult delivery)
- Hypoxic ischaemic encephalopathy (difficult delivery)
- Polycythaemia

PREMATURITY

Prematurity is birth at < 37 weeks' gestation. Many premature infants are small but appropriate for gestational age (AGA) due to prematurity.

Survival rates have increased dramatically over recent years but a significant proportion of extremely premature infants will have chronic disability if they survive.

SPECIFIC PROBLEMS ASSOCIATED WITH PREMATURITY

Temperature	Thermal instability. Temperature regulations mechanisms not fully developed and low body fat
Lungs	Apnoeas, respiratory distress syndrome (RDS), pneumothorax, pulmonary haemorrhage, broncho-pulmonary dysplasia (BPD)
Cardiac	Patent ductus arteriosus (PDA) (see p. 93), persistent pulmonary hypertension of the newborn (PPHN)
CNS	Apnoeas, hypoxic–ischaemic encephalopathy (HIE), intracranial haemorrhage, lack of primitive reflexes, e.g. sucking
Gastrointestinal	Intolerance of enteral feeds, gastro-oesophageal reflux, necrotizing enterocolitis (NEC)
Liver	Jaundice
Kidneys	Inability to concentrate urine, inability to excrete acid load
Immunity	Immature immune system, with susceptibility to infections
Eyes	Retinopathy of prematurity (see p. 384)
Metabolic	Hypoglycaemia, electrolyte imbalances, e.g. hypocalcaemia, osteopenia of prematurity
Haematological	Iron-deficiency anaemia, physiological anaemia
Surgical	Inguinal and umbilical hernia

RESPIRATORY DISORDERS

Features of respiratory distress in a neonate

- Tachypnoea (RR > 60/min)
- Expiratory grunting
- Nasal flaring
- Recession (intercostals, subcostal and suprasternal)
- Cyanosis

Investigations of respiratory distress

- Oxygen saturation (pulse oximetry and blood gas)
- Chest transillumination with cold light (? pneumothorax)
- Pass NG tube (if choanal or oesophageal atresia suspected)
- CXR
- Nitrogen washout test (to differentiate cause of cyanosis; see p. 97)
- Infection screen (blood, CSF, gastric aspirate for bacterial and viral culture; umbilical, ear and throat swabs). Also check maternal high vaginal swab result
- Other bloods: FBC, haematocrit and serology

RESPIRATORY DISTRESS SYNDROME

Respiratory distress syndrome (RDS) is a specific disease due to insufficient surfactant. In RDS the neonates lungs are non-compliant, or 'stiff'. A low alveolar compliance leads to hypoxia and acidosis and, if severe, causes PPHN

Surfactant

- Lowers surface tension and increases compliance in alveoli
- Is a phospholipid composed of lecithin and sphingomyelin
- Produced by type II pneumocytes
- Lecithin:sphingomyelin (LS) ratio is altered in RDS (less lecithin, LS ratio low, < 2)

LS ratio risk of RDS	
<1.5	70%
1.5–2	40%
>2	Very small

Predisposing factors	Prematurity, hypoxia, acidosis, shock, asphyxia
	Diabetic mother, APH, second twin, male
Protective factors	Prolonged intrauterine stress, e.g. IUGR), maternal drug addiction, maternal steroids

Clinical features

- Respiratory distress from 6 h of age
- Worsens over 2–3 days then improves over 1–2 weeks
- CXR: fine reticular **'ground glass'** appearance, air bronchograms

Management

Surfactant replacement	Administered via the ETT
	There are different formulations and more than one dose may be necessary
Ventilatory support	Oxygen, CPAP or positive pressure ventilation as needed
Antibiotics	If infection suspected
Minimal handling	
Complications	Pneumothorax, intraventricular haemorrhage, bronchopulmonary dysplasia (late)
Prevention	If early delivery is planned, maternal oral dexamethasone is commenced 48 h prior to delivery

PNEUMOTHORAX

Causes

- Idiopathic (1% term infants)
- Secondary to ventilation (especially if 'stiff' lungs in RDS or meconium aspiration)

Clinical features

- Mostly asymptomatic
- If large, causes respiratory distress (see above)
- NB: Rapid deterioration suggests a tension pneumothorax

Diagnosis

- Chest transillumination with fibre-optic 'cold' light (this does not damage the infant's skin)
- CXR

Management

Insertion of chest drain (anterior axillary line, 4th intercostal space).

> **Other air leaks**
> - Pneumopericardium
> - Pneumomediastinum
> - Pulmonary interstitial emphysema (PIE)
> - Pneumoperitoneum

PULMONARY HAEMORRHAGE

Haemorrhagic pulmonary oedema due to elevated pulmonary capillary pressure from acute left ventricular failure or lung injury.

Associations   Prematurity, RDS, asphyxia
Pneumonia, acute cardiac failure (PDA), coagulopathies

Clinical features

- Frothy pink sputum (in ET tube if ventilated)
- Acutely unwell neonate
- Low haematocrit

Management

- Ventilation
- Antibiotics
- Correct any coagulation defect

BRONCHOPULMONARY DYSPLASIA (BPD)

Bronchopulmonary dysplasia is a condition of chronic lung damage with persistent X-ray changes. It is defined as either an oxygen requirement on day 28 of life or at 36 weeks' gestation.

It occurs after:

- Severe RDS
- Other neonatal lung disease

Clinical features

- Chest hyperinflation, intercostals and subcostal recession
- Crepitations on auscultation
- Oxygen requirement

CXR

- '**Honeycomb lung**' (cystic pulmonary infiltrates in reticular pattern)
- Areas of emphysema and collapse, and fibrosis and thickening of the pulmonary arterioles

Management

- Steroids and diuretics if ventilator dependent. Steroids may have an adverse effect on long-term neurodevelopmental outcome
- Bronchodilators if wheezy
- May need long-term home oxygen

WILSON–MIKITY SYNDROME

Clinical features

Respiratory distress, hypoxia and apnoea developing slowly during the first month in premature infants who have no history of severe respiratory disease.

CXR

Streaky infiltrates and cysts.

Management

- Respiratory support, long-term oxygen may be required
- Resolves over weeks–months usually, with susceptibility to chest infections for the first few years of life

APNOEA

Apnoea is cessation of breathing for > 20 s. It may be accompanied by **bradycardia** and **cyanosis**. It may be due to:

- Central factors (chemoreceptor or respiratory centre failure)
- Airway obstruction
- Reflex protective mechanisms

Premature neonates have poorly developed central chemoreceptors and respiratory centres and therefore frequently have apnoeas.

Causes

Central	Obstructive	Reflex
Prematurity (usually resolves by 36 weeks)	Choanal atresia	Gastro-oesophageal reflux
Hypoxia	Laryngeal nerve palsy	Vagal response, e.g. suctioning, physiotherapy
Metabolic, e.g. hypoglycaemia	Foreign body	
Sepsis	Pierre–Robin sequence	
Hyper- or hypo-thermia		
Intracranial haemorrhage		
Convulsions		
Drugs, e.g. maternal intrapartum narcotics		
Developmental brain abnormalities		

Investigations

These depend on the clinical condition. Gastro-oesophageal reflux is important to exclude. Investigations may also include screen for sepsis, CXR, arterial blood gas, cranial USS, barium swallow and neurological investigations.

Management

- Treat the underlying cause
- *Acute episode*: stimulation, manual ventilation if necessary, apnoea monitoring
- *Recurrent episodes*: CPAP, methylxanthines, e.g. caffeine, theophylline
  - Intubation and ventilation if severe
  - Resuscitation skills for the parents
  - Home apnoea monitor if parents wish or hypoventilation syndrome

TRANSIENT TACHYPNOEA OF THE NEWBORN (TTN)

This is due to excessive retained fetal lung fluid and is a self-limiting condition. Incidence 1–2% of newborns.

Predisposing factors   Elective caesarean section (as no stress and fluid not squeezed out of lungs during delivery)
Heavy maternal analgesia, infant of diabetic mother

Clinical features

Respiratory distress from birth resolving over the first 24 h.

CXR

- Generalized streakiness
- Fluid in the fissures
- Pleural effusions

Treatment

- Oxygen (ambient, CPAP if necessary, rarely ventilation needed)
- Antibiotics until pneumonia and sepsis excluded

Causes

Common	Group B β-haemolytic strep. Gram-negative bacteria (*E. coli*, klebsiella, pseudomonas, serratia), *Staph. saprophyticus* aspirated blood/meconium and obstetric cream
Rarer	Listeria, chlamydia, mycoplasma, CMV, coxsackie, RSV, congenital surfactant deficiencies

Clinical features

Non-specific, respiratory distress features.

CXR

Patchy opacification.

Treatment

Antibiotics, physiotherapy and respiratory support.

MECONIUM ASPIRATION SYNDROME

Meconium is present in 10% of deliveries. If resuscitation is required, then the airway *must* be aspirated prior to ventilation.

Inhaled meconium can produce:

- Airway plugging with distal atelectasis, air leaks and secondary pneumonia
- Chemical pneumonitis (it is toxic to the lung tissue)
- Hypoxia, respiratory and metabolic acidosis, and PPHN if severe

Clinical features

- Respiratory distress from birth, worsening, hyperinflated chest (due to air trapping)
- Severe acidosis
- Signs of cerebral irritation

CXR

Hyperinflation and diffuse patchy opacification.

Management

- Respiratory support (high pressures or high-frequency oscillatory ventilation may be needed)
- Antibiotics and physiotherapy
- Management of PPHN

CARDIAC DISORDERS

For detail on congenital heart disease, see Chapter 13. General cardiac conditions are discussed below.

Causes of cyanosis

- Severe lung disease
- Cyanotic congenital heart disease
- PPHN
- Methaemoglobinaemia

- Others: Sepsis, airway problem
        Neurological, e.g. asphyxia, seizures, neuromuscular

See p. 93.

PERSISTENT PULMONARY HYPERTENSION OF THE NEWBORN (PPHN)

This is also known as persistent fetal circulation. It is the most difficult condition to distinguish clinically from cyanotic congenital heart disease.

In PPHN there is a failure of the pulmonary vascular resistance to fall after birth, and blood is therefore shunted away from the lungs via the ductus arteriosus (right to left) and the foramen ovale. This results in **central cyanosis**.

Predisposing factors   Hypoxia–ischaemia, acidosis
                         Metabolic disturbance
                         Severe lung disease, e.g. severe RDS, meconium aspiration syndrome
                         Hypothermia/acidosis

Clinical features and diagnosis

- Central cyanosis
- Loud P2 heart sound
- Arterial blood gases: PO_2 low, PCO_2 relatively normal
- Little improvement in saturations with 100% O_2
- Pre-ductal blood PO_2 is > 5 mmHg higher than postductal PO_2 (demonstrate by transcutaneous PO_2 measurements on right chest and lower abdomen)
- CXR: normal heart and well-expanded oligaemic lung fields
- Echocardiogram: structurally normal heart, high pulmonary artery pressures

Management

It is managed with PPV or HFOV and inhaled nitric oxide (a vasodilator), prostacyclin IV or tolazoline IV. ECMO may be necessary if ventilation fails.

PERSISTENT DUCTUS ARTERIOSUS (PDA)

Commonly seen in premature infants. For features and treatment, see p. 93.

CARDIAC FAILURE

Common complication of PDA. Seen in certain congenital heart diseases. For features and treatment, see p. 90.

DUCT-DEPENDENT CIRCULATIONS

Emergency treatment includes prostaglandin E_2 (see p. 104).

NEUROLOGICAL DISORDERS

HYPOXIA–ISCHAEMIA

Hypoxia is insufficient arterial oxygen concentration. **Ischaemia** is insufficient blood flow to the cells.

Fetal hypoxia–ischaemia can occur as an **intrauterine** or **intrapartum event** (a minority of cases are due to birth asphyxia). After birth, hypoxia may result from several causes including severe shock, failure to breath adequately and severe anaemia.

Intrauterine hypoxia	May be acute, presenting with **fetal distress**, or chronic presenting as **IUGR**
Intrapartum hypoxia	May be acute or acute on chronic (an elevated nucleated red cell count indicates that there has been an insult for long enough for the marrow to respond)

Signs of fetal distress

Fetal bradycardia, reduced beat-to-beat variability

Late decelerations (type II dips recovery of heart rate after the end of the contraction)

Reduced fetal movements

Meconium

Causes

Maternal	Pre-eclampsia, eclampsia, acute hypotensive episode
Placental	Placental abruption, cord prolapse, chronic insufficiency (many causes, e.g. pre-eclampsia)
Fetal	Prematurity, postmaturity, obstructed labour

After birth, hypoxia may result from several causes including severe anaemia, severe shock, failure to breathe adequately or cyanotic cardiac disease.

Effects of hypoxia–ischaemia

Hypoxia–ischaemia can result in damage to all organs, but initially there is preferential sparing of the brain at the expense of other organs. The effects of hypoxia–ischaemia in the different organs:

Kidneys	Acute tubular necrosis
Gut	NEC
CNS	Hypoxic–ischaemic encephalopathy
Heart	Ischaemic changes, heart failure
Lungs	RDS, pulmonary haemorrhage, PPHN
Metabolic effects	Metabolic acidosis, hypoglycaemia, hyponatraemia
Other	Adrenal haemorrhage, DIC

Hypoxic–ischaemic encephalopathy (HIE)

This is a disturbance of neurological behaviour due to ischaemic damage to the brain. The areas affected are the 'watershed zones' between the major arteries (those most susceptible to hypoperfusion). The condition can result in **cortical and subcortical necrosis** and cysts, and **periventricular leukomalacia (PVL)**. (In premature infants **germinal matrix haemorrhages** occur, with intraventricular haemorrhage.)

PVL is cystic changes in the white matter, with later reduction in myelin around the ventricles. Diagnosis is on USS, CT and MRI scan. A high risk of cerebral palsy follows.

HIE is classified as mild, moderate or severe. The condition develops over a period of a few days. The infants are floppy after birth, with seizures and irregular breathing, and may become hypertonic over a period of days. Mild disease generally resolves over a few days, but in severe HIE there is a 50% mortality and an 80% risk of cerebral palsy.

Clinical severity

Mild	Moderate	Severe
Irritability, hyperalert	Lethargy	Coma
No seizures	Seizures	Prolonged seizures
Normal tone	Differential hypotonia	Severe hypotonia
Jittery	(Legs > arms, neck extensors > flexors)	Need for ventilation
Weak sucking	Poor suck, NG feeds required	No sucking reflex
Sympathetic dominance	Parasympathetic dominance	Respiratory support needed

Management

- Initial resuscitation
- General support as necessary, e.g. metabolic balance, glucose homeostasis renal support
- Management of brain oedema (fluid restriction, ventilatory control)
- Seizure management
- Management of complications

PERIVENTRICULAR HAEMORRHAGE (PVH)

The term periventricular haemorrhage encompasses several types of intracranial haemorrhage. Neonates develop PVH as a result of an unstable cerebral circulation, most commonly into the germinal matrix at the head of the caudate nucleus.

Risk factors

- Prematurity
- Low birth weight
- Hypercapnoea
- RDS
- IPPV
- Metabolic acidosis
- Coagulation disorder

Clinical features

- Asymptomatic
- Subtle neurological signs, e.g. roving eye movements
- Slow deterioration – apnoeas, bradycardias, metabolic acidosis, seizures, anaemia
- Massive collapse – bulging fontanelle, hypotension

Diagnosis and grading

Made on cranial USS.

Complications

- Hydrocephalus
- Porencephaly
- Cerebral palsy

Management

Supportive shunt for hydrocephalus.

NEONATAL CONVULSIONS AND JITTERINESS

Neonates fairly commonly show signs of '**jitteriness**' with rapid fine shaking of the limbs, which must be differentiated from **seizures** (which have different causes and management).

Causes

Seizures	Jitteriness
Asphyxia	Hypoglycaemia
Infection (meningitis, sepsis, congenital)	Hypocalcaemia
Metabolic disturbance, e.g. glucose ↓, Ca ↓, Mg ↓	Sepsis
CVA, subarachnoid haemorrhage	Drug withdrawal (usually opiates or benzodiazepines)
Pyridoxine deficiency or other inborn error of metabolism	
Congenital brain anomalies	

Clinical features

NB: Neonatal seizures are not always obvious and may manifest, for example, as apnoea.

	Seizures	Jitteriness
Predominant movement	Multifocal, tone alteration, apnoea	Rhythmic movements
Conscious state	Altered	Alert or asleep
Eye movements	Eye deviation occurs	Normal
Do movements stop when limb held?	No	Yes

Investigations

Infection screen	Blood, CSF and urine microscopy and culture, and serology
	(NB: CSF is persistently blood-stained throughout the CSF in IVH)
Electrolyte disturbance	U&E, including Ca and Mg
Metabolic screen	Glucose, metabolic work-up if indicated
USS brain	
EEG	

Treatment

1. Treat the cause, e.g. IV glucose, IV calcium, IV magnesium, IV antibiotics, IV pyridoxine
2. Give anticonvulsants for seizures if necessary. Anticonvulsants used in neonatal seizures include:
   Phenobarbitone
   Phenytoin
   Paraldehyde
   Clonazepam and midazolam

DRUG WITHDRAWAL (MATERNAL DRUG ABUSE)

Clinical features

Wakefulness
Irritability
Temperature instability, tachypnoea
Hyperactivity, high-pitched cry, hypertonia, hyperreflexia
Diarrhoea, disorganized suck
Respiratory distress, rhinorrhoea
Apnoea, autonomic dysfunction
Weight loss, failure to thrive
Alkalosis
Lacrimation
Sneezing

Management

This includes close observation for the above signs. Naloxone contraindicated at delivery.

Conservative measures	Encourage mothers to breast feed, decrease sensory stimuli, swaddling
Drug treatment	These include opiates, e.g. morphine, and sedatives, e.g. diazepam, chlorpromazine. These are weaned over a few weeks

Consider immunization against Hep B and BCG. Screen mother for other blood-borne viruses (Hep C, HIV).

NB: Increased incidence of SIDS.

GASTROINTESTINAL DISORDERS

NECROTIZING ENTEROCOLITIS (NEC)

Necrotizing enterocolitis is a disease of bowel wall inflammation, ulceration and perforation due to many causes. It may be secondary to an **ischaemic or hypoxic insult** to the gut. There is mucosal damage leading to bacterial invasion and gastrointestinal gangrene and perforation.

Risk factors

- Prematurity
- Hypoxia
- Sepsis
- Hypovolaemia
- Hyperosmolar feeds
- Venous and umbilical catheters
- Exchange transfusion
- Polycythaemia

Clinical features

General   Apnoeas, lethargy, vomiting, temperature instability, acidosis and shock
Abdominal   Distended, shiny abdomen, bile aspirates, rectal fresh blood

Complications

Short-term   Perforation, obstruction, gangrenous bowel, intrahepatic cholestasis, sepsis, DIC
Long-term   Stricture, short bowel syndrome (due to resection of diseased bowel), lactose intolerance

Diagnosis

AXR   Fixed loops of bowel, **pneumostasis intestinalis** (intramural gas), portal vein gas, pneumoperitoneum, bubbles
        in portal vein on ultrasound
FBC   Neutrophils ($\uparrow$ or $\downarrow$), platelets ($\downarrow$), DIC

Management

- Manage shock, acidosis, electrolyte and clotting disturbance and anaemia, and ventilate if necessary
- Systemic antibiotics
- Gastrointestinal decompression (NG tube with aspiration)
- Only parenteral nutrition until gut recovered
- Surgical intervention (perforation, clinical picture not improving with medical management, and secondary strictures) if surgical complication occurs

Prognosis

There is a 10% mortality, and higher if perforation occurs.

INTESTINAL OBSTRUCTION

Causes

- Atresia: Oesophageal
          Duodenal
          Jejunal
          Colonic
          Imperforate anus
- Congenital hypertrophic pyloric stenosis
- Hirschsprung disease
- Volvulus neonatorum (malrotation)
- Meconium plug, e.g. cystic fibrosis
- Hernial obstruction (internal or external)
- Duplication cyst

- NEC (stricture, ileus)
- Annular pancreas

Clinical features

- Polyhydramnios
- Bile-stained vomiting
- Abdominal distension
- Visible peristalsis
- Delayed or absent passage of meconium
- Features of dehydration

Investigations

AXR and contrast studies, abdominal USS (and metabolic alkalosis in pyloric stenosis).

Management

Dependent on the condition (often surgical).

MECONIUM ILEUS

Intestinal obstruction of terminal ileum due to thick, inspissated meconium. There is failure to pass meconium within 48 h of birth and clinical features of obstruction; may perforate *in utero*. 10% of cases of cystic fibrosis present with meconium ileus.

Diagnosis

AXR	Foamy pattern seen around plug abdominal calcification with *in utero* perforation
Gastrograffin enema	Microcolon
Immune-reactive trypsin	NB: This falls after surgery
Sweat test	At 2–3 months to confirm diagnosis
Genetics	Genotype for cystic fibrosis

Management

1. Conservative
2. Gastrograffin enema or surgical decompression

NB: **Meconium plug syndrome** is a lower bowel obstruction or delayed passage of meconium due to a plug of meconium around 10 cm long. Seen in premature infants, Hirschsprung disease and cystic fibrosis.

OSTEOPENIA OF PREMATURITY

This is a generalized demineralization (osteopenia) seen in premature and low birthweight infants compared to a fetus of the same gestation. It is classically seen in immature infants who are solely breast fed.

Causes

Mineral deficiency, particularly phosphate due to placental insufficiency, and/or inadequate phosphate levels in breast milk, or low phosphate feeds.

Risk factors

- VLBW
- Severe IUGR and prematurity

- Inadequate milk intake or insufficient phosphate in feeds
- Chronic lung disease
- Drugs – steroids, long term diuretics

Clinical features

It is asymptomatic, diagnosed on long bone X-ray. Clinical rickets is rare, but rib fractures are not uncommon in babies with chronic lung disease.

Calcium normal, phosphate $\downarrow$, PTH $\uparrow$, alkaline phosphatase $\uparrow$.

Treatment

- Low birthweight formula (contain increased phosphate)
- Supplement breast milk with phosphate

HAEMATOLOGICAL DISORDERS

HYDROPS FETALIS

This is **severe oedema**, **ascites** and **pleural effusions** at birth.

Causes

Immune	Severe intrauterine anaemia, e.g. severe haemolytic disease of the newborn (rhesus, other blood group incompatibilities)	
Non-immune	*Severe anaemia*:	Chronic twin–twin transfusion
		Fetomaternal haemorrhage
		HB Barts
	Congenital infection, e.g. parvovirus B19	
	Cardiac failure, e.g. uncontrolled fetal SVT, severe CHD, premature closure of ductus arteriosus and foramen ovale	
	Hypoproteinaemia, e.g. congenital nephropathy Finnish, maternal pre-eclampsia	
	Congenital malformations, e.g. anomalies of lymphatics – lymphagiectasia (Turner syndrome), obstructive uropathy, pulmonary adenoma, fetal or placental angioma	

Investigations of cause

Establish cause is not haemolysis (Coombs' test).

If anaemic	Look for evidence of feto-maternal haemorrhage (Kleihauer test)
	Serum for parvovirus serology
If not anaemic	Chromosomes, metabolic studies and cardiac USS

The prognosis is significantly better if you can find a cause that can be treated.

Management

1. Resuscitation – transfusions, abdominal and chest drainage as necessary, ventilatory support
2. Treat the cause

HYPOGLYCAEMIA

Normal newborns can have intermittent low blood glucose levels but hypoglycaemia is frequently seen in small and premature infants, and also in unwell neonates. There is no accepted universal definition, however, blood glucose levels < 2.6 mmol/L at any age are hypoglycaemic. Persistent neonatal hypoglycaemia is unusual (see below).

TRANSIENT NEONATAL HYPOGLYCAEMIA

Causes

Substrate deficiency (ketotic)	IUGR, prematurity, asphyxia, hypothermia, sepsis, malformation
Hyperinsulinism (non-ketotic)	Diabetic mother, gestational diabetes, rhesus isoimmunization

Clinical features

- Asymptomatic
- Apnoeas, jitteriness, seizures, lethargy, hypotonia

Investigations

Check BMStix (immediate idea) and blood glucose (for accuracy).

If persistent and recurrent, screen for ketones, hormone levels and metabolic disorders.

Management

If able to feed	Oral glucose (breast milk or formula), then hourly feeds with monitoring of blood glucose levels
If unable to feed or reduced consciousness	IV 10% glucose 5 ml/kg bolus, then 10% glucose infusion 60–90 ml/kg/day, with frequent blood glucose monitoring
	If the glucose remains low, may need 15–20% glucose infusion

PERSISTENT NEONATAL HYPOGLYCAEMIA (RARE)

Causes

Hyperinsulinism	Persistent hyperinsulinaemic hypoglycaemia of infancy (PHHI, nesidioblastosis)
	Beckwith–Wiedemann syndrome
	Insulinoma
Metabolic disorder	Carbohydrate metabolism disorder, e.g. galactosaemia, hereditary fructose intolerance
	Organic acidaemia, e.g. maple syrup urine disease

Persistent hypoglycaemia is managed according to cause.

FURTHER READING

Levene M, Tudehope D, Sinha SK *Essentials of Neonatal Medicine*, 4th edn, Oxford: Blackwell Sciences, 2008

MacDonald MG, Mullet MD, Seshia MMK *Avery's Neonatology. Pathophysiology and Management of the Newborn*, 6th edn. Baltimore: Lippincott, Williams & Wilkins, 2005

Rennie JM *Roberton's Textbook of Neonatology*, 4th edn. Edinburgh: Churchill Livingstone, 2005

19
Surgical conditions

- *Neonatal surgical conditions*
- *Gastrointestinal conditions*
- *Genitourinary conditions*

- *Orthopaedic conditions*
- *Consent*

NEONATAL SURGICAL CONDITIONS

CONGENITAL ATRESIAS

Choanal atresia

This is a failure of the bucconasal membrane to cannulate during development. As babies are obligate nasal breathers unless they are crying, it presents as breathing difficulties from birth. It may be unilateral or bilateral.

Diagnosis

Inability to pass a nasogastric tube in the affected nostril(s).

Management

Provide an airway (pharyngeal or ETT) until surgery performed (urgently).

Oesophageal atresia and tracheo-oesophageal fistula

Overall incidence is 1:3000 live births.

A condition of oesophageal atresia usually associated with tracheo-oesophageal fistula. There are five different variations.

Associations   VACTERL = **V**ertebral, **A**nal, **C**ardiac, **T**racheo-o**E**sophageal, **R**enal and **L**imb abnormalities
VATER = **V**ertebral, **A**nal, **T**racheo-o**E**sophageal, **R**enal or **R**adial anomalies

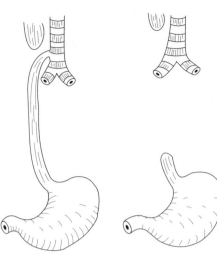

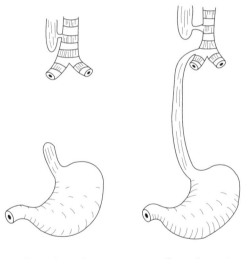

Figure 19.1 Types of oesophageal artresia and tracheo-oesophageal atresia

Clinical features

Presentation varies depending on the type:

- Maternal polyhydramnios (60%)
- Recurrent aspiration pneumonia
- Coughing episodes with cyanosis
- Abdominal distension (air passing into gut from lungs)
- Choking with feeds intermittently (H-type fistula) (these are notoriously difficult to diagnose)

Diagnosis

1. Inability to pass a radio-opaque catheter into the stomach (except for H-type)
2. AXR – no gas in stomach (types A and B)
3. CXR – areas of collapse
4. Non-irritant radio-opaque contrast study (to define the lesion)
5. Ciné contrast swallow with prone oesophagogram (for H-type fistula)

Management

1. Nurse head up and prone
2. Surgical correction: division of fistula and anastomosis of oesophageal segments. If large defect, temporary oesophagostomy and gastrostomy may be made, with definitive surgery later

Congenital intestinal atresias

These may occur anywhere along the gastrointestinal tract. Features are those of obstruction, which vary according to the level of obstruction.

Features of obstruction

- Polyhydramnios
- Bile-stained vomiting
- Abdominal distension
- Visible peristalsis
- Delayed or absent passage of meconium
- Features of dehydration

Diagnosis is made on imaging studies, in particular:

Duodenal atresia	'Double bubble' of air seen beneath diaphragm on plain AXR
Imperforate anus	Air bubble seen on AXR after first 12 h with baby held inverted

Duodenal atresia is associated with Down syndrome.

Management is with initial resuscitation and then surgical repair.

Imperforate anus

Incidence 1:2500.

- Low and high forms exist ± fistula to urethra or vagina
- Air bubble is seen on AXR after first 12 h of life with baby inverted
- Management is often with an initial colostomy with further repair later
- Rectal inertia is a long-term problem.

GASTROSCHISIS AND EXOMPHALOS

Exomphalos

Incidence 1:5000.

An evisceration of gastrointestinal contents **through the umbilicus** covered by peritoneum.

Associations (common)	Trisomy 13, trisomy 18
	Beckwith–Wiedemann syndrome
	Renal malformations including bladder exstrophy, Wilms tumour (40% incidence)
	Congenital heart disease

Gastroschisis

Incidence 1:30 000.

This is evisceration of gastrointestinal contents through a right **paraumbilical defect**. There is no peritoneal covering and hypoalbuminaemia occurs.

Associations	Bowel atresias adhesions
	Strictures
	Stenosis
Complications	Short bowel syndrome
	Faltering growth

Management

Pre-operative	Abdominal contents wrapped in moist antibiotic-soaked gauze
	Gastric decompression, resuscitation with IV albumin, antibiotics, TPN
Operative	Small lesions (< 5 cm) are surgically treated with primary closure. Larger defects treated with a staged repair, using a non-reactive silicon sheeting to cover bowel contents in gastroschisis

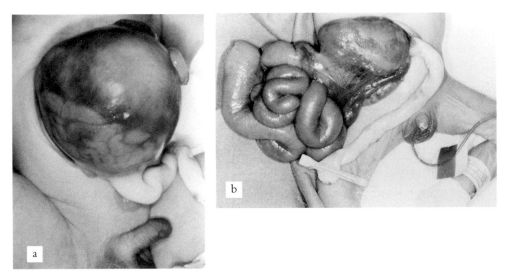

Figure 19.2 (a) Exomphalos (an umbilical defect) and (b) gastroschisis (a para-umbilical defect)

CONGENITAL DIAPHRAGMATIC HERNIA

This sporadic condition is seen in 1:4000 live births. They may be:

- Posterolateral (Bochdalek) type: common type, 80% on the left side
- Anteromedial (Morgagni) type

Clinical features

- Severe respiratory distress at birth
- Cyanosis
- Scaphoid abdomen (as intestine in chest)

- Apex displaced to the right
- Complications of pulmonary hypoplasia, pulmonary hypertension and PPHN may be present (due to lack of space for fetal lung development)

Diagnosis

CXR and AXR   Loops of bowel in the thorax

Management

Resuscitation   NG tube and aspiration
                    Intubation and ventilation (IPPV), and circulatory support
                    PPHN management
Surgical correction   When fully resuscitated

CONGENITAL LOBAR EMPHYSEMA

Uncommon condition due to a cartilaginous defect of a lobar bronchus. **Upper lobe** most commonly affected.

Clinical features

- Insidious onset respiratory distress in first few weeks
- Mediastinum displaced away from lesion
- Hyper-resonant with decreased breath sounds over affected lobe

Management

Lobectomy.

GASTROINTESTINAL CONDITIONS

THE ACUTE ABDOMEN

An acute abdomen is a clinical diagnosis indicating serious intra-abdominal pathology and requires urgent management through resuscitation and usually surgical intervention.

Peritonitis is an inflammation or irritation of the peritoneum resulting in clinical signs either localized to a specific area or generalized throughout the abdomen.

Clinical features

General   Unwell, fever, rigors (sometimes)
Abdominal   Abdominal pain – location, duration, severity, intermittent or constant?
Other   Anorexia, nausea, vomiting, dysuria, haematuria, altered bowel habit (diarrhoea, blood in stool, constipation)

Examination

Fever
Vital signs   Pulse (tachycardia), BP (hypotension?), RR (tachypnoea)
                  Peripheral shutdown with capillary refill time < 2 s

Abdominal signs	Tenderness (location and severity)
	Guarding
	Rebound tenderness
	Rigid abdomen (unable to 'blow out' abdomen to meet examiner's hand when held a few cm above) — Features of **peritonitis** (inflammation of the peritoneum)
	Abdominal mass
	Rectal examination to be done by experienced paediatric surgeon or physician (tenderness, blood, mucus)
General signs	Jaundice (gallstones)
	Anaemia (bleed)

Investigations

These will depend on the probable cause, but important investigations are:

Urine	Urinalysis and microscopy if indicated, pregnancy test
Bloods	FBC, U&E and creatinine, amylase, glucose, sickle cell status if indicated. Arterial blood gas, LFT. Bone profile (Ca and PO_4)
CXR	Erect (chest infection – usually lower lobe, gas under the diaphragm)
AXR	Supine (dilated loops of bowel)
USS abdomen	(Pyloric stenosis, intussusception, ovarian pathology)

Surgical causes of an acute abdomen

Upper GIT	Perforation (oesophageal, gastric or duodenal)
Hepatobiliary	Cholecystitis
	Ruptured liver, spleen or gallbladder (trauma)
Lower GIT	Acute appendicitis
	Inflamed Meckel diverticulum
	Incarcerated hernia causing ischaemia or obstruction
	Ischaemic bowel, e.g. intussusception, volvulus
	Inflammatory bowel disease causing obstruction, perforation, severe exacerbation or megacolon
Retroperitoneal	Pancreatitis
	Ureteric obstruction (renal colic from stones, trauma)
Pelvic	Ovarian cyst rupture or torsion
	Testicular torsion
	Pelvic inflammatory disease
	Ruptured ectopic pregnancy

Medical causes mimicking an acute abdomen

Respiratory	Right lower lobe pneumonia
Gastrointestinal	Mesenteric adenitis, gastroenteritis, constipation
Liver	Acute viral hepatitis
Haematological	Sickle cell disease crisis
	Congenital spherocytosis (haemolytic episodes)
Renal	Urinary tract infection (especially pyelonephritis)
	Henoch–Schönlein purpura (see p. 214)
Metabolic	Diabetic ketoacidosis
	Acute porphyries
	Lead poisoning

INTESTINAL OBSTRUCTION

Clinical features

- Features of an acute abdomen
- No passage of faeces or flatus per rectum
- Vomiting: Non-bile stained (high obstruction above bile duct entry)
  - Bile stained (obstruction below bile duct entry)
  - Faecal (very low obstruction large bowel)

Causes

Infants	Older children
Pyloric stenosis	Appendicitis
Intestinal atresia or stenosis	Inguinal hernia
Malrotation/volvulus	Malrotation/volvulus
Inguinal hernia	Inflammatory bowel disease
Intussusception	Intussusception
Appendicitis	Gastrointestinal malignancy (rare)
Hirschsprung disease	

ACUTE APPENDICITIS

Peak age 10–20 years. Rare < 5 years.

Typical clinical features

- Abdominal pain commencing para-umbilically and then moving to the right iliac fossa (McBurney's point). Worse on movement, gradually worsening. Guarding indicates peritonitis
- Nausea, vomiting and anorexia
- Low-grade fever, flushed, tachycardic, fetor
- Perforation is common in younger children
- In young children the pain is poorly localized and features of peritonism may be absent
- A retro-caecal and pelvic appendix may present with atypical signs

Investigations

- Diagnosis is *clinical* and difficult as classical signs are often not present. All the above causes of an acute abdomen (both medical and surgical) are in the differential diagnosis
- FBC (mild neutrophilia may be present)
- Urinalysis (to exclude UTI). NB: Pyuria may be seen in appendicitis, and so misdiagnosis of UTI should be avoided

Complications

Appendix mass, abscess or perforation.

Management

Urgent appendicectomy.

MESENTERIC ADENITIS

This inflammation of the mesenteric lymph nodes can mimic appendicitis with non-localized abdominal pain and is thought to be due to a viral infection, e.g. adenovirus or bacterial infection, e.g. *Yersinia enterocolitica*.

CONGENITAL HYPERTROPHIC PYLORIC STENOSIS

This is due to **hypertrophy of the muscle layer of the pylorus** of unknown cause.

Associations	Males > females
	Caucasian
	Positive family history (especially maternal)
	Syndromes: trisomy 18, Turner syndrome, Cornelia de Lange syndrome

Clinical features

- Usually presents at 4–6 weeks in first-born males
- Persistent vomiting (may be projectile, not bile-stained)
- Thin but hungry infant
- Abdominal examination: Visible peristalsis
                              Olive-shaped tumour in the right upper abdomen

Investigations

Diagnosis is made on a **test feed** or **USS**, both of which are operator-dependent.

Test feed	Palpate the abdomen while infant feeding milk for olive-shaped tumour and observe for peristalsis across upper abdomen from left to right $\pm$ vomiting
Abdominal USS	This may outline the tumour as a 'doughnut' ring (muscle thickness > 4 mm, pyloric length > 14 mm)

Blood electrolytes and pH must be done to look for:

- Signs of dehydration
- Jaundice (5–10%)
- **Hypochloraemic hypokalaemic metabolic alkalosis** (due to vomiting)
- NB: Serum K is usually maintained but total body K is depleted

Management

1. *Resuscitation*   Initial resuscitation with IV fluids is essential

                                  0.45% dextrose saline with 40 mmol KCl/L is given over the first 12 h until the bicarbonate is corrected and then standard fluid replacement

                                  Nasogastric tube with suction

                                  Regular U&E and ABG measurements

2. *Surgery*   When rehydrated and the alkalosis is corrected, a **pyloromyotomy** (Ramstedt's procedure) is performed

ACHALASIA

This is a motility disorder of the oesophagus with lack of normal peristalsis in the oesophagus and a relative gastro-oesophageal junction obstruction. It generally presents in adolescence or adulthood. The underlying pathology is of a decrease in the number of ganglion cells in the oesophagus, with an increase in inflammatory cells.

Associations   Chagas disease

                        Adrenal insufficiency

Investigations

Upright CXR   Air–fluid level in dilated oesophagus and/or absence of gastric air bubble

Barium swallow   Abnormal motility and dilatation of oesophagus

Oesophageal manometry   Abnormal

Management

Medical   Calcium-channel blockers, e.g. nifedipine   }

              Intrasphincteral botulinum toxin injection }   Temporary measures only

Surgical   Heller myotomy (division of the muscle fibres at gastro-oesophageal junction)

              Balloon dilatation (less effective than myotomy in childhood)

NB: Surgical management often results in gastro-oesophageal reflux.

MALROTATION

This is due to **incomplete rotation of the intestine** around the superior mesenteric artery during the third month of gestation. The most common type involves incomplete rotation with the caecum in the midline. In this case the duodenum does not pass posteriorly to the superior mesenteric artery. The base of the small bowel is not fixed from the ligament of Treitz to the caecum but is anchored on the superior mesenteric artery and the caecum is fixed in the right upper quadrant by fibrous tissue (Ladd's bands) crossing the second part of the duodenum. Obstruction may occur due to Ladd's bands crossing the second part of the duodenum or a volvulus occurring around the superior mesenteric artery.

Associations   Diaphragmatic hernia

                        Gastroschisis and exompholos

Clinical presentation

- Acute neonatal obstruction
- Intermittent childhood obstruction – distension, bilious vomiting, pallor, abdominal mass, bloody stools
- Midgut volvulus
- Protein-losing enteropathy (secondary to bacterial overgrowth)
- Asymptomatic to adolescence (up to 50%)

Investigations

Radiological   AXR (abnormal gas pattern, signs of obstruction)
Contrast studies (upper gastric series and enema)
A failure of the third part of the duodenum to cross the midline may be seen

Management

This is surgical, with release of Ladd's bands and fixation of the bowel. NB: If an asymptomatic malrotation is discovered, it should always be treated surgically to avoid volvulus in the future.

INTUSSUSCEPTION

Intussusception is invagination of a dilated segment of bowel into an adjacent proximal segment. The blood supply to the intussuscepted bowel is compromised and will become necrotic if not reduced rapidly. Usually occurs proximally to the ileo-caecal valve.

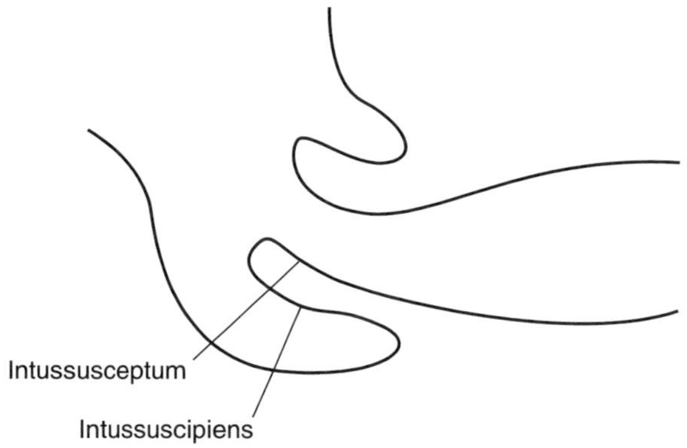

Intussusceptum

Intussuscipiens

Figure 19.3 Intussusception

Most common 6–9 months of age. Male > female.

Associations   Meckel diverticulum
Henoch–Schönlein purpura
Intestinal polyps
Lymphoma
Cystic fibrosis
Inflamed Peyer's patches

Clinical features

- Episodic abdominal pain with screaming and pallor, and infant draws their knees up. Often well in between attacks
- Abdominal distension, abdominal tenderness, sausage-shaped abdominal mass
- Blood stained mucus on rectal examination ('red-currant jelly stools') – a late sign
- Vomiting and diarrhoea
- Infant may be very unwell, dehydrated and progressing to shock

Investigations

Abdominal USS	May reveal the mass if the radiologist is skilled ('target' appearance)
Plain AXR	Signs of small bowel obstruction (fluid levels, dilated loops of small bowel)
Air enema	May be therapeutic as well as diagnostic

Management

- Initial fluid resuscitation as needed
- Air (or contrast) enema reduction (successful in 75%)
  Contraindications to enema: Rectal bleeding
                                                        Peritonism
- Surgical reduction ± resection if enema contraindicated or unsuccessful

MECKEL DIVERTICULUM

Meckel diverticulum is an ileal remnant of the vitellointestinal duct, which may contain ectopic gastric mucosa or pancreatic tissue.

Approximately:

- 2% of people are affected
- 2 inches long
- 2 feet from the ileocaecal valve

Clinical features

- Mostly asymptomatic
- May present with rectal bleeding, intussusception, volvulus or acute appendicitis

Investigations

Technetium scan	Increased uptake by gastric mucosa identifies 75%
	NB: Should be performed 4 weeks post-bleed to avoid false-negatives (as the gastric mucosa is often ulcerated post-haemorrhage)

Management

Surgical resection.

GENITOURINARY CONDITIONS

UNDESCENDED TESTES (CRYPTORCHIDISM)

The testes descend through the inguinal canal to the scrotum in the third trimester of pregnancy.

- Approximately 3.5% of boys have undescended testes at birth
- Approximately 1.5% of boys have undescended testes at 3 months of age (as some descend after birth)
- After 9 months of age they rarely descend spontaneously

Undescended testes have an increased rate of malignant transformation **even after orchidopexy**. They may be:

- Bilateral or unilateral
- Palpable or impalpable
- Somewhere along the normal line of descent or ectopic

NB: Undescended testes most commonly lie in the superficial inguinal pouch.

Undescended testes should not be confused with retractile testes, which can be massaged fully into the scrotum with no tension but retract back into the inguinal canal.

If possible, the testis is examined after massaging it gradually down the inguinal canal into the scrotum.

Karyotype should be done if bilateral impalpable testes or bilateral/unilateral impalpable testes associated with abnormal genitalia. Check β-hCG if bilaterally impalpable.

Investigations and management

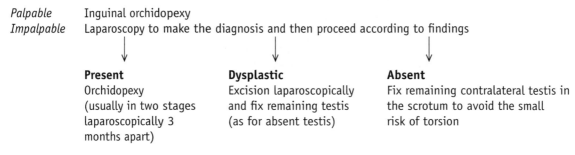

Palpable	Inguinal orchidopexy
Impalpable	Laparoscopy to make the diagnosis and then proceed according to findings

Present
Orchidopexy
(usually in two stages
laparoscopically 3
months apart)

Dysplastic
Excision laparoscopically
and fix remaining testis
(as for absent testis)

Absent
Fix remaining contralateral testis in
the scrotum to avoid the small
risk of torsion

Orchidopexy (surgical correction)

This is usually done before age 2 years, either as a one- or two-staged procedure, depending on the length of the testicular artery. It is done for:

- Cosmetic reasons
- To optimize testicular development and theoretically to increase fertility
- To allow early detection of malignant change

If the testis is abnormal or a unilateral intra-abdominal and unable to be corrected, it is removed (orchidectomy).

SCROTAL/INGUINAL SWELLINGS

Inguinal hernia

Males > females. Right side > left side.

Usually **indirect** in children, i.e. due to a wide patent processus vaginalis that allows omentum or bowel to pass into it.

Associations	Undescended testes
	Prematurity
	Connective tissue disorders, e.g. Marfan syndrome

Clinical features

- Intermittent scrotal swelling, more prominent on crying or straining
- If an **irreducible hernia**:   Painful
  Risk of bowel obstruction or strangulation
  Must be reduced urgently by a combination of *firm* pressure on the fundus, combined with control of the neck of the hernia. Alternatively, analgesia and Gollow's traction may be effective

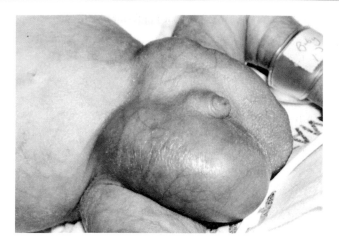

Figure 19.4 Inguinal hernia

Management

- Emergency repair – indicated if incarcerated (irreduceable), tender and any signs of bowel obstruction or bowel damage (perforation and peritonitis are rare but life-threatening complications). Children, especially babies, must be carefully resuscitated with fluids prior to the operation.
- Elective surgical repair once reduced (with *minimum delay* as incarceration may occur in the meantime)

HYDROCOELE

A hydrocoele in infancy is due to a narrow patent processus vaginalis that only permits peritoneal fluid to drain to the scrotum. It is common after birth.

Clinical features

- Scrotal swelling, usually fluctuant (may be tense)
- Variation in size of testes
- Transilluminates with a torch
- In an older child will characteristically increase in size during the day and reduce over night

Management

Small hydrocoeles	Usually observed for 1 year as most spontaneously resolve
Large and persistent hydrocoeles	Treated with surgical ligation of the processus vaginalis (herniotomy)

TESTICULAR TORSION

Testicular torsion is a rotation of the testis which causes vascular compromise by kinking the testicular pedicle.

Clinical features

- Acute scrotal pain, nausea and vomiting
- Firm dusky red scrotal swelling
- Pain may be a dull abdominal ache
- Usually tender on palpation
- Testis may be high in the scrotum and the spermatic cord feels thickened

The diagnosis is *clinical*. Doppler ultrasound of the testes can demonstrate the blood flow but it is relatively inaccurate and should not be relied on.

Management

- Any suspected testicular torsion should be taken to theatre to be *explored*
- Torted testis is untwisted and fixed. If it is non-viable it is excised
- *Other* testis should be fixed at the same time to prevent future torsion

NB: Testicular torsion is a surgical emergency and must be operated on within 6 h of onset of symptoms in order to save the testis.

TORTED TESTICULAR APPENDAGE (HYDATID OF MORGAGNI)

- Commonest cause of acute scrotum in younger boys
- Due to torsion of the appendix testis – at the upper pole of the testis
- Mimics torsion, so diagnosis is often made at exploration

Early examination may reveal the 'blue dot' sign, with a visible lump at the upper pole of the testis. When this is seen by an experienced surgeon, it may be treated conservatively.

IDIOPATHIC SCROTAL OEDEMA

- Oedema of the scrotal wall, extending to the groin and perineum
- Not tender although may mimic torsion
- Testes characteristically feel normal
- Important to exclude other causes of scrotal/testicular pathology

EPIDIDYMO-ORCHITIS

This is inflammation of the epididymis and/or testis.

Associations   UTI
                  Secondary to viral infection, e.g. mumps, or STD

The symptoms mimic testicular torsion but:

- More gradual onset of testicular pain
- Nausea and vomiting uncommon
- Usually associated with dysuria, pyuria and discharge
- Often febrile

Treatment is with antibiotics. In equivocal cases, surgical exploration must be performed to exclude torsion.

HYPOSPADIAS

Hypospadias is a common congenital abnormality due to a **failure in midline fusion of the urethral folds**. Degrees of severity are described according to the position of the urethral meatus.

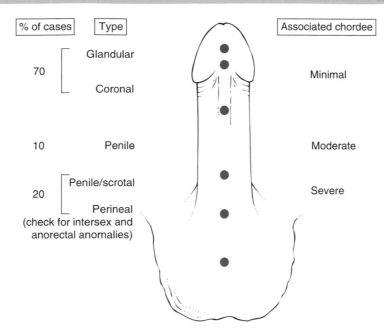

% of cases	Type		Associated chordee
70	Glandular		Minimal
	Coronal		
10	Penile		Moderate
20	Penile/scrotal		Severe
	Perineal		

(check for intersex and anorectal anomalies)

Figure 19.5 Hypospadias

There are three problems:

1. **Ventral urethral meatus** (this may lie anywhere from the base of the penis to just below the normal opening on the tip of the glans)
2. **Hooded prepuce** (due to a failure of the foreskin to form completely on the under surface of the penis)
3. **Chordee** (a ventral curvature of the penis)

Hypospadias is associated with a higher incidence of inguinal hernia and undescended testis. Unilateral or bilateral impalpable testis and hypospadias raise the possibility of an intersex condition so a karyotype and specialist review is indicated.

Surgical correction

- Based on straightening the penis and lengthening the urethra to the tip of the penis
- More severe forms are often repaired in two stages
- Foreskin hood is often used in the repair and boys are usually left with a circumcised appearance. NB: Parents must be told not to have their sons circumcised as the foreskin may be used in the repair
- Surgery is usually performed in the second year of life with a good long-term outcome from specialist centres

THE FORESKIN AND CIRCUMCISION

A non-retractile foreskin is *normal* in infants and young boys. In its early development the foreskin is **conical** in shape and cannot be retracted over the glans. In addition the under surface of the foreskin is **adherent** to the outer surface of the glans (physiological adhesions). During childhood the tip of the foreskin widens and the adhesions resolve at a variable rate, leading to retraction for around 70% by 5 years of age.

- **In young children** parents are reassured and advised that gentle retraction in the bath may help produce a retractile foreskin
- **Phimosis** (meaning muzzling) describes a tight foreskin which is non-rectractile

- Non-retraction may persist **at puberty** in around 1% of boys. In most of these there is a secondary scarring of the tip preventing its retraction. This is no longer a physiological narrowing but a pathological entity of the skin known as **lichen sclerosus et atrophicans** (also known as balanitis xerotica et obliterans [BXO] or posthitis [PXO]). This is the only true indication for medical circumcision which cures the condition. Other foreskin problems tend to be transient, with no long-term sequelae for foreskin development or general health, so they are only relative indications for circumcision

Balano-posthitis

Inflammation of the glans (balano) and foreskin (posthitis) – self-limiting. Rarely, severe cases may result in urinary retention but most resolve in a few days with bathing. Systemic or topical antibiotics and antifungals are non-contributory.

Ballooning

This is seen during voiding in young boys. The foreskin distends due to turbulence of urine beneath it. Although it may appear spectacular, it is rarely painful and resolves with foreskin retraction.

Paraphimosis

This occurs when a narrow foreskin becomes stuck behind the glans and restricts the venous and lymphatic drainage of the distal penis. The glans and inner prepuce swell and become quite painful. Urgent reduction is needed and is achieved after prior compression of the oedema, usually without anaesthetic. The foreskin may continue to develop normally after this.

Circumcision

Circumcision is performed for medical reasons and also by some religious groups.

Medical reasons

- True phimosis – usually BXO and an absolute indication due to the abnormal foreskin
- Recurrent balano-posthitis (dependent on severity and frequency of symptoms)
- Symptomatic ballooning
- Paraphimosis (rare)

In addition, recurrent UTIs may be resolved by circumcision, due to reduction of paraurethral organisms. This is indicated in boys with severe urinary tract anomalies.

ORTHOPAEDIC CONDITIONS

CAUSES OF LIMP

Painless	Painful
Missed congenital dysplasia of the hip (CDH)	Infection (septic arthritis, osteomyelitis)
Talipes	Trauma
Perthes disease	Neoplasia
Short limb	Slipped upper femoral epiphysis (SUFE)
Muscular weakness	Irritable hip (transient synovitis)
Neurological, e.g. ataxia, cerebral palsy	Juvenile idiopathic arthritis

NB: Any child with knee pain may have hip pathology presenting with referred pain to the knee.

INFECTIONS

Septic arthritis

- Infection in the joint space
- Usually occurs ≥ 2 years
- From haematogeneous spread, but also direct extension from osteomyelitis or abscess
- Serious joint destruction can occur if not promptly treated
- Neonatal disease may be multifocal

Organisms

Children	*Staphylococcus aureus* and streptococci are the most common agents
	Enterococci, salmonella (in sickle cell disease). Haemophilus now rare
	Meningococcus, yersinia (iron overload)
	TB (prolonged indolent arthritis with stiff joint)
Neonates	*Staph. aureus*, Group B streptococcus, *Escherichia coli*, gonococcus, enterobacteria

Clinical features

Joint	Hot, red, tender swollen joint
	Pain at rest and with movement
	Markedly reduced range of movement (pseudoparesis in infant)
	Joint position due to maximum joint relaxation or muscle spasm
Child	Toxic and febrile

NB: Osteomyelitis may have a sympathetic joint effusion, but tenderness is over the **bone**. Hip disease may present with referred pain to the knee.

Investigations

Bloods	Neutrophils ↑
	ESR, CRP ↑
	Serial blood cultures and antigens
X-ray	Normal initially but helpful to eliminate trauma
Joint USS	Useful for hips in infants
Bone scan	'Hot spots' at involved joints
Joint aspiration	Under USS guidance for M, C & S, and pain relief

Management

Antibiotics	Prompt and prolonged IV course, e.g. flucloxacillin + third-generation cephalosporin
Surgical	Athroscopic or open joint washout for hip disease and if delayed response to antibiotics
Physiotherapy	Initially joint immobilization for pain relief, then mobilized to prevent deformity

Osteomyelitis

- Acute, subacute and chronic depending on virulence of organism and efficacy of treatment
- Most commonly affects the proximal tibia and distal femur
- Usually due to haematogenous spread
- Occasionally multifocal
- Ineffective treatment results in discharging sinus and limb deformity

Organisms

Similar to those of septic arthritis, with *Staph. aureus* the most common.

Clinical features

- Site dependent with point tenderness
- Overlying skin is warm, red and swollen
- Toxic, febrile child
- Painful immobile limb ± muscle spasm
- May have adjacent sympathetic joint effusion or extension to joint
- Older children may present with limp or back pain

Investigations

Bloods	CRP, ESR ↑↑, neutrophilia
	Blood cultures and rapid antigen tests
X-ray/USS	Normal initially
	Periosteal reaction > 2 weeks
	Subsequent lucent areas in bone
Bone scan	'Hot spots'
Aspiration	In atypical cases or immunocompromised child to identify organism

Management

1. Prolonged course (several weeks) of IV antibiotics
2. Surgical drainage/decompression if rapid response to antibiotics not seen

CONGENITAL DYSPLASIA OF THE HIP (CDH)

Also known as developmental dysplasia of the hip (DDH), this condition is due to incomplete shallow development of the acetabulum, allowing the femoral head to dislocate. Optimal hip development *in utero* and postnatally requires abduction and external rotation. The following factors affect such positioning:

- Breech position (especially extended breech)
- Oligohydramnios
- Muscular or neurological problem, e.g. spina bifida
- Positive family history (polygenic inheritance. Recurrence risk 1:30)

Incidence 2:1000, female > male. Left side > right side.

Diagnosis

- Emphasis on screening by identifying risk factors and from examination (Ortolani and Barlow tests) at birth and 6-week check
- USS to confirm diagnosis ± orthopaedic examination
- Clinically obvious when walking develops, by which time too late

Management

Detected early, the hip is immobilized by casts or splints in abducted position with hips and knees flexed to keep the head of the femur in the acetabulum and allow development of the acetabulum and ligaments. Late diagnosis often requires major orthopaedic surgery.

OSTEOCHONDRITIDES

Boys > girls. Usual age 3–12 years.

A group of idiopathic acquired localized disorders of bone and cartilage, typically affecting the primary or secondary ossification centre in the growing child which undergoes aseptic necrosis with resorption of the dead bone and replacement by new osseous tissue. They are characterized by localized pain and are possibly associated with trauma of the affected area.

Disease	Osteochondrosis	Clinical features
Perthes disease	Femoral head	Painless limp, thigh or knee pain
Osgood–Schlatter disease	Tibial tubercle	Tenderness and swelling over the tibial tubercle
Kohler disease	Tarsal navicular	Foot pain and limp
Freiberg infarction	Second metatarsal head	Pain on weight bearing, swelling at 2nd metatarsal head
Thiemann disease	Phalangeal epiphyses	Painless enlargement of the PIP joints
		Irregularity of the epiphyses of the digits
Scheuermann disease	Midthoracic or lumbar	See below

Perthes disease (Legg–Calve–Perthes)

This is an osteochondrosis caused by avascular necrosis of the **femoral head**, often due to compromise of the nutrient artery.

Males > females, 5:1. Usually 4–10 years at presentation. 10–20% have bilateral disease.

Clinical features

- Intermittent referred pain to anterior thigh or knee
- Limp (may be painless)
- Decreased internal rotation, abduction and extension of the hip (at rest semi-flexed and externally rotated)
- Leg length inequality

Investigations

Hip X-rays   Fragmented, flattened femoral head, often of increased density
                       Increase in the medial joint space, subchondral fracture
MRI hip   May illustrate above features earlier
Radionucleotide scan Reduced femoral head uptake (but increased when neovascularization)

Management

Varies between centres and depends on severity.

If < 6 years   Conservative – splints and bed rest
If > 6 years   Abduction exercises and bed rest
                 Abduction casts and femoral osteotomy if necessary

Kyphosis

Postural kyphosis	Bad posture. Smooth back contour on examination. Correctable by child. X-rays normal
Idiopathic kyphosis	X-rays show kyphosis Scheuermann disease (this is not the same thing as such, but may be associated)
Congenital	Vertebral malformations, e.g. VATER/VACTERL. Often present in infancy

Scheuermann disease

- Osteochondritis of the spine occurring during pubescent growth spurt
- Pain in mid-thoracic (75%) or thoracolumbar spine, or
- Painless round shoulders and kypho(scolio)sis
- Due to wedging of vertebrae caused by loss of anterior vertebral height

X-rays

- Wedging of 1–3 adjacent vertebrae
- Schmorl's nodes (irregular end-plates)
- Kyphosis

Management

- Conservative management (physiotherapy) usually as generally self-limiting with good outcome
- Casting or surgical fusion may be necessary

SCOLIOSIS

Structural

Congenital	Due to vertebral malformations: Vertebral body anomaly Failure of segmentation
	Generally presents in infancy
	Associated with renal abnormalities in 20%
Idiopathic	Most common form
	Usually mild disorder (< 20°, M = F), often spontaneously corrects
	Severe and progressive in 1:20 cases (F > M, progressive in adolescence with growth)

Postural

No spinal rotation and normal alignment when flex spine.

May be secondary to:

- Neuromuscular disease, e.g. muscular dystrophy, unilateral paralysis
- Osteoid osteoma
- Leg length discrepancy

Management

- Enquire about bowel and bladder function and examine neurological system
- Management directed at any cause plus: Brace for moderate deformity (20–40°)
  Surgical intervention if more severe

SLIPPED UPPER FEMORAL EPIPHYSIS (SUFE)

The epiphysis of the femoral head 'slips' off the femoral neck. Seen in adolescence when growth plate at its weakest due to excess growth hormone relative to sex hormones.

Characteristically either   Fat boys with relative hypogonadism (small testes) but normal growth, or
Tall thin girls with increased growth hormone and normal sex hormone

Associations   Hypogonadism
Hypothyroidism
Pituitary dysfunction

Clinical features

- Acute presentation – pain on hip movement (possibly referred knee pain only) and limited hip movement
- Chronic presentation – antalgic limp, hip externally rotated
- 25% bilateral
- On examination, decreased internal rotation of the hip

Complications

- Osteonecrosis
- Chondrolysis (articular cartilage degeneration)
- Early arthritis

X-ray hip ('Frog-leg lateral view')

- Widened growth plate
- Femoral neck anteriorly rotated
- Femoral epiphyses slipped down and back

Management

Surgical pinning of the femoral head.

IRRITABLE HIP

- Self-limiting transient reactive synovitis associated with, e.g., gastrointestinal illness, EBV, influenza, mycoplasma, streptococcus
- Common cause of acute hip pain in children aged 2–6 years
- Diagnosis of exclusion and, if doubt regarding septic arthritis, aspirate joint

Clinical features

- Sudden onset joint pain (possibly referred to knee, but *no* pain at rest) or limp
- Decreased range of movement
- Child is well ± mild fever

Investigations

- ESR/CRP/neutrophils normal or mildly elevated
- Blood cultures negative
- Joint X-ray or USS – small effusion may be present

Management

Brief bed rest, NSAIDs and remobilize.

PULLED ELBOW

- Distal dislocation of radial head through the annular ligament
- Common injury in toddlers
- Caused by rapid pull/rotation on child's forearm, e.g. when lifting child by one arm
- Pseudo-paralysis at the elbow with arm extended, forearm pronated and held at the side
- Often non-tender but apparent 'paralysis' of limb
- X-rays – radial head away from socket and no fracture

Management

Treatment is manipulation back into socket (hold flexed elbow in one hand and forearm in other hand, supinate forearm and place thumb over radial head and push it into the elbow).

POSTURAL VARIANTS IN TODDLERS

Postural variants of the developing skeleton are attributable to different load bearing at different ages and so resolve with time. Pathological skeletal variations are fixed and associated with identifiable pathology.

Feature	Normal postural variant	Pathological causes/treatments
Flat feet (*pes planus*)	Normal in toddlers, due to a fat pad under foot and ligamentous laxity	**Arch support** if persists (hypermobility) ± pain CTDs, e.g. Ehlers–Danlos syndrome
Out-toeing	Common throughout childhood	
In-toeing	**Flat feet** **Metatarsus adductus** – mobile forefoot with adduction deformity. Resolves by 5 years **Medial (internal) tibial torsion**, esp. in toddlers and corrects by age 4–5 years. Bow legs or knock knees **Femoral anteversion** (ligamentous laxity), generally resolves by 8 years	Metatarsus varus may need surgery Persistence > 8 years may need surgery Spasticity, e.g. cerebral palsy
Toe-walking	Common and affects Achilles' tendon	Cerebral palsy and Duchenne MD
Bow legs (*Genu varum*)	Common in toddlers (May have medial tibial torsion)	Rickets Idiopathic (Blount disease, see below) Local damage (trauma, infection, tumour) Skeletal dysplasia, e.g. neurofibromatosis
Knock knees (*Genu valgum*)	Common in young children, usually improves with age	

BLOUNT DISEASE

Idiopathic disorder resulting from abnormal growth of medial proximal tibial epiphysis. Common in Africans.

If < 4 years	Females > males, 20% unilateral
If > 4 years	Males > females, 50% unilateral
Associations	Obesity

Clinical features

- Leg length discrepancy
- Internal tibial torsion

Investigations

X-ray legs	'Beaking' of the medial metaphysis of the tibia

Management

If < 4 years	Splinting or surgical treatment
If > 4 years	Surgical osteotomies

TALIPES

Talipes is a positional deformity of the foot of which there are two types.

Talipes equinovarus	The most common form
	May be positional or fixed
	Foot supinated with heel inwardly rotated
	Forefoot adducted
Talipes calcaneovalgus	Foot everted and dorsiflexed

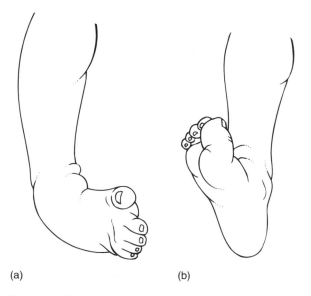

(a)   (b)

Figure 19.6 Talipes equinovarus (a) and calcaneovalgus (b)

Positional talipes	Will correct to normal anatomical position during manual examination and responds to physiotherapy
Fixed talipes	Requires diagnosis of underlying cause, e.g. muscular or neurological problems, oligohydramnios, and genetic conditions, and correction by conservative (serial plasters) or surgical means

NB: Congenital vertical talus causes 'rocker bottom' feet and is seen in Edwards syndrome.

CONSENT

THE COMPETENT CHILD

- Children over 16 years of age are regarded as adults for the purposes of consent
- A child under 16 years may *give* consent if they are deemed **competent**. However, a competent child *cannot withhold* consent (because a refusal to give consent can be countermanded by those with parental responsibility)
- A child under 16 years old will be considered competent to give consent to a particular intervention if they have 'sufficient understanding and intelligence to enable him or her to understand fully what is proposed' (known as **Frazer competence**)

THE INCOMPETENT CHILD

If a child does *not* have the **capacity** to provide consent a **proxy** may do so. The proxy is expected to act in the best interests of the child and they can include the following:

- A **parent** who has 'parental responsibility' for the child
- A **local authority** that has acquired 'parental responsibility' and the power of consent. A local authority can only usurp this power by restricting the parents' power
- The **court** can act as a proxy in wardship, under **inherent jurisdiction** or via **court orders**. In this way it can review a parent's decision, e.g. the refusal of a life-giving blood transfusion for a child of a Jehovah's Witness

FURTHER READING

Spitz L, Coran AG, eds *Paediatric Surgery*, 5th edn. London: Chapman & Hall Medical, 1995

20

Emergencies, accidents, non-accidental injury and the law

- *Resuscitation*
- *Reduced consciousness and coma*
- *Management of major trauma*
- *Head injury*
- *Shock*
- *Anaphylaxis*

- *Apparent life-threatening events*
- *Sudden infant death syndrome*
- *Childhood accidents*
- *Non-accidental injury*
- *The Law*

RESUSCITATION

Whatever the underlying cause, in a seriously unwell child the basic initial management is the same (see below). Any compromise of the Airway, Breathing or Circulation must be attended to immediately using basic resuscitation measures.

Advanced resuscitation is proceeded to when necessary and the equipment is available.

The procedures for basic and advanced life support are regularly updated by the European and the UK Resuscitation Committees, and thus the current guidelines should be checked.

MANAGEMENT OF A SERIOUSLY ILL CHILD (SUMMARY)

Rapid primary assessment and resuscitation

Check area is SAFE   **S**hout for help
                             Approach with care
                             Free from danger
                             Evaluate ABC
Assess responsiveness
Assessment and resuscitation:
     A   **Airway**
     B   **Breathing**
     C   **Circulation**
     D   **Disability**:
               Pupillary assessment (size and reaction)
               Conscious level   **AVPU** (see p. 508)
     E   **Exposure**

Basic life support

Secondary assessment

Detailed history

Detailed examination

Emergency investigations

Emergency treatment

Definitive further treatment (including investigations, monitoring and management as appropriate)

BASIC LIFE SUPPORT

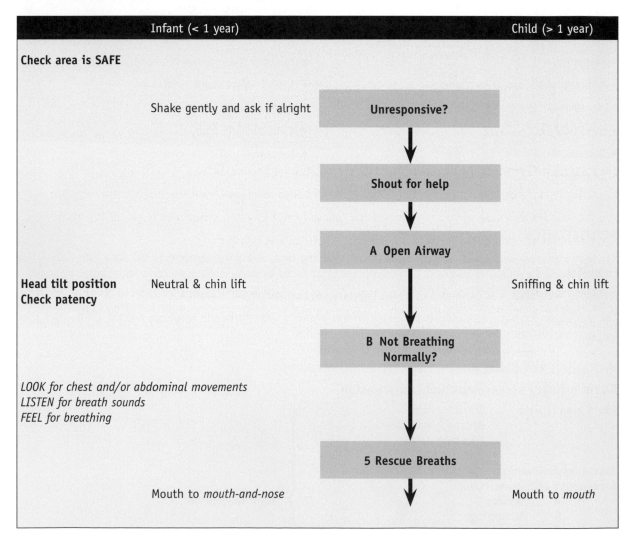

Infant (< 1 year)		Child (> 1 year)
Check area is SAFE		
Shake gently and ask if alright	**Unresponsive?**	
	Shout for help	
	A Open Airway	
Head tilt position **Check patency** Neutral & chin lift		Sniffing & chin lift
	B Not Breathing Normally?	
LOOK for chest and/or abdominal movements *LISTEN for breath sounds* *FEEL for breathing*		
	5 Rescue Breaths	
Mouth to *mouth-and-nose*		Mouth to *mouth*

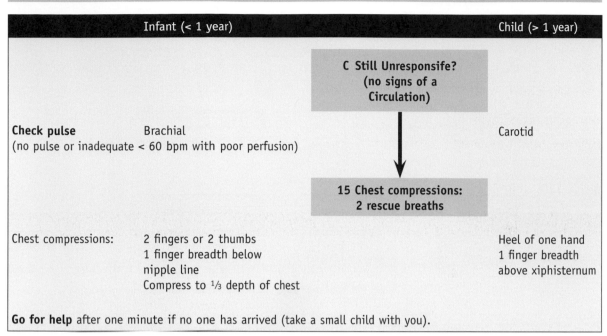

Infant (< 1 year)		Child (> 1 year)

**C Still Unresponsife?
(no signs of a
Circulation)**

**15 Chest compressions:
2 rescue breaths**

Check pulse   Brachial   Carotid
(no pulse or inadequate < 60 bpm with poor perfusion)

Chest compressions: 2 fingers or 2 thumbs   Heel of one hand
                       1 finger breadth below   1 finger breadth
                       nipple line   above xiphisternum
                       Compress to ⅓ depth of chest

Go for help after one minute if no one has arrived (take a small child with you).

Important differences between infants and children in resuscitation

Head position is **neutral** in infants (not sniffing) as this will keep the airway open (due to their different anatomy)

Mouth to **mouth-and-nose** in infants – because they are so small this is the easiest way to get air into them

Check **brachial or femoral pulse** (radial pulse is too difficult to feel in infants)

Choking

If a child is choking (foreign body aspiration suspected) back blows or chest thrusts are used to dislodge the object in an infant; abdominal thrusts are also used in a child 1 year old. (A finger sweep in the mouth used in adults is not recommended in children as the soft palate can easily be damaged or foreign bodies can be forced further down the airway.)

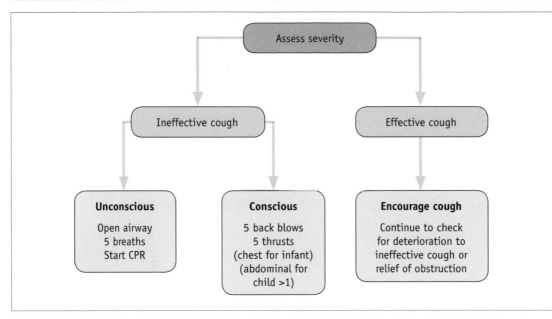

Figure 20.1 Protocol for management of choking
Adapted from Resuscitation Guidelines 2005. Resuscitation Council. www.resus.org.uk

ADVANCED LIFE SUPPORT

This involves basic life support with the addition of:

Airway	Oral airway or
	Nasal airway (not if risk of basal skull fracture) or
	Endotracheal intubation if necessary $\begin{cases} \text{ETT internal diameter} = [\text{age of} \\ \text{child}/4] + 4 \\ \text{ETT length} = [\text{age}/2] + 12 \end{cases}$
	Suctioning and nasogastric tube insertion
Breathing	Bag and mask/mechanical ventilation with 100% oxygen
	Monitor with pulse oximeter and ECG leads
Circulation	Assessment of cardiac output and rhythm (clinically and on ECG monitor)
	Give drugs and defibrillate as per protocols
	Fluid replacement (intravenous or intra-osseous)

Cardiac arrest protocols

Most cardiac arrests in children are **respiratory** in origin, with a secondary cardiac arrest.

Three basic cardiac arrhythmias are seen in cardiac arrest:

- Ventricular fibrillation (and pulseless VT)
- Asystole
- Pulseless electrical activity

The blood sugar must be monitored during cardiac arrest as children have low glycogen stores and thus rapidly become hypoglycaemic.

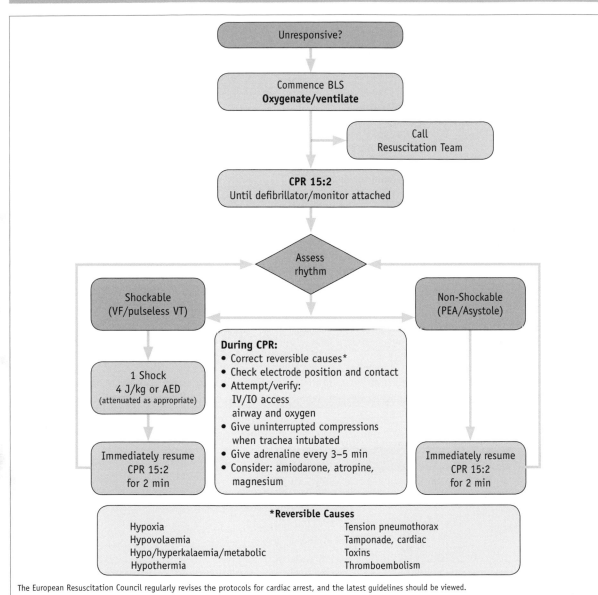

Figure 20.2 Cardiac arrest protocols for VF/pulseless VT and asystole/pulseless electrical activity
Adapted from Resuscitation Guidelines 2005. Resuscitation Council. www.resus.org.uk

REDUCED CONSCIOUSNESS AND COMA

Consciousness is awareness of oneself and surroundings in a state of wakefulness.

Coma is a state of unrousable unresponsiveness.

Causes of reduced conscious level/coma

CNS	Epilepsy (post-ictal)
	Traumatic brain injury (accidental or NAI)
	Infection, e.g. meningoencephalitis
	Subarachnoid haemorrhage
	Hypoxic ischaemic brain injury
	Acute ↑ ICP, e.g. intracranial mass, CSF obstruction; coning
	Brainstem neoplasm, trauma or infarction
Toxins	E.g. alcohol, glue, CO, lead, salicylates
Metabolic imbalance	E.g. glucose, Ca, Na (↑ or ↓)
Temperature instability	Hypothermia or hyperthermia
Systemic organ failure	E.g. sepsis, liver failure, Reye syndrome, renal failure, respiratory failure
Inborn error of metabolism	

COMA SCALES

These are important rapidly to assess depth of coma in a consistent way. A very rapid assessment is the AVPU coma scale, but the Glasgow and Children's Coma Scales are more comprehensive. The Children's Coma Scale (unlike the Glasgow Coma Scale) has not been validated.

AVPU – Rapid consciousness assessment in primary assessment	
A	Alert
V	Voice responsive
P	Pain responsive
U	Unresponsive
And pupillary size and reaction should be noted	
If P or U intubate and ventilate	

Children's Glasgow Coma Scale (< 4 years)		Glasgow Coma Scale (> 4 years)	
Response	**Score**	**Response**	**Score**
Eye opening		*Eye opening*	
Spontaneous	4	Spontaneous	4
To speech	3	To speech	3
To pain	2	To pain	2
None	1	None	1

Children's Glasgow Coma Scale (< 4 years)		Glasgow Coma Scale (> 4 years)	
Response	**Score**	**Response**	**Score**
Best motor response		*Best motor response*	
Spontaneous or obeys command	6	Obeys command	6
Localizes pain	5	Localizes pain	5
Withdraws from pain	4	Withdraws from pain	4
Abnormal flexion to pain	3	Abnormal flexion to pain	3
Abnormal extension to pain	2	Abnormal extension to pain	2
None	1	None	1
Best verbal response		*Best verbal response*	
Alert, babbles as usual	5	Orientated and converses	5
Fewer sounds/words than usual, irritable cry	4	Disorientated and converses	4
Cries to pain only	3	Inappropriate words	3
Moans to pain	2	Incomprehensible sounds	2
None	1	None	1

MANAGEMENT OF DECREASED CONSCIOUS STATE

The initial management of an unconscious child is to assess and stabilize them. While this is being done, further history, examination and investigations to establish the **cause** of the coma can be performed.

Rapid primary assessment (ABCDE) and resuscitation

Pay particular attention to:

- Securing the airway (give 100% oxygen and intubate and ventilate if necessary)
- Establish IV access, check glucose stick (and treat any hypoglycaemia)
- Initial blood samples
- Give IV fluids 20 ml/kg initial bolus if in shock
- Give broad-spectrum antibiotic if meningitis or sepsis suspected
- Rapid coma scale (AVPU), pupillary assessment, posture
- Check all over for other signs including temperature and rash

Secondary assessment

History	*Specific points*:
	Where discovered and by whom. Any witnesses?
	Resuscitation history with accurate timings
	Enquire about trauma, poisons, possible self-harm, infectious disease exposure, travel, preceding fit, febrile illness, pre-existing disease (neurological, metabolic) and social history (NAI)
Further examination	Check for any 'medic alert' bracelet
	Detailed neurological examination (including full coma scale score)
	Signs of injury (including nasal discharge)
	Signs of meningism (fundi – retinal haemorrhages, papilloedema, neck stiffness)
	Skin rash (petechial rash, bruising, jaundiced)
	Abnormal smell, e.g. ketones, organic solvents, metabolic disorder
	General examination – signs of other systemic disease

Investigations

Blood	BMStix, blood cultures, FBC, clotting studies, cross-match, U&E, creatinine, LFT, glucose, CRP, toxicology, lactate, ammonia and blood gas.
Urine	Glucose, protein, microscopy and culture, toxicology, amino and organic acids
	Keep sample for rarer inborn errors of metabolism especially if hypoglycaemic at time of presentation (store at − 70°C).
Brain scan (CT or MRI)	If no identifiable cause found
CXR ± AXR	(Post intubation)
Lumbar puncture	Should *not* be done on a comatose child. It can be performed later when the condition allows

Further treatment

- Monitor vital signs (pulse, temperature, BP, respiration, oxygen saturation, neurological observations)
- Treat on paediatric intensive care unit if GCS < 8.
- Site NG tube and aspirate (keep initial contents for analysis)
- Catheterize
- Monitor and stabilize blood sugar and electrolytes
- Treat any epileptic seizures with anticonvulsants
- Consider aciclovir (if herpes encephalitis a possibility)
- Monitor and treat any ↑ ICP (mannitol IV ± hyperventilation to induce hypocapnoea)
- Further detailed investigations to establish the cause and treat specific conditions as necessary

BRAIN DEATH

Brain death is the irreversible **loss of consciousness** and the **capacity to breathe**. This is accepted to occur when there is permanent functional death of the brainstem.

- Diagnosis of brain death requires the absence of brainstem function (no brainstem reflexes) for at least 24 h
- Child must be unconscious with no drugs acting that affect consciousness or respiratory function
- Coma state must: Be apnoeic despite hypercapnoeic drive, i.e. $PaCO_2$ > 6.7 kPa

    Be of diagnosed cause

    Exclude drugs, poisons, hypothermia (< 35°C), and biochemical disturbance

    There must be no treatable metabolic or endocrine cause
- Assessment of brainstem reflexes, tested by two senior physicians working independently. The reflexes must be retested at least ½ h apart

Brainstem reflexes

Pupils	Fixed, dilated. No direct or consensual reflexes
Corneal reflex	Absent
Oculocephalic reflex	Absent ('doll's eye reflex')
Caloric tests	(Vestibulo-ocular reflexes). Absent
Painful stimulus	No response to central and peripheral stimuli (primitive reflexes may be present)
Gag reflex	Absent
Apnoea	10 min disconnected from the ventilator, with 100% high flow oxygen, and arterial blood gas PCO_2 > 6.7 kPa (50 mmHg)

MANAGEMENT OF MAJOR TRAUMA

Primary survey and resuscitation (ABCDE)

Life-threatening conditions are identified and treated immediately.

Pay particular attention to:

- Securing airway with **cervical spine** control (assume spinal injury until excluded)
- Check for **pneumothorax** and **haemothorax**
- Estimation of **blood loss** (heart rate, BP, capillary refill, respiratory rate, temperature, skin colour and mental status)
- IV access and give 20 ml/kg fluid bolus, repeat if necessary. If > 40 ml/kg needed, give blood and obtain urgent surgical opinion
- Rapid **neurological status** assessment (AVPU and pupillary size and reactivity)
- Complete examination to check for **other injuries** (and then cover with blanket)

During the resuscitation take a more detailed history and basic investigations.

Detailed history of accident and medical history

Allergies
Medications
Previous illness / injury (PMH)
Last oral intake
Environment in which the injury occurred

Investigations

X-rays   CXR, pelvis, C-spine
Blood tests   ABG, FBC, Cross-match, glucose, U&Es

Further treatment

- Catheterize if necessary
- NG tube and aspiration (pass tube orally if basal skull fracture suspected)
- Give analgesia if necessary (IV morphine)

Secondary survey

When the child is stabilized a detailed secondary survey can be done, from top downwards:

- Head ⎱ Assess for injuries
- Face ⎰
- Neck – assume spinal injury until excluded
- Chest – open wound, tension pneumothorax, haemothorax
- Abdomen – ruptured organs (kidneys, liver, spleen, bowel)
- Pelvis ⎱ Assess for injuries
- Spine ⎰
- Extremities – open wounds, fractures

Emergency treatment

Treatment of any injuries discovered during secondary survey.

HEAD INJURY

This is the single most common cause of trauma death in children. Minor head injuries are common.

Causes

- Road traffic accidents
- Falls, e.g. windows, trees, walls
- NAI (usually infants)

Forms of head injury

Concussion	A brief reversible impairment of consciousness
Extradural haematoma	A bleed in the middle meningeal space due to rupture of the middle meningeal artery or dural veins
	A convex lesion is seen on CT scan
Subdural haematoma	A bleed between the dura and cerebral mantle, due to rupture of cortical veins
	Seen in **shaken infants** (NAI)
	May be **chronic**, with gradual enlargement and a history of irritability, poor feeding and lethargy
	A concave lesion is seen on CT scan
Intracerebral contusions	An insult to the brain substance

NB: A skull fracture is not always present with severe cerebral injury. Subdural haematoma is most common in head injuries without skull fracture.

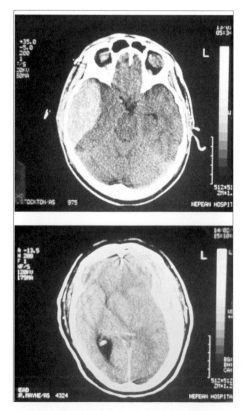

Figure 20.3 Extradural (top) and subdural (bottom) haematoma

512

Skull fractures

Non-depressed, linear	Most common fracture seen
Depressed	Need surgical treatment if $\geqslant$ 3–5 mm depressed
Basal skull fracture	CSF rhinorrhoea (can check with dextrostix to differentiate from mucus) and bilateral eyelid ecchymoses ('panda eyes')
	Difficult to demonstrate on SXR, CT views helpful

Suspect severe head injury if:

- Substantial injury, e.g. RTA, fall from great height
- Loss of consciousness at time of injury
- Impaired level of consciousness
- Neurological signs
- Penetrating injury

Management

Primary survey and resuscitation (as for major trauma)

- Immobilize neck until cervical spine injury ruled out
- AVPU, pupil size and reactivity, temperature and glucose

Secondary survey

Head examination	Lacerations, compound or depressed fractures
	Check for basal skull fracture ('panda eyes', CSF leak from ear or nose – check glucose level, bruising over mastoid [**Battle's sign**])
Full neurological	Glasgow coma scale, neurological examination, fundi
examination	Especially check for localizing signs
Investigations	FBC, U&E, cross-match, ABG ⎫ During primary survey
	C-spine, CXR, pelvis ⎭
	Do CT brain scan once stable if indicated (GCS < 12, loss of consciousness at time of incident, skull fracture, retrograde amnesia or neurological symptoms or signs, significant injury). If GCS < 12, an anaesthetist should assess for elective intubation for the CT

Emergency treatment

- Monitor closely to detect any change in clinical state and conscious level, recording regular neurological observations using the appropriate coma scale
- Treat seizures and raised ICP as necessary
- Check for and treat any other injuries
- Assessment for surgical intervention by neurosurgeons if necessary (focal neurology, deteriorating neurological signs, ICP ↑, abnormal CT, penetrating injury, basal skull fracture, depressed skull fracture)

SHOCK

Shock is the failure of adequate perfusion of the tissues.

Causes

- Hypovolaemic, e.g. blood loss, gastrointestinal fluid loss, ketoacidosis, skin loss (burns)
- Distributive, e.g. **septicaemia**, anaphylaxis, spinal cord injury
- Cardiogenic, e.g. arrythmias, cardiac failure, myocardial infarction

- Obstructive, e.g. tension pneumothorax, cardiac tamponade, pulmonary embolism
- Dissociative, e.g. profound anaemia, carbon monoxide poisoning

Three stages of shock

It is important to recognize the early stages (compensated) shock because early treatment of shock is vital.

1. *Compensated shock*	Perfusion to vital organs is maintained at the expense of non-essential tissues (capillary refill time (CRT) may be normal or poor, core–peripheral differential of < 2°C)
2. *Uncompensated shock*	Mechanisms start to fail, tissue hypoxia and acidosis occur. Poor CRT. Core–peripheral differential of > 2°C
Preterminal	Situation is becoming irreversible

Clinical features of the stages of shock

	Compensated	Uncompensated	Preterminal
Heart rate	↑	↑↑	↑ then ↓
Systolic BP	N	N or ↓	Falling
Respiratory rate	N or ↑	↑↑	Sighing
Pulse volume	N or ↓	↓	↓↓
Capillary refill time	N or ↑	↑	↑↑
Skin	Pale, cool	Mottled, cold	Pale, cold
Mental status	Agitation	Lethargic	Deeper coma
Urine output	↓	Absent	Absent
Peripheral temperature	Low	Low	Low
Core:peripheral temp. diff.	< 2°C	> 2°C	> 2°C
Estimated fluid loss	< 25%	25–40%	> 40%

Estimated blood volume	
Age	**EBV (ml/kg)**
Neonate	90
Infant up to 1 year	80
> 1 year	70

Management

Immediate management is the same for all types of shock:

Primary assessment and resuscitation (ABCDE)

Pay particular attention to cardiovascular status:

- Pulse rate, pulse volume, capillary refill, blood pressure

514

Effects of circulatory compromise on other organs (sighing respirations, pale skin, mental status, urine output)
Features of heart failure

- Give 100% oxygen via face mask
- Obtain IV or IO access. Fluid replacement in boluses of 20 ml/kg (crystalloid or colloid, then blood) as required.
- Low threshold for broad-spectrum antibiotics as **sepsis** is the most common cause in children

Secondary assessment (including detailed neurological status with detailed history and examination)

If there is no improvement, or if improvement requires > 40 ml/kg fluid, then consider mechanical ventilation, inotropic support, intensive monitoring, catheterization and correction of any biochemical and haematological abnormalities as necessary.

ANAPHYLAXIS

This is a severe, life-threatening, generalized systemic hypersensitivity reaction. It is an IgE mediated acute reaction to an allergen. The clinical features and severity are variable and include:

Airway and breathing	Bronchospasm, upper airway obstruction (stridor, wheeze, cyanosis), respiratory arrest
Circulation	Tachycardia, shock, cardiac arrest
Skin	Urticaria, flushing, angioedema, facial swelling

Management

Anaphylactic reaction?

Airway, Breathing, Circulation, Disability, Exposure

Diagnosis – look for: Acute onset of illness
Life-threatening Airway and/or Breathing and/or Circulation problems[1]
And usually skin changes

- **Call for help**
- Lie patient flat
- Raise patient's legs

Adrenaline (IM unless experienced with IV)

When skills and equipment available:
- Estabilish airway
- High flow oxygen   **Monitor:**
- IV fluid challenge (crystalloid)   Pulse oximetry
- Chlorphenamine (IM or slow IV)   ECG
- Hydrocortisone (IM or slow IV)   Blood pressure

1 Life-threatening problems:
   Airway: swelling, hoarseness, stridor
   Breathing: rapid breathing, wheeze, fatigue, cyanosis, SpO_2, <92%, confusion
   Circulation: pale, clammy, low blood pressure, faintness, drowsy/coma

APPARENT LIFE-THREATENING EVENTS (ALTE)

Apparent life-threatening events are unexpected episodes in infants that may involve:

- Apnoea
- Unresponsiveness
- Choking
- Central cyanosis or pallor

There are often no other obvious symptoms. A serious underlying disorder needs to be excluded but no cause may be found.

Causes

- Infection – sepsis, viral infection
- Seizure
- Gastro-oesophageal reflux
- Hypoglycaemia
- Central apnoea
- Cardiac – arrhythmia, cyanotic spell
- Encephalopathy – metabolic upset
- Suffocation (fictitious or induced illness)

Management

- Initial survey (ABCDE) and resuscitation as necessary
- Secondary survey: Thorough history (in particular check social situation)
                       Full examination
- Admit to hospital for close monitoring (oxygen saturations, ECG, respiration)
- Investigate further as appropriate: ABG, glucose, FBC, U&E, creatinine
                                         Infection screen
                                         Reflux investigations (pH study)
                                         Cardiac screen (CXR, ECG, echocardiogram)
                                         Metabolic screen
                                         Toxicology screen
- Teach parents resuscitation

SUDDEN INFANT DEATH SYNDROME (SIDS)

Sudden infant death syndrome is the sudden unexplained death of a previously well infant in whom no cause is found after postmortem examination.

It most commonly occurs at 2–4 months. The risk of SIDS for subsequent children is increased.

There has been a significant decrease in the numbers of SIDS cases with the advice:

- Put the baby to sleep on their back
- Avoid overheating the baby
- Tuck the baby in with their feet to the base of the cot (so the risk of slipping under the cover is reduced)
- Use blankets with holes in them and not duvets for infants
- Avoid smoking while pregnant and after pregnancy
- Avoid smoking in the house
- Have the baby sleep in the parents' bedroom for the first 6 months at least
- Do not put the baby in the parents' bed when the parents are tired or have taken drugs or alcohol

Basic resuscitation skills should be taught to parents of children at risk. Home apnoea monitoring for infants at risk may be considered, though in some cases this can prove anxiety-provoking for the parents and has not been proven to be of benefit.

CHILDHOOD ACCIDENTS

Accidents are the commonest cause of death in children aged 1–14 years, and they are broadly predictable and therefore often preventable.

Causes of fatal accidents

- Road traffic accidents (50%)
- Fire (30%)
- Drowning (10%)
- Suffocation and choking
- Falls
- Poisoning

ROAD TRAFFIC ACCIDENTS

Road traffic accidents are the cause of most accidental childhood deaths in the UK. They may involve:

Car passenger	Well fitting car seats and seat belts are preventative
Pedestrian	Young school boys at highest risk. Environmental measures most preventive
Bicyclist	Most common in boys. Crash helmets significantly reduce severity

For management, see Major Trauma and Head Injury, p. 511.

NEAR DROWNING

The third commonest cause of accidental death in children in the UK. Up to 70% will survive if basic life support is provided at the scene.

Near drowning	If any recovery following immersion
Drowning	No recovery after immersion

Effects of submersion:

- Breath-holding $\rightarrow$ bradycardia (diving reflex) $\rightarrow$ hypoxia $\rightarrow$ tachycardia, BP $\uparrow$, acidosis
- Then breathing movements occur (< 2.5 min) $\rightarrow$ laryngeal spasm and secondary apnoea
- Then involuntary breathing efforts, bradycardia, arrythmias, cardiac arrest
- Hypothermia common (this protects against hypoxic brain damage)
- Fresh water and salt water both cause (via different mechanisms) pulmonary oedema and hypoxaemia, and have the same prognosis

Management

- Initial survey (ABCDE) and resuscitation. Assume cervical spine injury. Early intubation and nasogastric tube placement with aspiration to remove swallowed water
- Rewarming (**passive**, e.g. blankets and **active**, e.g. radiant lamps, warm IV fluids)
- Do not stop resuscitation if core temperature < 32°C
- Secondary survey (full history and examination). Commence advanced life support when able
- Investigations: ABG, U&Es, glucose, blood cultures, CXR
- Definitive care in hospital
- NB: Initial examination may be normal (including CXR and blood gas) as progressive pulmonary oedema and respiratory failure can develop over 72 h
- Good prognostic indicators: Short time to first gasp on resuscitation (< 3 min)
                                  Hypothermia < 33°C core temperature

BURNS

Causes of burns and scalds

- Hot liquids
- Fire

- Smoke inhalation
- Electrical injury
- Chemical burns

Electrical burns

Lightning	Direct current (DC), very high voltage (200 000–2 billion V) over milliseconds
	Causes asystole, respiratory arrest, minimal tissue damage
High voltage wires	Alternating current (AC) usually < 70 000 V over longer time
	Causes ventricular fibrillation, deep tissue injury, muscle necrosis, renal failure
Low voltage household	AC: causes tetanic muscle contractions, victim unable to let go, and thus sustains substantial damage
	DC (or high voltage AC): causes single forceful muscle contraction, throwing the victim away

Assessment

Burns are assessed by:

Depth	**Partial thickness** (pink or mottled skin, blistering, painful)
	Full thickness (white or charred skin, painless)
Extent	Expressed as a percentage of body surface area
Location	Airway involvement in smoke inhalation must be checked for
	Hand and face burns are of particular cosmetic and functional significance

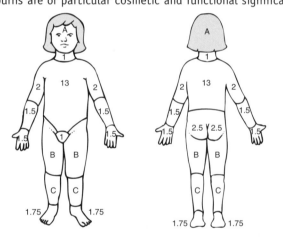

Figure 20.4 Assessment of burns

Percentage surface area at different ages					
Area	0 years	1 year	5 years	10 years	15 years
A	9.5	8.5	6.5	5.5	4.5
B	2.75	3.25	4.0	4.25	4.5
C	2.5	2.5	2.75	3.0	3.25

Management

Burn management is coordinated by the plastic surgical team, and if treated as an inpatient this should be on a burns unit.

Primary survey and resuscitation (ABCDE)

Pay special attention to:

- Airway – if inhalation injury intubation by expert may be necessary.
- Exposure – rapid heat loss occurs from burnt areas

Secondary survey

Assess the burn (as above).

Emergency treatment

Analgesia	Burns are very painful so strong IV analgesia required for all but minor burns
Initial shock	IV fluids via two large cannulae as skin fluid loss may be extensive
	Burns > 10% body surface area will need additional IV fluid replacement:
	Additional fluid requirement = percentage burn x weight (kg) x 4
	Monitor urine output
Wound care	Removal of dead tissue, then placement of sterile dressings
	Significant burns must be managed on a burns unit, i.e. full thickness burns, > 10% body surface area, inhalational burns, hand and face burns

Definitive care

Carried out on a paediatric burns unit.

POISONING

Poisoning in young children is usually accidental, though deliberate poisoning is seen in adolescents and in fictitious or induced illness (FII).

General management

Take history	Including:
	Substance(s) ingested
	Amount
	Exact timing
Examination	ABCDE assessment and resuscitation
	In particular: Level of consciousness
	Orophayrnx
	Features specific to various poisons (see below)
Investigations	Drug levels, e.g. salicylates, paracetamol
	U&Es, creatinine, LFTs, clotting profile, ABGs, FBC
Elimination	Contact the Regional Poisons Information Centre for advice

Specific antidotes, investigations and therapy for particular poisons

There are two methods of elimination:

Activated charcoal	This is considered if ingestion is recent
	Charcoal is given orally (via nasogastric tube if necessary), and works by absorbing the drug itself, thereby reducing the intestinal absorption of drugs
Gastric lavage	Rarely indicated in children
	Most effective <1 h of ingestion
	Airway must be protected during the procedure
	Contraindicated after ingestion of corrosives and hydrocarbons due to potential for aspiration pneumonitis

Clinical features and possible causes	
Small pupils	Opiates, organophophates
Large pupils	Amphetamines, tricyclics, cocaine, cannabis
Tachycardia	Amphetamines, cocaine, antidepressants
Bradycardia	β-blockers
Hypotension	β-blockers, antidepressants, opiates, iron, tricyclics
Hypertension	Cocaine, amphetamines
Tachypnoea	Aspirin, carbon monoxide
Bradypnoea	Alcohol, opiates
Convulsions	Tricyclics, organophosphates

Specific poison remedies

Substance	Clinical effects	Specific management
Bleach	Local erosions	Give oral milk and antacids (may help) Avoid emesis Place of systemic steroids is contentious Ventilatory support if necessary Endoscopy to assess damage if necessary
Button batteries	Gastointestinal upset Gut wall corrosion Oesophageal stricture Mercury release if batteries broken	CXR and AXR to assess progress along the gut Remove if there are signs of disintegration or not moving, and consider if not passed within a few days
Paracetamol	Gastric irritation Liver failure after 2–3 days	Check plasma levels 4 h after ingestion If plasma concentration high or > 150 mg/kg, IV acetylcysteine as per protocol Monitor liver function over next few days (PT prolongation is best predictor of need for liver support or transplant)
Salicylates	Nausea and vomiting Dehydration Tinnitus, deafness Disorientation Hyperventilation Respiratory alkalosis Metabolic acidosis Hypoglycaemia	Check plasma salicylate level Empty stomach if < 12 h of ingestion Correct dehydration, electrolyte and fluid imbalance Forced alkaline diuresis if severe Dialysis if severe
Alcohol	Hypoglycaemia	Monitor blood glucose regularly Give IV glucose if necessary
Iron	Vomiting and diarrhoea Haematemesis and melaena Gastric ulcerations and later gastric strictures Drowsiness, convulsions Liver failure, coma within hours	AXR to view the number of tablets Serum iron levels Management of shock Gastric lavage Iron chelation (IV desferrioxamine)

Lead poisoning

This is usually chronic poisoning from the ingestion of lead-containing paint or water in lead pipes. Rare in the UK. It may result in permanent mental retardation.

Chronic illness	Bone features, developmental delay, gum involvement, constipation, neuropathy
Acute	Vomiting, ataxia, seizures, coma, anaemia, renal involvement

Clinical features

Gastrointestinal	Anorexia, nausea, vomiting, constipation, abdominal pain
Haematological	Hypochromic microcytic anaemia with basophilic stippling on red cells
Neurological	Peripheral neuropathy, e.g. wrist drop, foot drop
	Lead encephalopathy (seizures and reduced consciousness)
Skeletal	Dense metaphyseal bands at the growing end of long bones – 'lead lines'
Renal	Fanconi syndrome
Other	Blue line on gums

Diagnosis

Serum	Lead levels
	FBC (basophilic stippling, hypochromic microcytic anaemia)
Urine	Proteinuria, glycosuria, aminoaciduria

Management

Chelation therapy with dimercaptosuccinic acid (DMSA). Calcium EDTA and dimercaprol may be used instead. Removal of source.

NON-ACCIDENTAL INJURY (NAI)

Types

- Physical abuse
- Sexual abuse
- Emotional abuse and neglect
- Fabricated or induced illness (FII) (used to be termed Munchausen syndrome by proxy)

PHYSICAL ABUSE

Following accidental injury, parents would normally be very concerned and bring their child straight to medical attention and give a consistent and plausible history of events. The following features of the history should raise suspicion of physical abuse:

- Unexplained or multiple injuries
- Inconsistent history
- Late presentation
- Unusual parental behaviour, e.g. hostile, unconcerned
- Anxious withdrawn child (termed **'frozen watchfulness'**)

Injuries seen in physical abuse:

Lacerated oral frenulum	(Due to carer forcing bottle in infant's mouth)
Cigarette burns	

Bruises	Finger tip bruises
	Belt mark bruises
	Bite marks
	Unexplained multiple bruises (especially when *not* occurring over bony prominences)
Head injuries	Retinal haemorrhages (caused by shaking injury 'shaken baby', see p. 385)
	Subdural haematoma (from shaking injury)
	Wide skull fractures (> 3 mm displacement)
Fractures	Unexplained or multiple fractures
	Spiral fractures
	Old fractures not previously brought to medical attention

Differential diagnosis

Bruising	Fractures	
Coagulation disorders (family history?)	Osteogenesis imperfecta	
Leukaemia	Copper deficiency	NB: All rare
Immune thrombocytopenic purpura (ITP)	Rickets	
Henoch–Schönlein purpura	Local bone tumour	
Mongolian blue spot		

SEXUAL ABUSE

In most cases of sexual abuse the perpetrator is male and the abused child female, although all variations exist. Features of sexual abuse include:

- Sexually transmitted infection
- Genital injury with no plausible explanation
- Urinary tract infection, enuresis
- Anal fissure, pruritis ani, constipation, encopresis
- Inappropriate sexual behaviour, i.e. sexualized behaviour
- Behavioural disturbance
- Direct allegation of abuse

EMOTIONAL ABUSE AND NEGLECT

This can be difficult to identify. Features include general neglect, dirty child, scruffy clothing, a miserable child and growth faltering.

FABRICATED OR INDUCED ILLNESS (FII)

This is an uncommon form of abuse in which illness in the child is fabricated by the parents(s) or carer.

Features of the disorder include:

- Condition which is difficult to diagnose
- Features are only present when the parent is present
- Multiple hospital admissions
- Mother often has healthcare connections, e.g. a nurse

Examples	Feeding salt to the child
	Putting blood in the urine, stool or vomit
	Putting sugar in the urine

The child can come to serious harm from these activities, not least from protracted unnecessary medical investigations to determine the source of the fictitious symptoms.

MANAGEMENT OF NON-ACCIDENTAL INJURY

There are national guidelines regarding the management of NAI, emphasizing the team approach between hospital- and community-based professionals, and dedicated child protection teams including paediatricians, social workers, health visitors, GP, police, teachers and lawyers. Important points to remember in suspected cases are:

- Involvement of **senior child protection paediatrician** early
- **Detailed history** should be taken including direct 'quotes'. Remember to record date and time and sign notes. Include detailed family and social history
- **Full examination with consent** (ideally only once by senior paediatrician(s) and if necessary a forensic physician from the child protection team to minimize distress to the child). Observe child–parent interaction
- **Detailed documentation** of the injuries with chronology (if possible photographs with consent)
- Relevant **investigations** (X-rays, blood tests) and treatment of injuries
- In suspected or confirmed abuse, all cases are managed by a **dedicated multidisciplinary child protection team**. The team decide whether any emergency and/or long-term action is needed
- If necessary **immediate protection** with admission to hospital for observation, treatment and investigation. (Parental consent usually obtained for this but if not, legal enforcement is necessary using a child protection order).
- Every child at risk or referred for abuse should now have a Laming Checklist in the notes, and all sections should be signed by the responsible consultant
- A **child protection conference** is scheduled to decide whether further action is necessary and what. From this there may be a decision to place the child on the Child Protection Register, and/or the development of a child protection care plan. In some cases placement in care is necessary (in severe cases long-term foster care and/or adoption)

If a practitioner has concerns about a child's welfare

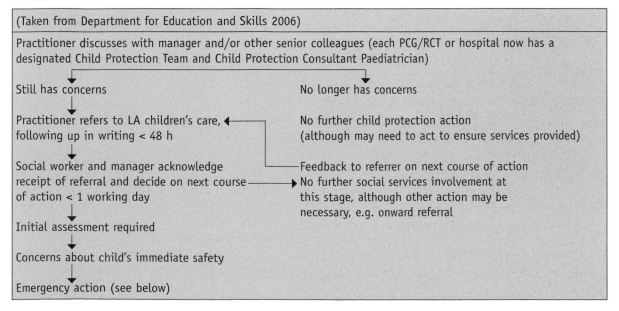

Emergency action to safeguard a child

(Taken from Department for Education and Skills 2006)

Decision made that emergency action may be necessary to safeguard a child

↓

Immediate strategy discussion between LA children's social care, police and other agencies as appropriate

↓

Relevant agency seeks legal advice and outcome recorded

↓

Immediate strategy discussion makes decision about:
- Immediate safeguarding action
- Information giving, especially to parents

↓

Relevant agency sees child and outcome records outcome

No emergency action taken   Appropriate emergency action taken,

   Child in need   Strategy discussion and s47 enquiries initiated

   Initial assessment
   (to be completed within 7 days)

With family and other professionals, agree plan for ensuing child's future safety and welfare and record decisions

THE CHILDREN'S ACT

The Children's Act is a document designed for the protection of children. It was fully implemented in 1991 (and given royal assent in 1989). The act includes the following features:

- Child's welfare is the Court's paramount consideration, so any Court order made should contribute positively to the child's welfare
- Prime responsibility for bringing up children lies with the parents
- Local authorities should provide supportive services to help parents in bringing up children
- Local authorities should take reasonable steps to identify children and families in need
- Every local authority should have a register of children in need
- Every local authority should work in partnership with the parents

The Children Act 1989 also provides protection orders for children 'at risk'. These are:

1. **Emergency protection order (EPO)**. Any person may apply to a magistrate's court for an EPO and then would have parental responsibility for the child if granted. The order lasts 8 days and an extension of a further 7 days is possible. An appeal can be made after 3 days
2. **Police protection provision**. A police constable may take a child into police protection without assuming parental responsibility. This lasts up to 3 days only
3. **Child assessment order**. This allows proper assessment of a child to be done over a period of up to 7 days. (Removal of the child from the family home does not necessarily occur)
4. **Care and supervision orders**. These allow a child to be placed in the care of or under the supervision of the local authority. Maximum duration is 8 weeks

STATEMENTING

As part of the **Education Act 1981** (updated 1993) the local education authority must provide a statement for a child with special education needs to outline the special needs of the child and the consequent services that the education authority will provide.

- An **initial assessment** is made of the child's particular needs and disabilities by interested professionals (including as necessary teacher, paediatrician, educational psychologist, occupational therapist, physiotherapist and speech therapist)
- Then a **statement of special educational needs**, i.e. plan of help, of the child's educational and non-educational needs is made, which includes information given by the parents and professionals The special services to be offered to the child are included within the statement, e.g. one-to-one tuition, special transport to school
- It is important that the statement be regularly reviewed and revised or cancelled as necessary

WARDSHIP

If a child is a '**ward of court**': 'the court is entitled and bound in appropriate cases to make decisions in the interests of the child which override the rights of its parents'.

Wardship may not be invoked by the local authority or while the child is in care, but may be made by other interested parties, e.g. a health authority, and it ends when a child ceases to be a minor. This is a major step to take as, when evoked, 'no important step in the life of that child can be taken without the consent of the Court'.

INHERENT JURISDICTION

This is most commonly used in medical law cases. The court does not take all the decisions relating to the child's life, but only in certain issues, e.g. medical care. It can be invoked in an emergency and also by a local authority even while the child is in care.

COURT ORDERS

The court has the power to make **specific issue orders** and **prohibited step orders**.

- A **prohibited step order** means that no step (specified in the order) can be taken by any person (including the parent) without the consent of the court
- A **specific issue order** gives directions to determine a **specific question** in connection with any aspect of parental responsibility for a child

These orders cannot be made if a child is in care, or in an emergency, and are rarely made if the child is 16 years old. They do not represent a true order as they only allow a local authority to authorize and supervise a policy. As with all treatment, the final decision and duty of care still rests with the doctor in charge of the case.

FURTHER READING

Meadows R, ed *ABC of child abuse*, 3rd edn. London: BMJ Publishing Group, London, 1997

Resuscitation Council (UK) Guidelines July/Sept 2008

Index

1590